The Path We Tread
Third Edition

The Path We Tread

Blacks in Nursing Worldwide,
1854–1994

Third Edition

Mary Elizabeth Carnegie,
DPA, RN, FAAN
Editor Emerita, *Nursing Research*

Foreword by
Josephine A. Dolan,
RN, MS, PdD
Professor Emerita and Special Lecturer
University of Connecticut
Storrs, Connecticut

National League for Nursing Press • *New York*
Pub. No. 14-2678

Copyright © 1995
National League for Nursing Press
350 Hudson Street
New York, NY 10014

ISBN 0-88737-640-1

The views expressed in this publication represent the views of the author and do not necessarily reflect the official views of the National League for Nursing.

Library of Congress Cataloging-in-Publication Data

Carnegie, Mary Elizabeth.
    The path we tread : blacks in nursing worldwide, 1854–1994 / Mary Elizabeth Carnegie : foreword by Josephine A. Dolan. — 3rd ed.
        p.   cm.
    Includes bibliographical references and index.
    ISBN 0-88737-640-1
    1. African-American nurses—United States—History.   2. Nursing—United States—History.   3. Nurses, Black—Caribbean, English-speaking—History.   4. Nurses, Black—Africa, English-speaking—History.   I. Title.
    [DNLM: 1. History of Nursing. 2. Blacks—history. WY 11.1 C289p 1995]
    RT83.5.C37   1995
    610.739089996073—dc20
    DNLM/DLC
    for Library of Congress   94-49183
                                                                                CIP

This book was set in Bembo by Publications Development Co., Crockett, Texas. The editor was Maryan Malone. The designer was Nancy Jeffries. The printer was Clarkwood Corp., Totowa, New Jersey.

Cover photo of Sojourner Truth, 1864. Courtesy of the United States Army Center of Military History. Adapted by designer Lauren Stevens.

Printed in the United States of America

To my late cousin, Iola Melbrook,
who through the years had been supportive of me
in all my endeavors

Foreword

Despite the rapidly expanding professional role of nursing, the need to reflect on the people and events that formed the basis of our rich historical heritage demands our reflection and appreciation. It is with pride that one observes the current resurgence of interest in the documented history of our profession, as well as the emergence of significant historical research. One area that has needed strengthening has been research and delineation of the accomplishment of our Black nurse leaders. *The Path We Tread* provides a valuable contribution to the dearth of those historical data.

Dr. M. Elizabeth Carnegie is eminently qualified to have undertaken the research and writing of this historical publication. The author's education, the positions of great responsibility she has held especially in the key editorial roles of our leading nursing journals (*American Journal of Nursing, Nursing Outlook,* and *Nursing Research*) have brought her in touch with events and those who are molding our professional achievements. Dr. Carnegie's own contributions to our professional enrichment have been praised and honors have been showered upon her. Among these tributes, the Nursing Archives at Hampton University has been named in her honor. Dr. Carnegie has held many board offices in association with institutions of higher learning, as well as in professional associations, such as the past presidency of the American Academy of Nursing.

In this book, the long and constant struggle to gain a rightful position in the health care system for black nurses has been identified by Dr. Carnegie. Through her efforts, a gold mine of information and illustrations not available previously have been vividly portrayed.

The Path We Tread should highlight an awakening of interest in the historical evolution of black nurses, and the impact of their leadership should be understood. Pride in their achievements and their education should be elicited on the part of all nurses. All black nurses should glow with pride and gratitude to those who have achieved and to Dr. Carnegie, who brings it forth for all to view.

Josephine A. Dolan, RN, MS, PdD

Preface to First Edition

Black nurses, like blacks in many other professions, have had a long and difficult history. Whereas many books have been written about blacks in this country, no comprehensive history of black nursing exists. Most books on black history have excluded the nursing profession.

Despite there being many general books on the history of nursing, until recently, only a few have devoted more than a sentence or two to black nurses and their contributions to health care. The one typical sentence found in nursing history texts is, "Mary Mahoney was the first trained black nurse in America, having been graduated from the New England Hospital for Women and Children in 1879." All nursing history books, for example, refer to Florence Nightingale, the Founder of Modern Nursing, and her work in the Crimean War, but omit the fact that a black woman nursed along with her. Another example of how black nursing history has been ignored: All history books credit the University of Minnesota as having established the first nursing program in a university setting in 1909, but Howard University, a black school in Washington, DC, had established one 16 years before, in 1893.

In 1980, the U.S. registered nurse population was estimated to be 1,662,382. Of this number, 60,845, or 3.7 percent were black (*Facts About Nursing*, 82–83, 1983). In the four years since 1980, graduates of the 1,422 basic nursing programs have added to this pool. These nurses, both black and white, have been deprived of historical data on the heritage of their profession, and thus their education has been incomplete. A book on black nursing history is not only timely, but also highly relevant to professional education in contemporary society.

The Path We Tread is organized into six chapters, the content of which spans 130 years—from 1854 to 1984. No attempt has been made to interpret the facts presented or to make philosophical projections.

The first chapter, "Answering the Call," is about black nurses in the early wars. It begins with the Crimean War in which Mary Seacole, a black woman from Jamaica, is depicted as having served as a nurse on the battlefield along with Florence Nightingale. Of the many women and men who served as nurses during the Civil War (also called the War Between the States), the work of three black women is referred to: Sojourner Truth, Harriet Tubman, and Susie King Taylor. During the Spanish-American War in 1898, blacks served as contract nurses, an outstanding one being Namahyoke Sockum Curtis who was given a government pension for her services and was buried in Arlington National Cemetery, along with other famous war dead.

In collecting data on black men and women who served as nurses during the Civil and Spanish-American Wars, extensive use was made of the National Archives in Washington, DC. Records of those blacks who nursed in the Civil War were kept in a separate journal, which facilitated the research. Information of all nurses who served in the Spanish-American War was recorded on alphabetically arranged Personnel Data Cards which had an item requesting the person to indicate his or her "color." The responses to this question included "light," "dark," "medium," "fair," "black" (only one), "blond," "brunette," "colored," "light skinned," "brownish," "mulatto," and "octoroon"; a few did not answer the question. Because both black and white people commonly refer to themselves as "fair," "light," and "dark," it was difficult to determine race; therefore, other demographic information was considered, such as place of birth, address, school of nursing attended, and the like.

The second chapter, "The Foundation Is Laid," is devoted to formal education programs—basic and advanced. The basic programs at historically black institutions are divided into diploma, baccalaureate, and associate degree, with two tables—one listing the 75 known diploma programs that existed between 1886 and 1982, when the last one closed; and the other listing baccalaureate and associate degree programs at historically black colleges and universities as of 1984. The advanced programs include two in public health nursing and two in nurse-midwifery that were conducted in the South exclusively for black registered nurses and three master's programs that are offered at historically black institutions of higher education.

The third chapter, "From Dreams to Achievements," describes the Cadet Nurse Corps that was in operation during World War II and explores three special education projects: one to recruit minorities for all types of nursing programs; one to help recruit and retain disadvantaged students in baccalaureate programs; and one to increase the number of doctorally prepared nurses from ethnic/racial minority populations.

The fourth chapter, "Struggle for Recognition," is devoted to those national nursing organizations that have or have had relevance for black nurses, including those established by and for black nurses themselves. Special attention is given to the role of the National Association of Colored Graduate Nurses in its fight for integration of the black nurse in the American Nurses' Association and into the mainstream of professional nursing. Included, also, are biographical sketches of each of the Black regular and honorary Fellows of the American Academy of Nursing.

The fifth chapter, "Stony the Road," highlights black nurses who pioneered in the profession in the late 19th and early 20th centuries, paving the way for black nurses of today.

The final chapter, "So Proudly We Hail," deals with black nurses in the federal government—the military, the U.S. Public Health Service, and the Veterans Administration.

The terms *Negro* and *colored* have been used when appropriate to maintain the historical perspective of the resources used.

Mary Elizabeth Carnegie, DPA, RN, FAAN
1984

Preface to Second Edition

The first edition of this book spanned 131 years—from 1854 through 1984. This second edition extends the time frame through 1990, noting the progress made by black nurses.

The popularity of the first edition has convinced me that black nurses take pride in their heritage and accomplishments and non-black nurses have learned about the contributions of black nurses to health care in this country. It shows how black nurses have had to work, sometimes desperately, to create, against tremendous odds, a place in the mainstream of the profession.

The first chapter, "Answering the Call," an account of the contributions of black women who nursed in the early wars—the Crimean War, the Civil War, and the Spanish-American War, has only a few additions that include reference to a black man, James Derham, who nursed while a slave, earning enough money to buy his freedom. He later became a prominent physician in Philadelphia, recognized by the well-known Dr. Benjamin Rusk.

The second chapter, "The Foundation Is Laid," devoted to basic and advanced programs in nursing, lists an additional 15 black diploma programs that had been in existence from 1886, when the first one was established, to 1982 when the last one was closed, bringing the total to 90. Nursing programs at historically black colleges and universities are identified: baccalaureate—23; associate degree—6; master's degree—4.

The third chapter, "From Dreams to Achievements," which presents special educational projects, includes a new component to the American Nurses Association (ANA) Minority Fellowship Program—one which focuses on leadership training for minority women nurses who have earned doctorates.

The number of professional nursing organizations, discussed in Chapter 4, "Struggle for Recognition," has increased from 12 in the first edition to

24, including two regional bodies. This large increase is due not only to the growing number of new organizations that have or have had blacks in leadership roles, but to old, well-established ones that have had elected or appointed black officials since the first edition went to press. Included, also, are biographical sketches of the 38 black nurses who have been inducted into the American Academy of Nursing, an increase of ten.

Nothing was added to the fifth chapter, "Stony the Road," because of its nature—biographical sketches of the black pioneers in nursing, all of whom are deceased.

The last chapter, "So Proudly We Hail," devoted to blacks in the federal government—the Military, the Public Health Service, and the Veterans Administration—has a number of changes, due primarily to the reorganization of the Public Health Service and the identification of more black nurses in key positions.

The chronology has been broadened to include not only additional nursing events, but those that have relevance for blacks in nursing, for example, the 1954 Supreme Court Decision, ending segregation in public schools.

Because members of other disciplines and those teaching or engaged in research on women have used the book as a resource, the bibliography has been broadened to include more sources related to the content.

My thanks goes to the many readers and to those faculty in schools of nursing who have adopted the book as a text in their courses on issues and trends.

Acknowledgments have been enlarged to express special appreciation to Memphis State University in Tennessee and Indiana University in Indianapolis for providing staff and other resources needed to complete this second edition.

Mary Elizabeth Carnegie, DPA, RN, FAAN
1990

Preface to Third Edition

Because the second edition had won two awards in 1992—one from the American Academy of Nursing for its positive portrayal of nurses; the other from the *American Journal of Nursing* as book of the year, the publisher suggested that I consider writing a third edition. Shortly, thereafter, while attending the quadrennial congress of the International Council of Nurses in Madrid, Spain, I noticed the large number of member associations from black English-speaking African and Caribbean countries. So the idea was conceived to expand the scope of the third edition to include these 26 countries—17 from Africa and 9 from the Caribbean.

Demographic information on the African and Caribbean countries was obtained from the U.S. Department of State, Bureau of Public Affairs, Office of Public Communications.

To gather information about nursing in the selected African and Caribbean nations, the archives of the International Council of Nurses in Geneva, Switzerland, were searched. Other literature examined included volumes of the *International Nursing Review,* issues of journals of those African and Caribbean nursing associations that publish such journals, and a few relevant doctoral dissertations.

This third edition, which spans the years 1854 through 1994, has two additional chapters—one on the Caribbean; the other Africa. To verify the authenticity of the content, copy was sent to the president of the national nurses association of each country.

The old chapters, 1 through 6, have been updated. The first chapter, "Answering the Call," an account of black nurses in the early wars, beginning with Crimean, recognizes two black women in Baltimore, Maryland, who were listed as nurses in the City Directory as early as 1840.

The second chapter, "The Foundation Is Laid," devoted to basic and post-basic nursing programs, lists two additional diploma programs that existed between 1886 and 1982, making the total 92. One baccalaureate program closed after the second edition was published and another was established, making the total still 23; two associate degree programs have been added; and the additional masters program brings the total to five. Added, also, is reference to the nurse midwifery program that existed at Meharry Medical College in Nashville, Tennessee, from 1973 to 1982.

Chapter 3, "From Dreams to Achievements," has an additional project titled FACE—Faculty and Community Enhancement.

Chapter 4, "Struggle for Recognition," has four additions and two deletions because they no longer exist. The four additions are the International Council of Nurses, the Association of Black Seventh-Day Adventist Nurses, the Caribbean American Nurses Association, and the Coalition of African Nurses. The Society for Nursing History ceased to exist in 1989 and the Mid-Atlantic Regional Nurses Association has merged with the North East Organization for Nursing.

To Chapter 5, "Stony the Road," has been added reference to the American Nurses Credentialing Center.

Chapter 6, "So Proudly We Hail," devoted to blacks in the military, the Public Health Service, and the Department of Veterans Affairs, has some additions, which include black nurses in the Persian Gulf War and the Women's Vietnam Memorial.

Books and journal articles on nurses and nursing in Africa and the Caribbean have been added to the bibliography.

Hopefully, this edition will inform all about the contributions of black nurses and strengthen the ties between nurses not only in the United States of America but throughout the world.

Mary Elizabeth Carnegie, DPA, RN, FAAN
1995

Acknowledgments

Acknowledgment is made to the following individuals, associations, and institutions for generously contributing their knowledge, making suggestions, and giving encouragement and support, and for the use of their resources in the preparation of this edition: Hattie Bessent, Director, Project FACE; Doris Bloch; Patricia Moccia, NLN; Donna Richardson and Carla Serlin, ANA; Constance Holleran, Nancy J. Vatré, Sarojini Patel, and Taka Oguisso, ICN; Carol Raphael, Visiting Nurse Service of New York; Nancy Dickenson-Hazard, Sigma Theta Tau International; Catherine Binns, Chi Ete Phi; Robert Piemonte, NSNA; Barbara Butler, NEF; Geraldine Bednash, AACN; Alicia Georges; Sallie Tucker-Allen, ABNF; Pamela Maraldo, Planned Parenthood Federation of America; Joyce Elmore, Deborah Parham, CDR; Russell Green, RADM; Julia Plotnick, U.S. Public Health Service; Brig. Gen. Adams-Ender (ret.) and Brig. Gen. Nancy Adams, Army Nurse Corps; Brig. Gen. Sue Turner, Air Force Nurse Corps; Rear Adm. M. Stratton, Navy Nurse Corps; Col. Iris West, Army Center for Military History; Evelyn Moses, DHHS; Marie Mosley; Kenneth Niles and Dorothy Moore, National Library of Medicine; Nancy Valentine, Department of Veterans Affairs; Anne Davis, Nan Green, and William Holzemer, University of California; Mary Ellen Doona and Joellen Hawkins, Mass. Nurses Association; Syringa Marshall-Burnett and Angela Morgan, Jamaica, West Indies; Jesus Incarnacion, Puerto Rico, for sharing his stamp collection; U.S. Embassy of Mozambique; Library, Teachers College, Columbia University, New York; Library, American Journal of Nursing Company; Frederick Hinson; Eleanor Herrmann; Gloria Smith, Kellogg Foundation; Dorothy Powell and Bernardine Lacey, Howard University; Cynthia Capers; Pearline Gilpin; Jennie S. Bernard, Liberia; Margaret Phin and Ann M.M. Phoya, Malawi; Yvonne Pilgrin and Bernice Avis-Parris, Trinidad and Tobago; Helen Frett-Georges, British Virgin Islands; Lelia Harrocksingh and Ester Felix, St. Lucia; Joyce

O. Musandu, Kenya; Emma Banga, Ghana; Theresa Munkonge and T. Pensulo, Zambia; Lillian German, House of Representatives, Congress of the United States; Ancylin Morgan, Jamaica; Anita Furbert, Bermuda; Atheline Haynes, Barbados; Grace Madubuko, West African College of Nursing; P. P. Mella, Tanzania; Joyce Fitzpatrick, Doris Modly, and Joette Clark, Case Western Reserve University; R. M. Kakande, East, Central, Southern African College of Nursing; Edith Quartey, Ghana; Nonceba Lubanga, Uganda; Claudia LaTouche, Grenada; Emawayish Gerima, Ethiopia.

A very special thanks to Dr. Nancy F. Langston, Dean, School of Nursing, Medical College of Virginia of Virginia Commonwealth University, Richmond, VA, who made it possible for me to write this third edition while serving as Visiting Professor during the second semester of the 1993–1994 academic year; Dr. Gloria Francis, a friend of many years who came out of retirement to be my research associate; and Jackie Jackson, Assistant to the Dean, who did all of the word processing for the book and tolerated me.

Contents

Chapter
1

Answering the Call

Long before nurses were trained to care for the sick, many women—black and white—volunteered their services during crises. Black men were also nurses; for example, James Derham working as a nurse in New Orleans in 1783, was able to save enough money to buy his freedom from slavery. Within six years, he had become an outstanding physician. After he moved to Philadelphia, he won the highest respect from his colleagues in the medical profession, especially that of the eminent Benjamin Rusk (Quarles, 1969). Derham has been credited with having been the first black physician in America (Lincoln, 1967).

Historically, nursing was a role assigned to black women. During the time of slavery, black women were expected to take care of the sick in the families that owned them, breast-feed the white babies, and care for their own families and fellow slaves. Although the term nurse was not applied to them, their activities were clearly within the definition of nursing. Thus, in situations of great crisis, it was natural for many black women with such practical experience to volunteer as nurses.

Not all blacks in the United States were enslaved. Among the free blacks were some who worked as nurses. African-American women of Baltimore, Maryland, for example, have a long, proud tradition of providing health care and social services in their community. As early as 1840, Mary Williams and Frances Rose, free black women, were listed as nurses in the City Directory (Bloom, 1990). During the 1820s, Jensey Snow became widely known in Petersburg, Virginia. After earning her freedom,

1

she opened a hospital and provided health care for more than 30 years (*The Power Within,* 1993).

This chapter is limited to the stories of five black women who served as nurses in three wars: Mary Seacole, who nursed along with Florence Nightingale in the Crimean War; Sojourner Truth, Harriet Tubman, and Susie King Taylor who nursed in the Civil War, or War Between the States; and Namahyoke Sockum Curtis, who served under contract with the federal government in the Spanish-American War.

THE CRIMEAN WAR

In the Crimean War (1853–1856), Great Britain, France, and Turkey fought against Russia for control of access to the Mediterranean from the Black Sea. The immediate causes of the war were more complicated than this, but of a pattern familiar enough today—the "protection of oppressed minorities" in the target country and reprisals for the death of nationals in religious riots. The war on land was fought in three main theaters: the Danube Valley, Asia Minor, and the Crimea (Blake, 1971).

Russia and France had members of religious orders to care for their armies, but England had only untrained men to care for the sick and wounded. Ugly rumors of deplorable medical and sanitary neglect and mismanagement of casualties began to reach England. A famous letter from Sir Sidney Herbert, secretary of state for war, to Florence Nightingale, printed in the *Daily News* on October 28, 1854, contained a plea for Nightingale to supervise the military hospitals in Turkey:

> There is but one person in England that I know who would be capable of organizing and superintending such a scheme . . . My question simply is, Would you listen to the request to go out and supervise the whole thing? You would of course have plenary authority over all the nurses, and [cooperation] from the medical staff, and you would also have an unlimited power of drawing on the Government for whatever you think requisite for the success of your mission . . . I must not conceal from you that I think upon your decision will depend the ultimate success or failure of the plan. Your own personal qualities, your knowledge and your power of administration, and among greater things your rank and position in Society give you advantages in such a work which no other person possesses. (Cook, 1913, p. 153)

On October 21, 1854, Nightingale set out for the Crimea with 38 women volunteers to serve as nurses, among whom were Roman

Catholic, Anglican sisters, and lay nurses. She and her band were assigned to the base hospital at Scutari, across the strait from Constantinople (Dolan, 1968).

There may have been other black women who nursed in the Crimean War, but the services of only one, Mary Seacole, have been documented in the literature.

Mary Seacole

Mary Grant Seacole (1805–1881) (Fig. 1–1) learned the caring and healing arts from her mother, who, in her native Jamaica, British West Indies, was nicknamed "the Doctress" because of her ministrations to the sick in her lodging house in Kingston. There she nursed many of the British army officers and their families from Up-Park Camp. Although no formal training in nursing existed at that time, Mary Seacole served in Panama and Cuba during cholera and yellow fever epidemics. In order to learn more about the effects of the disease, she performed a postmortem examination on an infant who had died of cholera in Panama (Burnett, 1981).

When Mary Seacole learned that hostilities had broken out in the Crimea, she wrote the British government asking to be allowed to join Florence Nightingale in the Crimea as a nurse, but her request was denied. She was especially concerned when she learned that many of the regiments she had known in Jamaica were being sent to this area where disease killed more soldiers than did wounds. She was convinced that her knowledge of tropical diseases was vital to Britain's war effort. So, at her own expense, Mary Seacole sailed to England with a letter of introduction to Nightingale, but her attempts to join the group of recruited nurses were blocked because she was black, even though she had personal credentials written by British army doctors. When her services were

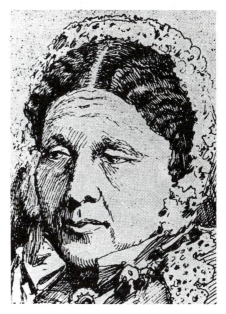

Figure 1–1 Mary Grant Seacole, black nurse in the Crimean War. (Courtesy Moorland-Spingarn Research Center, Howard University)

rejected, she appealed to the War Office. Mrs. Sidney Herbert, wife of the secretary of war, petitioned on her behalf, but the Crimean Fund would not reverse its decision. Undaunted, Seacole purchased supplies and traveled 3,000 miles to the Crimea. There she built and opened a lodging house on the road between Balaklava and Sebastopol for the comfort of the troops, naming it "The British Hotel." On the lower floor was a restaurant and bar; the upper floor was arranged like a hospital ward with her supply of medicines, many of which she concocted herself and used to nurse the sick among the officers (Alexander & Dewjee, 1981).

Seacole still hoped to secure a position as an army nurse, but when she met with Florence Nightingale, the response was the same—no vacancies. However, each night at 7:00, after having worked in her provisions store on the outskirts of the camp, she made her way to the hospital and worked as a volunteer side-by-side with Nightingale. Seacole attended not only the British casualties, but French, Sardinian, and Russian soldiers as well. She saved the lives of countless soldiers, both those wounded and others with cholera, yellow fever, malaria, diarrhea, and a host of other ailments.

Although her services in the Crimea went unheralded by the British government, Seacole had won the admiration, respect, and love of many of the English people. Public resentment brought attention to those whose prejudice had prevented her official enlistment (King, 1974). At the end of the war, news of her heroic efforts spread throughout England. London *Times* correspondent, William Howard Russell, bore testament to her services: "trust that England will not forget one who has nursed her sick . . . ." (Swaby, 1979, p. 9). Long after the war ended, the government bestowed a medal upon her for services rendered the sick and injured.

In the Institute of Jamaica is a terra-cotta bust of Seacole modeled by Count Gleichen, a nephew of Queen Victoria; and two of her Crimean War medals. Seacole had nursed Gleichen in her canteen-hotel-hospital during the Crimean War (Rogers, 1947). On the campus of the University of the West Indies is Mary Seacole Hall. In 1954, the nurses of Jamaica named their headquarters Mary Seacole House. The building was opened in 1960, and a life-sized bust was placed in the foyer where it stands today. The bust was reproduced by a Jamaican sculptor, Curtis Johnston, from the original in the Institute. At the Kingston Public Hospital is Mary Seacole Ward. All these tributes have been made in a conscious attempt to perpetuate the name of a great Jamaican and an even greater nurse, one whom the Cubans called "The Yellow Woman from Jamaica with the Cholera Medicine," and the Crimean soldiers, "The Florence Nightingale of Jamaica."

The British Commonwealth Nurses War Memorial Fund and the Lignum Vitae Club, an organization of Jamaican women in London, provided funds to restore Seacole's grave (Swaby, 1979). On November 20, 1973, there was a ceremony of reconservation of the grave of a nurse who had served in the Crimean War, who had returned to England, who had received rapturous acclaim, but who, after her death on May 14, 1881, had been totally forgotten in England—although not in her own country. According to her wish, Seacole was buried in the Catholic portion of the cemetery at Kensal Green, London, where her restored headstone today says simply, in letters of gold and blue, "Here lies Mary Seacole (1805–1881) of Kingston, Jamaica, a notable nurse who cared for the sick and wounded in the West Indies, Panama, and on the battlefield of the Crimea, 1854–1856" (Gordon, 1975).

In 1990, the Nurses Association of Jamaica received the Order of Merit conferred posthumously on Mary Seacole for distinguished services to nursing and the international community. Seacole is the first nurse to be so honored with the country's highest national award and the only person recognized with the Order of Merit on the 1990 National Honors List.

In 1992, the Royal College of Nursing (RCN) in England launched a series of "Seacole Seminars." The program at the second seminar that year included a paper, "The Role of Gatekeeping in Accessing Participants," by Vina Mayor, a black British nurse, based on her research on career patterns of black nurses in senior positions in nurse education, nursing practice, and nurse management. In addition, key members of RCN laid a wreath in Mary Seacole's memory. In the spring of 1993, RCN played host to a Mary Seacole Memorial Day, which had been organized by the Mary Seacole Memorial Association. At the Florence Nightingale Museum, a special exhibition on Seacole was mounted in collaboration with the Black Cultural Archives.

THE CIVIL WAR

The Civil War (1861–1865) has been called the second American Revolution, the War of the Rebellion, the War Between the States, the War for Southern Independence, the Rich Man's War and the Poor Man's Fight, the War to Save the Union, and the War for Freedom. It was also called a struggle between national sovereignty and states' rights. It has been referred to as a contest between profiteers, northern and southern. We know it was a revolution in which slaves and owners were freed, for both were enslaved by the system of forced labor. James Ford Rhodes, Civil War historian, stated in 1913, "Of the American Civil War it may safely be asserted that there was a single cause, slavery" (Wesley & Romero, 1967, p. 2).

> Slavery was the underlying cause of the War, despite the economic and political questions which were involved. The North contended that its fight was to preserve the Union, while the South rested its defense on states' rights. Each section declined to recognized slavery publicly as a cause of the War—until the issuance of the Emancipation Proclamation. (p. xi)

When the Civil War began with the Confederate attack on Fort Sumter, South Carolina, April 17, 1861, there were no formally trained nurses in the country. However, thousands of men and women from the North and South volunteered almost immediately for nursing assignments in field hospitals and on hospital transports.

On June 8, 1861, Dorothea Lynde Dix, a school teacher from New England, already well known as a humanitarian on behalf of the mentally ill, and a group of women friends journeyed to Washington and offered to assist the War Department by providing care for sick and wounded soldiers. On June 10, 1861, Dix was appointed by Secretary of War Simon Cameron to superintend the women nurses. This was a post of honor, but one that carried no official status and no salary. Dix's wide-ranging authority, dated April 12, 1861, theoretically gave her the power to organize hospitals for the care of the sick and wounded soldiers; to appoint nurses; and to receive, control, and disburse special supplies donated by individuals or associations for distribution among the troops (Brockett & Vaughan, 1867). Many nursed all through the war without official recognition or financial compensation; those who had been regularly appointed received $12 a month from the government, or 40 cents a day and rations (Piemonte & Gurney, 1987).

No accurate records of the appointment of nurses, their number, where they served, or the number who died, can be found. However, the records show that women serving in hospitals during the Civil War were:

> . . . regularly appointed nurses, about 3,214; Sisters of Charity, number not known; women of middle age and no training acting as cooks, etc; women who gave time without pay; women accompanying regiments, wives, etc.; and colored women . . . . (Stimson & Thompson, 1928)

Twenty journals in the National Archives in Washington, D.C., contain information about contract nurses in the Civil War, one of which is devoted to black nurses. According to these records kept on nurses at 11 hospitals in 3 states, 181 black nurses—men and women—served between July 16, 1863, and June 14, 1864: Convalescent Hospital, Baltimore, Maryland—16; Contraband Hospital, Portsmouth, Virginia—14; Flag of

Truce Boat, from Fort Monroe, Virginia—3; Contraband Small Pox Hospital, New Bern, North Carolina—44; Jarvis USG Hospital, Baltimore, Maryland—46; Chesapeake Hospital, Virginia—21; Green Heights Hospital, Virginia—1; McKims Mansion Hospital, near Alexandria, Virginia—3; and Patterson Park, US General Hospital, Baltimore—7 (Colored Nurses, 1863–64).

The stories of three black women who played significant roles as nurses in the Civil War—Sojourner Truth, Harriet Tubman, and Susie King Taylor—are presented here, although they were not contract nurses.

Sojourner Truth

Born a slave in New York, where slavery had been officially recognized as legal since 1684, and freed by the New York State Emancipation Act of 1827, Sojourner Truth (1797–1883; Fig. 1–2) was not only a famous abolitionist and underground railroad agent, itinerant preacher, lecturer, women's rights worker, and humanitarian, but also a nurse during the Civil War and immediately thereafter. When she gained her freedom in 1827, she changed her name from Isabella to Sojourner Truth to reveal the nature of her mission—"Sojourner" because she would travel and "Truth" because she would tell the truth about slavery wherever she went (Wesley & Romero, 1967). In fact, she was the first black woman in the United States to give antislavery lectures (Ortez, 1974).

Of the slaves who were freed in New York on July 4, 1827, Truth was one of the most remarkable. An abolitionist and an advocate of women's rights, she remained a lifelong illiterate, but made a deep impression by her commanding figure. With a hopeful heart and an unshakable confidence in ultimate justice and the goodness of God, she bore pity rather than bitterness toward the slaveholders (Quarles, 1969).

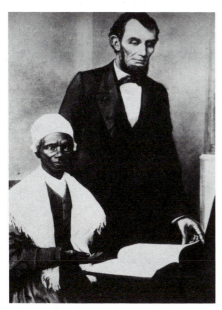

Figure 1–2   Sojourner Truth visits President Abraham Lincoln, 1864. (Courtesy U.S. Army Center of Military History)

The newly freed slaves—many sick, decrepit, mentally ravaged, and destitute—poured into Washington, D.C., from the South during and after the war (slavery had been abolished in Washington in 1862) with the hope that their needs would be provided for. Because of this problem, the War Department of the United States decided to establish the Freedmen's Bureau and to create an emergency facility. Started by the concerned citizens, the endeavor was quickly ratified by an act of the 38th Congress, dated March 3, 1865, "to Establish a Bureau for the Relief of Freedmen and Refugees."

Truth worked as a nurse/counselor for the Freedman's Relief Association during Reconstruction in the Washington area, helping freed men who had migrated from the South find homes and employment in Northern states. Many of her activities were sanctioned by President Lincoln, whom she visited in 1864, traveling from Battle Creek, Michigan, to do so. Lincoln is reported to have told her during their meeting that he had heard of her activities before being elected president. He autographed her book of names of interesting people she had met, writing, "For Aunty Sojourner Truth, October 29, 1864, A. Lincoln" (Wesley & Romero, 1967).

While in Washington, Sojourner Truth spent much time in Freedmen's Village providing care to patients in the hospital. She organized a corps of women to clean Freedmen's Hospital because, she contended, "the sick can never be made well in dirty surroundings." Truth also visited Congress to urge that funds be provided to train nurses and doctors. In 1986, as part of the Black Heritage series, the commemorative Sojourner Truth postage stamp was issued. Truth is also in the National Women's Hall of Fame, Seneca Falls, New York.

Harriet Tubman

Harriet Ross Tubman (1820–1913; Fig. 1–3), a woman of unusual capabilities and great courage, was born to slave parents in Bucktown, Dorchester County, Maryland. In addition to being an abolitionist, she had the unofficial title, "Conductor of the Underground Railroad." Before and during the Civil War, she made 19 secret trips below the Mason–Dixon Line, leading more than 300 slaves north to freedom. To join her rescue party meant to remain with it, for she threatened to kill anyone who attempted to turn back.

Tubman also volunteered her services as a nurse. By 1858, Tubman was known in abolitionist circles in England, Ireland, Scotland, Liberia, and Canada and had received financial aid from Great Britain and Canada.

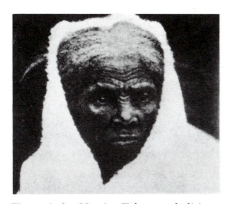

Figure 1–3 Harriet Tubman, abolitionist and nurse in the Civil War.

During the Civil War, Harriet Tubman served as a nurse in the Sea Islands off the coast of South Carolina, caring for the sick and wounded without regard to color. She also held the position of matron or nurse at the Colored Hospital, Fort Monroe, Virginia (Bradford, 1961). Acting Assistant Surgeon General Henry K. Durrant was so moved by her warmth and generous attitude that he wrote a note, addressing it, "To Whom It May Concern," commending her for "kindness and attention to the sick and suffering" (Wesley & Romero, 1967, p. 107).

Citing her for outstanding work as a nurse, a Union general urged Congress to award Harriet Tubman a pension. Like all Civil War nurses, she did not receive it until nearly 30 years after the close of the war by an act of Congress (27 Stat. 348). However, unlike the white Civil War nurses, whose pensions were only $12 a month, Harriet, along with a select few, was awarded $20 a month for the remainder of her life. In addition to her husband's pension, which she received, she was compensated by Congress for her work as a spy and a scout for the Union Army. It is reported that Tubman was the first woman to lead American troops into battle. It was reported that "Col. Montgomery and his gallant band of 300 black soldiers, under the guidance of a black woman, dashed into the enemy's country, struck a bold and effective blow, destroying commissary stores, cotton and lordly dwellings . . . ." (Bennett, 1970, p. 4).

In 1914, a bronze plaque containing a portrait of Tubman with an inscription was erected next to the entrance of the Cayuga County Courthouse in Auburn, New York. On February 1, 1978, the U.S. government honored Tubman with a commemorative postage stamp, the first in a new Black History Heritage series. The fact that Tubman was chosen to inaugurate this new series, in recognition of the contributions of black Americans to the growth and development of the United States, is of great importance. Though she was only 5 feet tall, the stamp depicts a strong face matched by her great physical strength, endurance, and a commanding presence. Unable to read or write, she developed remarkable skill planning activities as a fugitive slave, while avoiding arrest as she acted upon her single driving passion—freedom for herself and others.

The original art work of the Tubman commemorative stamp was presented to Hampton University for Placement in the M. Elizabeth Carnegie Nursing Archives during a ceremony at the University on April 15, 1978. The program was co-sponsored by the American Nurses' Association (ANA), and Joyce Elmore, Director of ANA's Department of Nursing Education, described the impact that Harriet Tubman's nursing practice had on both the military and civilian population. Earlier that year, NBC Television Network had aired a two-part special program on the life of this famous black Civil War nurse and freedom fighter, *A Woman Called Moses,* in which Cicely Tyson portrayed Tubman.

The House of Representatives passed and cleared S.J. Resolution 257, to designate March 10, 1990, as "Harriet Tubman Day." The resolution included her service "in the Civil War as a soldier, spy, nurse, scout, and cook, and as leader in working with newly freed slaves . . . whose courageous and dedicated pursuit of the promise of American ideals and common principles of humanity continues to serve and inspire all people who cherish freedom—died at her home in Auburn, New York, on March 10, 1913 . . ." (Congressional Record, 1990, p. H672). Tubman has also been inducted into the National Women's Hall of Fame, Seneca Falls, New York.

Susie King Taylor

Susie King Taylor (1848–1912; Fig. 1–4) was born into slavery on the isle of Wight in Liberty County, about 35 miles from Savannah, Georgia. When she was only 14 years old and had learned surreptitiously to read and write, a Union officer placed her in charge of a school for black refugee children at Fort Pulaski, after it fell to the Union army. Wife of a noncommissioned officer in Company E of the First South Carolina Volunteers, King was employed as a laundress for the company, but served as both teacher and nurse in her free time. When the hospital needed additional competent women to nurse the growing number of wounded Union troops, she quickly volunteered her services (Wesley & Romero, 1967).

At Beaufort, South Carolina, during the summer of 1863, Taylor met Clara Barton, a former New England school teacher, later to be the great "moving spirit" in the founding of the American Red Cross. Taylor frequently accompanied Barton, who treated her very cordially, on rounds in the hospitals at the front (Roberts, 1954). As the Civil War continued in the South, Taylor assumed duties as a volunteer nurse on the battlefront, and for four years and three months she witnessed horror, pain, suffering, and death. On April 9, 1865, Confederate General Robert E. Lee surrendered to General Ulysses S. Grant at Appomattox Court House in Virginia, ending the Civil War. During her service with the Union, she received no pay, and later, because she was not classified as an official Army nurse, she received no pension or government recognition, although her services were witnessed and had been documented. (Only contract nurses, regardless of color, received a pension.)

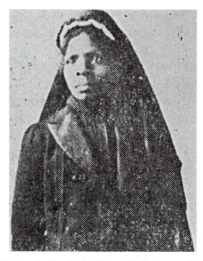

Figure 1–4   Susie King Taylor served as both teacher and nurse in the Civil War.

In 1902, Taylor published her book, *Reminiscences of My Life in Camp.* In it, she refers to having cooked, carried out physicians' orders, and taught. "I taught," she said, "a great many of the comrades in Company E to read and write . . . Nearly all were anxious to learn" (Taylor, 1902).

In 1914, a large bronze statue, "a tribute of honor and gratitude" to Civil War nurses, was erected in the rotunda of the State Capitol Building, Boston, Massachusetts, by the Massachusetts Daughters of Veterans Organizations. The statue depicts a woman caring for a wounded Union Army soldier. The inscription on the base of the statue reads: "To the Army Nurses from 1861 to 1865, Angels of Mercy and Life Amid Scenes of Conflict and Death" (Piemonte & Gurney, 1987).

THE SPANISH-AMERICAN WAR

Shortly after the Civil War ended in 1865, Cuba, then a Spanish colony, began experiencing internal unrest. Repression and rigid control of every aspect of life in Cuba had inspired numerous revolts against Spain, and between 1868 and 1878 there was a full-blown uprising. Toward the end of the century, the Cubans had become determined to have their independence. By that time, the United States had begun to assume a role in world affairs, considering herself the guardian of civilization in the New World (Franklin, 1967).

In January 1898, the American battleship, USS *Maine* was ordered to Havana to protect American life and property and to demonstrate to Spain that the government of the United States was willing to take energetic action. On February 15, an explosion of undetermined origin sank the *Maine* in the Havana harbor, killing over 250 officers and men, including 30 black sailors (Stillman, 1968). This incident set off a train of events that culminated in war two months later. On April 24, Spain declared war on the United States; the next day, the United States declared war on Spain, and hostilities continued until August 12, 1898, when the armistice protocol was signed.

The American and Spanish peace commissioners met in Paris, and on December 10, 1898, the Treaty of Paris was signed. The treaty provided that Spain was to relinquish all claim to sovereignty over Cuba. In lieu of war indemnity, Spain ceded to the United States the island of Puerto Rico and the other Spanish insular possessions in the West Indies. Upon the payment of $20 million by the United States, Spain was to relinquish the Philippines to the victor (Franklin, 1967).

At the onset of the Spanish-American War, the surgeon general requested and promptly received congressional authority to appoint women nurses under contract at the rate of $30 a month and a daily ration. Three days after the United States declared war on Spain, Anita Newcomb McGee, a medical doctor who was also vice-president of the National Society of the Daughters of the American Revolution (DAR), approached the assistant surgeon general of the army with a plan to provide nurses for the army (McGee, 1898). McGee's plan was accepted, and she was placed in charge of selecting graduate nurses for the army. She also suggested that the DAR act as an application review board for military nursing services. Thus, the DAR Hospital Corps was founded, with McGee as its director (Shields, 1981).

The epidemics of typhoid fever, malaria, and yellow fever, which were rampant during the Spanish-American War, killed many more American soldiers than did Spanish bullets. Although there were 400 training schools for nurses and more than 2,000 trained nurses in the country, there were difficulties in recruiting a sufficient number of trained nurses. During the summer of 1898, some 1,200 nurses were contracted to care for patients in the general and field hospitals in the United States and Cuba (Flanagan, 1976).

As in the Civil War, black women served. One such woman was Namahyoke Sockum Curtis (1871–1935), who played a leadership role, although she was not a trained nurse.

Namahyoke Curtis

When yellow fever appeared among troops in Santiago, McGee contacted Namahyoke Curtis (Fig. 1–5), wife of Austin M. Curtis, surgeon-in-chief at Freedmen's Hospital in Washington, D.C. Curtis, who had had yellow fever herself and was thus immune to it, was sent on July 13 under contract by the surgeon general of the army to New Orleans, Louisiana, and cities in Alabama and Florida to secure the services of blacks, both male and female, who were immune to yellow fever. Curtis was able to register 32 immune blacks to work as nurses (Kalisch & Kalisch, 1978). According to Stimson (1937), 80 colored women served as nurses during the Spanish-American War.

Curtis also served under Clara Barton, head of the American Red Cross, during the Galveston flood in Texas in 1900. During the San Francisco earthquake in 1906, she carried a commission from William H. Taft, then secretary of war. Because of her wartime service, she received a government pension. At her death on November 25, 1935, Curtis was buried in Arlington National Cemetery with the nation's military dead. A newspaper article dated November 26, 1935, recorded that, "Her work with the nurses during the Spanish-American War won her high official commendation."

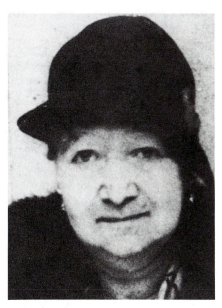

Figure 1–5 Namahyoke Sockum Curtis, contract nurse during the Spanish-American War. (Courtesy Moorland-Spingarn Research Center, Howard University)

According to the records of Tuskegee University, a black school in Alabama, five of its nursing graduates served in the camps during the war (Washington, 1910). Personnel data cards in the National Archives in Washington, D.C., show that other black, trained nurses had served: two 1898 graduates of Freedmen's Hospital—Sarah Jane Ennies Brooks and Lillian May Sumley; Nellie Singleton, an 1898 graduate of Provident in Chicago; Sarah L. Stowall, an 1897 graduate of Massachusetts General Hospital in Boston; and May Williams, who indicated that she was a graduate of Phillis Wheatley Training School, 1896, and Charity Hospital in New Orleans. One black man who volunteered as a contract nurse indicated that he was a dentist by profession.

Although the Spanish-American War was of short duration, it gave the army nurses ample time to become indispensable to the service (Stimson, 1937). It was the distinguished service of contract nurses during and following the war in the United States, Cuba, Puerto Rico, the Philippines, Hawaii, China, and

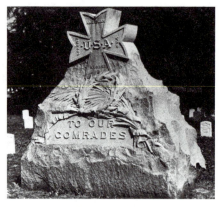

Figure 1–6   Memorial to the Spanish-American War nurses at Arlington National Cemetery. (Courtesy U.S. Army Center of Military History)

briefly in Japan, and on the hospital ship *Relief,* that paved the way for a permanent nurse corps in the army, established on February 2, 1901 (Shields, 1981).

On May 22, 1902, a monument to the Spanish-American War nurses who gave their lives in 1898 was dedicated in the nurses' section of Arlington National Cemetery (Fig. 1–6). The memorial was given by surviving Spanish-American War nurses who paid tribute "To Our Comrades" (Shields, 1981).

SUMMARY

Between 1853 and 1898, three wars were fought in which it is known that black women, most of whom were untrained, served as nurses: The Crimean War, the Civil War, and the Spanish-American War. Although there may have been other black nurses in the Crimean War, Mary Seacole is the only one documented in the literature.

Serving in the Civil War were Sojourner Truth, Harriet Tubman, and Susie King Taylor. These women's stories are only illustrations of the contributions made by many in the course of the war. Throughout the South, on untold battlefields and in many camps, black women worked with the Union army as spies, scouts, nurses, and teachers. They served in their way, as did their menfolk, to show the willingness of blacks to sacrifice for freedom (Wesley & Romero, 1967).

The only black woman cited by name in the literature for service in the Spanish-American War is Namahyoke Sockum Curtis, an untrained contract nurse, who not only received a pension from the War Department but, when she died in 1935, was buried in Arlington National Cemetery with other famous war dead. Of the 80 black women who served as nurses in the Spanish-American War, 32 (mostly untrained, but immune to yellow fever) were recruited by Curtis.

REFERENCES

Alexander, A., & Dewjee, A. (1981). Mary Seacole. *History Today, 31,* 45.

Bennett, L. (1970). *Before the Mayflower: A history of the Negro in America, 1619–1964,* (7th ed.). Chicago: Johnson Publications.

Blake, R. L. V. F. (1971). *The Crimean War.* London: Leo Cooper.

Bloom, N. D. (1990). *Annie M. Barnes Hitchens.* Baltimore, MD: Hen House Productions.

Bradford, S. (1961). *The Moses of her people.* New York: Corinth Books.

Brockett, L. P., & Vaughan, M. C. (1867). *Women's work in the Civil war: A record of heroism, patriotism, and patience.* Philadelphia: Seigler, McCurdy.

Burnett, S. M. (1981). Jamaica: Professional progress, case for all are goals. *American Journal of Nursing, 81,* 13–14.

Colored Nurses—Contract Nurses, 1863–64. Record Group 94, Entry 591. Washington, DC: National Archives.

Congressional Record (1990) Proceedings and Debates of the 101st Congress Second Session, Vol. 136, No. 22. Washington, DC: U.S. Government Printing Office.

Cook, E. (1913). *The life of Florence Nightingale* (Vol. 19). London: Macmillan.

Dolan, J. (1968). *History of nursing* (12th ed). Philadelphia: W.B. Saunders.

Flanagan, L. (1976). *The story of the American nurses' association.* Kansas City: The Association.

Franklin, J. H. (1967). *From slavery to freedom* (3rd ed). New York: Alfred Knopf.

Gordon, J. E. (1975). Mary Seacole—a forgotten nurse heroine of the Crimea. *Midwife, Health Visitor & Community Nurses, 11,* 47–50.

Kalisch, P., & Kalisch, B. (1978). *The advance of American nursing.* Boston: Little Brown & Co.

King, A. (1974, April). Mary Seacole, Part II, the Crimea. *Essence.* pp 68, 94.

Lincoln, C. E. (1967). *The Negro pilgrimage in America.* New York: Bantam Books.

McGee Journal. (1898). Washington, DC: The National Archives.

Ortez, V. (1974). *Sojourner Truth, a self-made Woman.* Philadelphia: J.B. Lippincott.

Piemonte, R. V., & Gurney, C. (1987). *Highlights in the history of the Army Nurse Corps.* Washington, DC: U.S. Army Center of Military History.

Quarles, B. (1969). *The Negro in the making of America.* New York: Macmillan.

Roberts, M. M. (1954). *American nursing: History and interpretation.* New York: Macmillan.

Rogers, J. A. (1947). *World's great men of color: 3000 B.C. to 1946 A.D.* (Vol. II). New York: The Author.

Shields, E. A. (1981). *Highlights in the history of the army nurse corps.* Washington, DC: U.S. Government Printing Office.

Stillman, R. J. (1968). *Integration of the Negro in the U.S. armed forces.* New York: Praeger.

Stimson, J. D. (1937). *History and manual of the army nurse corps.* Carlisle Barracks, PA: Medical Field Service School.

Stimson, J. D., & Thompson, E. C. S. (1928). Women nurses with the union forces during the Civil war. *The Military Surgeon, 62,* (Jan–Feb).

Swaby, G. (circa 1979). The story of Mary Seacole. *The Profession of Nursing,* 19–20.

Taylor, S. K. (1902). *Reminiscences of my life in camp.* Boston: The author.

The power within: The legacy of Dr. Daniel Hale Williams. The 1993 Calendar of African-American History, Aetna.

Washington, B. T. (1910). Training colored nurses at Tuskegee. *American Journal of Nursing, 10,* 167–171.

Wesley, C., & Romero, P. (1967). *Negro Americans in the Civil war.* New York: Publishers Co.

Chapter
2

~

The Foundation Is Laid

This chapter is devoted to the history of basic and post-basic nursing programs at historically black institutions. Basic programs include those awarding the diploma, bachelor's, and associate degree; post-basic programs include five nondegree programs—two in public health nursing and three in nurse-midwifery, and five master's degree programs. The master's program at Meharry Medical College, Nashville, Tennessee, reported in the first edition, was short lived, opening in 1982 and closing in 1985.

When the early schools of nursing were established in the United States, quota systems tended to restrict the admission of black students. The New England Hospital for Women and Children in Boston, Massachusetts, founded by a group of women physicians, was incorporated on March 18, 1863, with a charter calling for the admission of one "Negro and one Jew" to each nursing class. The purposes of the hospital were "(1) to provide for women medical aid of competent physicians of their own sex; (2) to assist educated women in the practical study of medicine; (3) to train nurses for the care of the sick; and (4) to prove to the world that a woman can be a good physician and a skillful surgeon" (Annual Report for 1878). Although the first formal program in nursing at the hospital was not begun until 1872, nursing students were accepted as early as 1866, receiving only six months of training. Those who completed the course were given neither a diploma nor a certificate. Later, the course was increased to one year, and to 16 months by 1878 (Chayer, 1954).

On March 23, 1878, the first black student, Mary Eliza Mahoney (Fig. 2–1) was admitted to the 16-month course at the New England Hospital for Women and Children; she was graduated on August 1, 1879. Of a class of 42, Mahoney was one of four students who successfully completed the course. The opportunity given to Mahoney was also extended to a few other blacks. Before the school closed in 1951, six other blacks had completed the program: Lavinia Holloway, Josephine Braxton, Kittie Toliver, Ann Dillit, Roxie Dentz Smith, and Laura Morrison Bayne. Throughout her life, Mahoney, America's first black, trained nurse, gave unselfishly of herself in professional and community affairs. In 1920, the Nineteenth Amendment to the Constitution was ratified to enfranchise women. At the time Mahoney cast her vote, she was 76 years old.

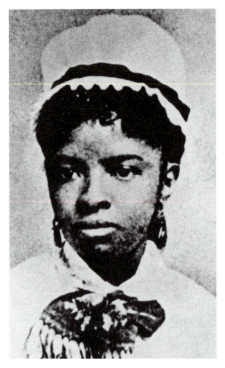

Figure 2–1 Mary Eliza Mahoney, America's first trained black nurse.

In 1926, Mahoney died at the age of nearly 81. A hallmark of her more than 40 years of service included the furthering of intergroup relations. Among her many honors conferred posthumously was the Mary Mahoney Award established in 1936 by the National Association of Colored Graduate Nurses (NACGN) for presentation to a person(s) for outstanding contributions in the area of intergroup relations. The first recipient of the Mary Mahoney Award was Adah B. Thoms, a black nurse who devoted her time and energies during 1917 and 1918 to gaining admittance for black nurses to the American Red Cross, which would make them eligible for service in the U.S. Army Nurse Corps. Since 1952, the Mary Mahoney Award has been given by the American Nurses' Association (ANA) at each biennial convention. In 1944, the Recreation Hall at Camp Livingston, Louisiana, was named in her honor. In 1970, the city of Boston honored Mahoney by the naming the Area 2 Family Life Center in Roxbury the Mary Eliza Mahoney Family Life Center.

In 1973, Chi Eta Phi, a national black sorority, and ANA restored Mahoney's grave in Woodlawn Cemetery, Everett, Massachusetts, and a granite monument bearing a sculpture of her head was erected. In 1976, along with 14 other outstanding nurses, Mahoney was admitted to the ANA Hall of Fame. In September 1984, nurses from across the nation traveled over the Labor Day weekend to join Chi Eta Phi Sorority and ANA as they made the first National Pilgrimage to the gravesite of Mary Mahoney, where a service of commemoration was held. This service was repeated in June, 1990 during the ANA convention, which was held in Boston. The Community Health Project, Inc., a nonprofit corporation funded by the Department of Health, Education, and Welfare (DHEW), has established a center in her memory. It is located in Oklahoma and provides health care services to isolated communities (Grippando, 1983).

Only two other black women in this country had been honored with a gravesite ceremony—in Battle Creek, Michigan, Sojourner Truth, an abolitionist and Civil War nurse, and Mary McLeod Bethune, a renowned educator, who was interred in Daytona, Florida, where she had founded a black school, Bethune-Cookman College, which currently has a baccalaureate program in nursing. Bethune, founder of the National Council of Negro Women and the first black woman to receive a major appointment from the U.S. government, directed the Division of Negro Education during the life of the National Youth Administration, one of the federal agencies of the Great Depression, and had given practical assistance and effectively promoted the aspirations of the National Association of Colored Graduate Nurses.

Nominated by Joellen W. Hawkins for the Lucy Lincoln Drown Nursing History Society of Massachusetts Nurses Association, on October 9, 1993, Mary Mahoney was among the 35 distinguished American women inducted into the National Women's Hall of Fame at Seneca Falls, New York. The honor was accepted by Nettie Birnbach, President, New York State Nurses Association for the American Nurses Association.

In addition to those black nurses who completed the course of study at the New England Hospital for Women and Children, a few other black women were graduated, along with whites, from other schools—New York Infirmary in New York City and Washington General Hospital and Asylum Training School for Nurses in the District of Columbia were among them. Martha Franklin from Connecticut, who was to found the National Association of Colored Graduate Nurses, completed the course in 1897 at the Women's Hospital in Philadelphia, which had been established in 1861 by a group of Quaker ladies of Philadelphia who announced their intention of opening a school "for training of a superior class of young women" (Jamieson & Sewall, 1944). Franklin was the second and last black nurse to be graduated from the Women's Hospital. The first one, Anne Reeves, was graduated in April, 1888 (West, 1931).

Gertrude Voorhees was graduated from Blockley Hospital Training School (renamed Philadelphia General). Rose Snowden finished the course of study at Jefferson Polyclinic in Chicago. Sarah L. Stowall, who served as a contract nurse during the Spanish-American War, indicated on her personnel data card that she had been graduated from McLean Hospital School of Nursing in 1896 and Massachusetts General Hospital, Boston in 1897 (Personnel Data Cards, 1898). Three black women graduated from the nursing program at Berea College in Kentucky in 1902: Sarah Belle Jerman, Mary Eliza Merritt, and Margaret Jones (Peck & Pride, 1982). Mossell (1908, p. 178) reports, "It is also said that Johns Hopkins (in Baltimore) has twenty-four Afro-American women graduates."

BLACK BASIC PROGRAMS

By the early part of the twentieth century, America had started developing rigid patterns of segregation and discrimination in all sections of the country. Nursing, along with other kinds of education, was affected. Black codes were set up in the South by law and in the North by custom. In 1904, a bill was passed in Kentucky declaring it "unlawful for any person, corporation, or association of persons to maintain or operate any college, school, or institution where persons of the white and Negro races are both received as pupils for instruction" (Peck & Smith, 1982, p. 51). This law caused Berea College to end its practice of admitting blacks and they would not attend Berea College again until the 1950s after the Supreme Court Decision outlawing segregation in public schools. During the time when it was unlawful to admit black students, Berea College gave financial support to Lincoln Institute, a black private school in Frankfort, Kentucky. Currently, Berea College has blacks on its Board of Trustees (Alex Haley, a black author of note, served until his death in 1993) and the dean of its school of nursing is black—Dr. Cora Newell Withrow. Hospitals and nursing schools followed the segregated pattern, which forced the establishment of hospitals and schools of nursing for blacks.

Diploma

Like the typical nursing school that emerged in this country in the late 1800s, most of those established exclusively for blacks had their origins in hospitals and led to a diploma. The few nursing schools established outside of the hospital also led to a diploma.

Founded in 1881, The Atlanta Baptist Female Seminary (renamed Spelman College in 1924 after Lucy Henry Spelman, the mother-in-law of John D. Rockefeller) was the first college for black women in the country. Spelman College grew from a school started in the basement of Friendship Baptist Church, a black church. The founders were two white women from New England, Sophia B. Packard and Harriet E. Giles, who, deploring the lack of educational opportunities for black women, went to the South during the post-Civil War period to establish a school for young black women who had been freed from the bondage of slavery. John D. Rockefeller had given a large grant to the school.

Feeling the need to open to black women a wide field of honorable, lucrative, and helpful employment, as part of the missionary course, a 2-year nursing program leading to a diploma was added at Spelman in March 1886 (*Spelman Messenger,* 1908). This was the first nursing program exclusively for blacks in the country. In 1901, Dr. Malcolm MacVicar raised funds and built the 31-bed MacVicar Hospital on the campus of Spelman Seminary as a department of the school for the benefit of black women and children (*Spelman Messenger,* 1914). It also served as a practice facility for the nursing students. Before then, clinical practice had been limited to the school's infirmary (Fig. 2–2). The program which had expanded to three years, was closed in 1928 so that students could be exposed to more

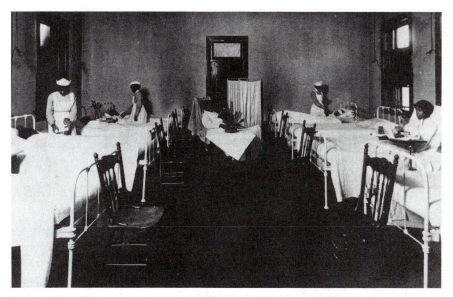

Figure 2–2   Early nursing students at Spelman College gaining clinical experience in the school's infirmary. (Courtesy Spelman College)

extensive clinical experiences available in larger institutions. During its lifetime, Spelman had graduated 117 nurses.

Howard University was conceived in 1866 by members of the Missionary Society of the Congregational Church of Washington, DC. The original educational objectives were to provide instruction for "colored men for the ministry; later, for the education of teachers and preachers; finally, for the preparation of anyone who might contemplate any vocation or profession whatever" (Dyson, 1921, p. 9). The university was formally approved by President Andrew Johnson on March 2, 1867.

By 1893, the School of Medicine at Howard University had decided to train nurses in theory and practice and so established an 18-month program. The students enrolled in this program gained clinical experience at Freedmen's Hospital. As of July 1, 1894, 75 nursing students were in attendance. Seven of the women who were admitted in 1893 were graduated in 1895. The diplomas were signed by the medical faculty and the officials of the University. Although this first program at Howard University was short lived—discontinued when Freedmen's Hospital School of Nursing assumed the responsibility for the nurse training program in 1894—it is significant to note that it did exist, with the unique feature of having been established under the aegis of a university. Two factors may have been responsible for the demise of the Howard University program: economic conditions that followed the panic of 1873, which created budgetary problems for all colleges and universities, and the general consensus that higher education for women was neither necessary nor practical (Davis, 1976).

Like most nursing schools in the beginning, black schools were established by hospitals because of the need to have patients receive nursing care at no, or little, cost to the hospital. Formal education for nurses was not the primary goal. Unlike most diploma schools in this country, when Lincoln School for Nurses in New York was established in 1898, it was operated independently of the hospital—one of the principles upon which the Nightingale system was based. Lincoln was supported by a group of white philanthropists. The major purpose was to train black women to care for the black sick people. During its lifetime of 64 years, this nationally accredited school graduated 1,864 nurses. Its sphere of influence was both national and international, with students coming from just about every state in the Union and 16 foreign countries, including Canada, Bermuda, the British West Indies, British Guiana, the Bahamas, Haiti, Panama, Liberia, and Nigeria. Before Lincoln closed in 1961, the charter had been changed to permit the admission of white students. Esther Eshelman, who was graduated in 1957, was the only white student who received a diploma from Lincoln.

In the North, for the most part, schools of nursing were segregated. Only 39 of the 1,708 schools of nursing existing in 1928 had a policy to admit blacks. Because blacks were denied admission to most of the white schools in the North, schools were created just for blacks. Provident Hospital School of Nursing in Chicago was established in 1891 by a black physician, Dr. Daniel Hale Williams, because a black woman, Emma Reynolds from Kansas City, had been denied admission to every school of nursing in Chicago.

Between 1891 and 1924, 11 nursing schools for blacks were established in five northern states: Illinois, Kansas, Pennsylvania, New York, and Michigan (Table 2–1). The vast majority of blacks, however, attended only six of these schools: Provident in Chicago, Lincoln and Harlem in New York, Douglass in Kansas City, Kansas, and Mercy and Douglass in Philadelphia. In 1949, Mercy and Douglass merged, becoming Mercy-Douglass Hospital School of Nursing.

Both Lincoln and Harlem were controlled and administered by whites in the beginning; both had black directors before they closed: Ivy N.

Table 2–1 Diploma Nursing Programs for Blacks, 1886–1982

Institution	Location	Established	Year Closed
Alabama			
Tuskegee Institute	Tuskegee	1892	1948*
Hale Infirmary	Montgomery	1917	1932
Fraternal Hospital	Montgomery	1919	1941
Tuggle Institute	Birmingham	1925	1930
Burwell Hospital	Selma	1927	1933
Stillman College	Tuscaloosa	1930	1948
Tennessee Coal & Iron	Birmingham	U	1931
Oakwood College	Huntsville	1909	1923
Arkansas			
United Friends	Little Rock	1918	1932
Bush Memorial (Royal Circle)	Little Rock	1918	1933
Great Southern Fraternal	Little Rock	1921	1930
District of Columbia			
Howard University	Washington	1893	1895
Freedmen's Hospital	Washington	1894	1973
Florida			
Brewster Hospital	Jacksonville	1902	1954
Brewster Hospital	Jacksonville	1961**	1963
Daytona Hospital	Daytona Beach	1922	1939
Florida A & M College	Tallahassee	1925	1936*

U–Unknown
*Converted to baccalaureate program
**Reopened

(Continued)

Table 2–1   *(Continued)*

Institution	Location	Established	Year Closed
Georgia			
Lamar Wing, University Hospital	Augusta	1894	1957
Lamar Wing, University Hospital	Augusta	1960★★	1965
Spelman College	Atlanta	1886	1928
Charity Hospital	Savannah	1901	U
Lula Grove Hospital	Atlanta	1913	U
Grady Hospital	Atlanta	1917	1982
John Archbold	Thomasville	1925	U
Morris Brown College	Augusta	1930	U
City Hospital	Columbus	U	U
McKane Hospital	Savannah	U	U
Illinois			
Provident Hospital	Chicago	1891	1966
New Home Sanitorium	Jacksonville	1922	1930
Hinsdale Sanitarium and Hospital	Hinsdale	1922	1969
Kansas			
Douglass	Kansas City	1898	1937
Protective Home & Mitchell Hospital	Leavenworth	1909	1911
Kentucky			
Citizens National Hospital	Louisville	1888	1912
Red Cross Hospital	Louisville	1898	1938
Louisiana			
Flint Goodridge Hospital	New Orleans	1896	1934
Providence Sanitarium	New Orleans	1907	1917
Maryland			
Provident	Baltimore	1895	1976
Crownsville State Hospital	Crownsville	1917	1930
Maryland Tuberculosis Sanitorium	Henryton	1926	1962
Michigan			
Battle Creek Sanitarium	Battle Creek	1910	1934
Dunbar Memorial Hospital	Detroit	1924	1931
Mississippi			
Mississippi Baptist Hospital	Jackson	1911	1960
Missouri			
University Medical College	Kansas City	1895	1897
Provident Hospital	St. Louis	1899	U
Kansas City General Hospital, No. 2	Kansas City	1911	1973
Wheatly-Provident Hospital	Kansas City	1914	1934
Homer G. Phillips Hospital	St. Louis	1919	1968
People's Hospital	St. Louis	1921	1928
St. Mary's Infirmary	St. Louis	1933	1958
Perry Sanitorium	Kansas City	1910	1929
New York			
Lincoln School for Nurses	New York	1898	1961
Harlem Hospital	New York	1923	1977

Table 2-1 *(Continued)*

Institution	Location	Established	Year Closed
North Carolina			
Good Samaritan Hospital	Charlotte	1891	1960
St. Agnes Hospital	Raleigh	1896	1959
Lincoln Hospital	Durham	1902	1971
Community Hospital	Wilmington	1920	1936
Community Hospital	Wilmington	1940★★	1966
Negro Division, State Sanitorium	Sanitorium	1926	1953
L. Richardson Memorial Hospital	Greensboro	1927	1953
Kate Bitting Reynolds Hospital	Winston-Salem	1938	1971
Pennsylvania			
Douglass Hospital	Philadelphia	1895	1923
Mercy Hospital	Philadelphia	1907	1949
Mercy-Douglass Hospital	Philadelphia	1949	1960
South Carolina			
Cannon Street Hospital	Charleston	U	U
Hospital & Training School for Nurses	Charleston	1897	1959
Good Samaritan Waverly	Columbia	1910	1953
Benedict College	Columbia	1917	U
Waverly Fraternal	Columbia	1924	U
Columbia Hospital	Columbia	1935	1965
Tennessee			
Meharry Medical College	Nashville	1900	1947★
University of West Tennessee	Memphis	1900	1923
Mercy Hospital	Nashville	1900	U
Terrell Memorial Hospital	Memphis	1907	U
Collins Chapel Hospital	Memphis	1907	1940
Negro Baptist Hospital	Memphis	1912	U
Millie Hale Hospital	Nashville	1916	1928
Mercy Hospital	Memphis	1918	U
Royal Circle Hospital	Nashville	1921	U
City of Memphis Hospital	Memphis	1956	1968
Texas			
Prairie View A & M University	Prairie View	1918	1952★
Negro Baptist Hospital	Fort Worth	1919	1930
Houston Negro Hospital	Houston	1927	1933
Houston Negro Hospital	Houston	1943★★	1944
Virginia			
Dixie Hospital	Hampton	1891	1956
Richmond Hospital	Richmond	Circa 1899	Circa 1923
Burell Hospital	Roanoke	1915	1933
Piedmont Sanitarium	Burkeville	1918	1960
Whittaker Memorial Hospital	Newport News	Circa 1918	Circa 1930
St. Phillip Hospital	Richmond	1920	1962
West Virginia			
Lomax Sanitarium	Bluefield	1906	1928
Brown Hospital	Bluefield	1919	1937
Barnette Hospital	Huntington	Circa 1920	Circa 1930

Tinkler at Lincoln and Alida Dailey at Harlem, followed by Edith Benoit. From their inception, Provident and Mercy-Douglass were administered and controlled by blacks. From the beginning, Provident had an interracial board and treated patients regardless of race, creed, or nationality. By 1893, Provident Hospital had gained fame when Dr. Daniel Hale Williams, its founder, performed the first recorded operation on the human heart. In later years, the Julius Rosenwald Fund made possible many improvements in the school of nursing (Staupers, 1961).

In the South, a typical pattern emerged: the dual system, in keeping with the doctrine of "separate but equal" as an outcome of the Plessy vs. Ferguson Supreme Court Decision of 1896. This decision supported the constitutionality of a Louisiana law requiring separate but equal facilities for whites and blacks in railroad cars. As a result, schools of nursing were established in all-black institutions—hospitals and colleges. Some white hospitals conducted two programs—one for whites and one for blacks. Theory was usually given by the same white faculty in separate classrooms; practice was also gained separately—for black students in separate buildings, wings, or wards for black patients. Separate, yes, but in no way equal! A case in point: St. Philip Hospital School of Nursing in Richmond, Virginia, was opened in 1920 as a program for blacks under the aegis of the Medical College of Virginia (MCV) which had had a school for whites since 1893. Until 1941, when the first black faculty were hired for St. Philip, whites had taught both black and white students separately—in the classroom and in the clinical facilities. The black students and faculty were housed in a separate dormitory, where the classrooms and library were located, and ate their meals in a separate dining room. The black faculty, of which the author was one, also had the responsibility for supervising the extracurricular activities of the students; for example, the glee club, drama club, and basketball team.

With the advent of integration in the 1950s, and its accompanying increase of black students being accepted at previously all-white institutions (MCV School of Nursing admitted its first black student in 1958), and the decline in enrollment of blacks at these dual-system institutions, it was no longer necessary or economically feasible for an institution to support two racially distinct programs. Hence the decision by MCV to phase out its program for blacks (Francis, 1967). When St. Philip School of Nursing closed in 1962, it had graduated 688 black nurses, among whom was Elizabeth Lipford Kent, Class of 1944. In 1955, as far as can be determined, she became the first black nurse in the country to earn a doctoral degree, conferred on her by the University of Michigan, Ann Arbor. For a number of years, until retirement, Dr. Kent was Director of Nursing and Psychiatric

Nurse Executive, Lafayette Clinic, Detroit, Michigan and Adjunct Assistant Professor, Wayne State University, College of Nursing, Detroit.

In 1924, The Hospital Library and Service Bureau conducted a survey of the black schools of nursing in the country to determine management of these Schools—control of budget, amount of white cooperation, number of students, number of instructors, entrance requirements, length of course, working hours per week, division of service, postgraduate courses, housing, and recreation. Regarding the quality of these schools, one white director of a southern school commented:

> The type of training the average colored nurse receives in this part of the country is far inferior to that given to white nurses. Even the best training for colored nurses hardly approximates the poorest training given to white nurses. From another standpoint, their educational background is not so good . . . (Educational Facilities, 1925)

In 1917, Julius Rosenwald, a Jewish immigrant and President of Sears Roebuck and Company, created the Julius Rosenwald Fund as a philanthropic corporation to promote better black education and American race relations (Kessel, 1989). In 1928, the Fund was reorganized and modeled after the Rockefeller Foundation and management was turned over to a professional staff. The Fund continued to work on behalf of blacks, developing programs in medical economics, fellowships for the professions, library service, social studies, general education and race relations (Jones, 1981). By the time of his death in 1932, Rosenwald had contributed over $4 million to the building of more than 5,000 Rosenwald schools.

Under aegis of the Rosenwald Fund, Nina D. Gage, a highly respected nurse educator, and Alma C. Haupt, associate director, National Organization for Public Health Nursing, made a survey in 1932 of black schools of nursing in six southern states: Alabama, Georgia, Louisiana, Mississippi, Tennessee, and Texas. They reported:

> The schools of nursing themselves are of many varieties—some so poor as to make one question how they can possibly meet the standards of a State Board of Nurse Examiners . . . In . . . one, two shabby houses were used as a hospital of 35 beds and a nurses' home for 12 students. A colored nurse is superintendent of nurses and the sole member of the faculty. A three-year course is given, every subject being taught by the one nurse . . . No public health subjects are included in the curriculum . . . but the students are frequently sent out to homes as private duty nurses, and the wages thus earned help to run the hospital. (Gage & Haupt, 1932, p. 678)

Twelve years after the Gage and Haupt survey, Estelle Massey Riddle Osborne, then consultant for the National Nursing Council for War Service, and Rita E. Miller Dargan, then part-time consultant for the U.S. Public Health Service, conducted a survey at the request of Surgeon General Parran to determine the status of black nursing schools in the country and to elicit trends relating to the employment and professional participation of black nurses. They found that conditions in the schools, especially in the South, had not changed to any great extent. They also reported that in black nursing schools having white directors, with the exception of one, the interest and knowledge of these directors in the broader aspects of black life ranged from apparent indifference to hostility. These attitudes, they said, were definitely reflected in the programs for the nurses and the communities' reaction to the group (Newell, 1951).

Although Riddle and Miller made specific recommendations for upgrading the educational situation in the poorer schools, no formal steps were taken at that time to implement the recommendations (Newell, 1951). It should be noted that not all black schools were poor in quality. Many were excellent, meeting all national standards. The 1949 interim classification of state-approved schools offering basic programs, based on data voluntarily submitted by 1,156 schools in the United States, Hawaii, and Puerto Rico, consisted of two groups. Group I included the upper 25 percent of all basic programs; group II included the middle 50 percent. Of the 29 black schools in existence at that time, 16 were included in groups I and II—9 in group I and 7 in group II. Of the 9 in group I, 6 were baccalaureate programs and three were diploma programs. Of the 7 in group II, only 1 was a baccalaureate program, whereas the other 6 were diploma programs (West & Hawkins, 1950).

After the midcentury, the number of black diploma programs steadily decreased. From 1886 to 1982, when the last black diploma program closed, 91 black diploma programs in 87 institutions (four hospitals had had two programs over the years, i.e., they closed, reopened, and closed again) in 20 states and the District of Columbia had been in existence, graduating the vast majority of black nurses in the country up to that time (Table 2–1). Four diploma schools located in academic institutions were converted in time to baccalaureate programs: Tuskegee University in Alabama (the oldest continuing historically black program in the country), Florida A&M in Tallahassee, Meharry in Nashville, Tennessee; and Prairie View A&M University in Texas.

Tuskegee University, which had had a diploma program since 1892, began a baccalaureate program in 1948. Florida A&M University, whose diploma program had been state-approved since 1925, established a baccalaureate program in 1936. Prairie View A&M University in Texas had had a diploma program since 1918 and initiated a baccalaureate program in 1952. Meharry Medical College, which began its diploma program in 1900, changed to a baccalaureate program in 1947, but closed it in 1962. Tuskegee's first graduating class in 1894 included a man—Oscar R. Gayle, who had an admirable career as a nurse in Army hospitals.

After the famous May 17, 1954 Supreme Court Decision on school desegregation (*Brown v. the Board of Education of Topeka*), which nullified the *Plessy v. Ferguson Decision of 1896,* establishing the separate-but-equal doctrine, all types of educational discrimination were considered, including nursing. The unanimous decision read by Chief Justice Earl B. Warren, asserted that "separate educational facilities are inherently unequal, making racial segregation in public schools unconstitutional." It was also around this time that schools of nursing were being accredited according to national standards; and many schools were forced to close. Not all of the black schools closed because they did not meet standards, however, some closed because of financial difficulties.

With integration permitting black students to be admitted to formerly all-white schools—North and South—good black schools often had difficulty attracting the number of qualified students who otherwise might have applied; hence, many closed. It should be noted that not all formerly all-white schools voluntarily opened their doors to black students. For example, Esther McCready, a black resident of Baltimore, brought suit against the University of Maryland School of Nursing because her application for admission had been denied. She had also been advised by the officials of the University to apply to an all-black school. McCready instituted legal proceedings in 1950, the result of which was her eventual admission to the University of Maryland School of Nursing by an order of the Maryland Supreme Court.

It is interesting to note that in 1955 when the master's program was being established at the University of Maryland School of Nursing, Dean Florence Gipe contacted the author by telephone to inform her that the decision had been made to include blacks in the enrollment and to request that a qualified black nurse be sent for admission to the program. As a result, Juanita Franklin Wilson who had a diploma from Homer G. Phillips Hospital School of Nursing in St. Louis, Missouri, and a bachelor's degree from Florida A&M University, enrolled and was the first in her class to complete the requirements for a master's degree, with a major in psychiatric nursing. This was an annual request for several years thereafter.

To obtain official data on the diploma programs, Boards of Nursing in those states with known historically black schools of nursing were contacted by the author. Because registration laws were not in effect until 1903, and only four states had such laws in that year, many records do not exist for schools established before then. In one state, North Carolina, the records had been destroyed by fire; in some, the data were just not available. From the data available, however, a profile emerges in terms of location, administrative control, financial support, length of program, life span of the program, state approval, enrollment, number of graduates, and reasons for closing.

All but 6 of the schools were located in urban areas. As for administrative control, 10 were in colleges and universities, 3 were under medical schools, and 1 was independent. Six were supported by the state, 5 of which were in tuberculosis sanitariums, 1 was supported with federal funds, and the rest were financed with private funds, mostly by religious organizations, but some by physicians. The programs ranged in length from 18 months to three years, and the life span was from 1 to 81 years. Most of those existing after state registration laws were passed had state approval. The enrollment was as few as one (in one school), and the number of graduates ranged from one to nearly 2,000. The reasons given for closing were many, among which were financial difficulties, insufficient applicants, integration (i.e., white and black units in the same institution combined to one school or black students were admitted to formerly all-white schools in the same area); student strikes due to poor living and working conditions; and loss of state board approval or national accreditation.

In 1965, the nursing profession took the position that all education for nursing should take place in institutions of higher education and that by 1985 the bachelor's degree would be required for entry into practice (American Nurses' Association, 1965). By 1965, 71 of the 91 black diploma programs had closed, and after 1982 there were no black diploma programs left. The black diploma programs served a valuable purpose, and most of the black nurses who have successfully completed programs in higher education and now occupy top level positions in the profession are graduates of these schools. Without their existence, the percentage of black professional nurses in the total nurse population, although low, would have been even lower.

Although there are no more black diploma programs, many of those that did exist still have active alumnae associations and hold reunions. Attending the 1993 reunion of the St. Philip Alumnae Association was Dr. Nancy Langston (Fig. 2–3), Dean of the School of Nursing at the Medical College of Virginia, Virginia Commonwealth University, of which St. Philip had been a part from 1920 to 1962.

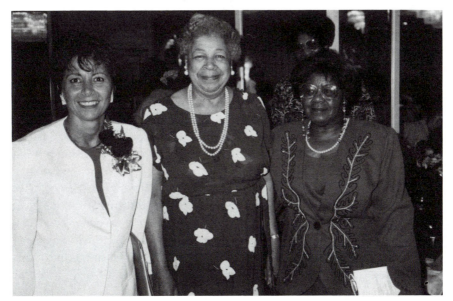

Figure 2–3   L–R: Dr. Nancy F. Langston, Dr. Mary Elizabeth Carnegie, a former St. Philip faculty member (1942–1943), and Marian Shoffner, attending the banquet at St. Philip Alumnae reunion, Newark, NJ, 1993.

Baccalaureate

Entry of nurses to institutions of higher education did not begin until 1899, with the establishment of a course for graduate nurses at Teachers College, Columbia University, New York. At that time, this was not a degree-granting program, but the course marked a new recognition that nurses needed advanced education to prepare them for leadership positions in hospitals and schools of nursing. It was also an indication of the acceptance of nursing by the university as an academic discipline.

In 1916, the University of Cincinnati established a five-year program leading to a bachelor's degree in nursing—the first in the country (Roberts, 1954). For many years, the pattern followed had consisted of two years of liberal arts courses and three years of nursing. Six years later, in 1922, Howard University, a black school in Washington, DC, established a five-year program leading to a bachelor of science degree in nursing in cooperation with Freedmen's Hospital, which was already operating a diploma program. The graduate would then have both the degree from Howard and a diploma from Freedmen's. The plan was to have students spend two years in the College of Liberal Arts and three years in the School of Nursing at Freedmen's. The Nursing Department at Howard was part of the School of Public Health and Hygiene. This program was not popular and because of an insufficient number of applicants, it was discontinued three years later, in 1925.

The oldest continuing baccalaureate nursing program at a historically black institution is at Florida A&M University in Tallahassee. As long ago as 1897, attempts had been made by the first president of the State Normal College for Colored Students (now Florida A&M University) in Tallahassee to convince the Florida legislature of the need for establishing a training program for nurses in Florida to give women "one additional field in which they may develop their capacity, and put money in their purses, while soothing back to health and usefulness the suffering patient." After several unsuccessful attempts, in 1909 the school began offering such training in its Department of Mechanical and Domestic Arts. Finally, on April 11, 1911, the legislature approved the Florida A&M Hospital and Nurse Training program and appropriated funds to construct a 19-bed facility on the campus. The new hospital opened its doors on October 12, 1911.

By 1925, the hospital at Florida A&M College had expanded to 25 beds and extended its facilities to serve both white and black patients in Tallahassee and the surrounding areas. The early nursing program was two years long, until 1925 when the school was established as a three-year diploma program, completely controlled by the hospital and administered by the medical director, who even signed the diplomas. In 1936, the diploma program was discontinued, and the College began offering a bachelor's degree in nursing (Fig. 2–4). With financial assistance from the General Education Board of the Rockefeller Foundation, which had placed emphasis on the South and education of blacks since its establishment in 1903 by John D. Rockefeller, Jr., the program was reorganized in 1945 with the appointment of a dean of the school of nursing (Carnegie, 1948). This school still exists, is now an integral part of the university and is fully accredited by the National League for Nursing. Other baccalaureate

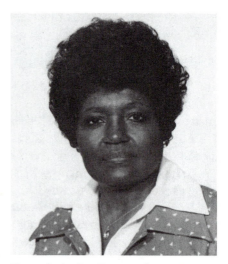

Figure 2–4   Dr. Eunice Johnson Burgess, one of the first three baccalaureate nursing graduates of Florida A&M College, 1941.

nursing programs at historically black colleges and universities have been developed, making a total in 1994 of 23, located in 17 states and the District of Columbia (Table 2–2). Black deans and directors of baccalaureate and higher degree programs in nursing are listed in Appendix A.

Innovative aspects of some of the nursing programs at historically black universities merit attention. Hampton University in Virginia is a comprehensive institution of higher education whose curricular emphasis, both scientific and professional, is undergirded by a strong liberal arts program. The University's mission reflects activities integral to research and public

Table 2–2   Baccalaureate and Associate Degree Programs at Historically Black Schools, 1994

Institution	Location	Program (AD, Bacc)	Year Established	Accreditation
Alabama				
Bishop State Community College	Mobile	AD	1976	NLN
Tuskegee University	Tuskegee	Bacc	1948	NLN
Oakwood College	Huntsville	AD	1987	State
		Bacc★	1991	
Arkansas				
University of Arkansas at Pine Bluff	Pine Bluff	Bacc	1976	NLN
Delaware				
Delaware State University	Dover	Bacc	1974	NLN
District of Columbia				
Howard University	Washington	Bacc	1969	NLN
Florida				
Florida A & M University	Tallahassee	Bacc	1936	NLN
Bethune-Cookman College	Daytona Beach	Bacc	1977	State
Georgia				
Albany State College	Albany	Bacc	1961	NLN
Kentucky				
Kentucky State University	Frankfort	AD	1967	NLN
Louisiana				
Dillard University	New Orleans	Bacc	1942	NLN
Grambling University	Grambling	Bacc	1984	NLN
Southern University	Baton Rouge	Bacc	1986	NLN
Maryland				
Coppin State College	Baltimore	Bacc	1974	NLN
Bowie State University	Bowie	Bacc★	1979	NLN
Mississippi				
Alcorn State University	Natchez	Bacc	1979	NLN
		AD	1963	NLN
Missouri				
Lincoln University	Jefferson City	AD	1970	NLN

(Continued)

Table 2–2　*(Continued)*

Institution	Location	Program (AD, Bacc)	Year Established	Accreditation
North Carolina				
North Carolina A & T State University	Greensboro	Bacc	1953	NLN
North Carolina Central University	Durham	Bacc	1969	NLN
Winston-Salem State University	Winston-Salem	Bacc	1954	NLN
Fayetteville State University	Fayetteville	Bacc★	1992	—
Oklahoma				
Langston University	Langston	Bacc	1980	NLN
South Carolina				
South Carolina State University	Orangeburg	Bacc	1988	NLN
Tennessee				
Tennessee State University	Nashville	Bacc	1980	NLN
		AD	1974	NLN
Texas				
Prairie View A & M University	Houston	Bacc	1952	NLN
Virginia				
Hampton University	Hampton	Bacc	1944	NLN
Norfolk State University	Norfolk	AD	1955	NLN
		Bacc	1990	NLN
		Bacc★	1981	NLN
West Virginia				
Bluefield State College	Bluefield	AD	1967	NLN
		Bacc★	1987	—

Notes: Baccalaureate Program, Howard University, Washington, DC, 1922–1925; Baccalaureate Program, Meharry Medical College, Nashville, TN 1947–1962; Associate Degree Program, Mississippi Valley College, Itta Bena, Mississippi, 1964–1979

★For RNs only

service. The vision statements, as part of the current strategic plan for the year 2000, further indicate that students will be actively engaged in research, scholarship, creative expression, and all forms of the creation and dissemination of knowledge (Davis et al., 1993).

In 1977, Dr. Patricia Sloan (Fig. 2–5), professor in the Graduate Department of Hampton University School of Nursing, established the M. Elizabeth Carnegie Nursing Archives. She had collected historical information by and about black nurses and early black nursing schools and interviewed nurses about their education. She presented the rationale for the development of a separate collection to the university president and received final approval on April 9, 1977. These were the first archives

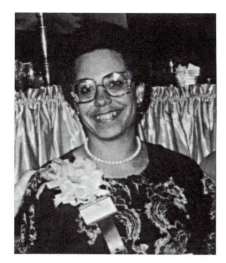

Figure 2–5   Dr. Patricia Sloan, Director, M. Elizabeth Carnegie Nursing Archives, Hampton University.

designed to centralize historical data by and about black nurses and their educational institutions, categorized under oral histories, trends and correspondence, and photographs. The archives are used extensively by historians in many disciplines.

After about 10 years of planning under the leadership of Elnora Daniel (Fig. 2–6), then Dean of the School of Nursing (now vice president for health), and with a grant from the W. K. Kellogg Foundation, a nurse-managed clinic was initiated at Hampton University in 1986 by the School of Nursing.

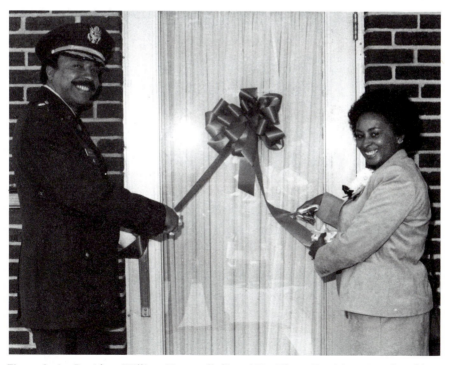

Figure 2–6   President William Harvey (left) and Dr. Elnora Daniel cutting the ribbon for the opening of the nurse-managed clinic, Hampton University.

The clinic, named Hampton University School of Nursing Interdiscipli-
nary Nursing Center for Health and Wellness is equipped with a mobile
unit that provides health care services to medically unserved and underserved residents of communities in and around the city of Hampton. A
multidisciplinary team of faculty and students from the School of Nursing, Education, Arts and Letters, and Business conduct programs designed to promote and maintain optimum levels of health. The Nursing
Center also serves as a site for faculty practice, consultation, and clinical
research.

Howard University College of Nursing, Washington, DC, operates a
nurse-managed health care service for the homeless at the Federal City

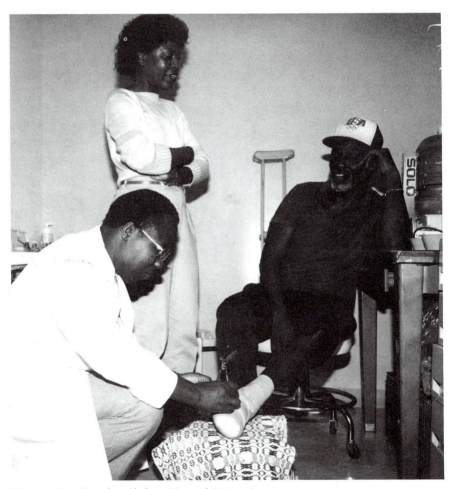

Figure 2–7   Homeless Shelter, Howard University.

Shelter. The project was started as a health care delivery model and for several years was funded with a grant from the W. K. Kellogg Foundation. It now operates with a grant from the District of Columbia government. Nursing students are given an opportunity to work with homeless persons as part of their curriculum (Fig. 2–7).

To acknowledge the establishment in 1893, of the first school of nursing at Howard, a black university, Dr. Charles Sanders, an alumnus, established an endowed chair in 1988 at the College of Nursing in honor of Dr. Mary Elizabeth Carnegie whose academic studies began at Howard in 1939. Under the chairmanship of Dr. Joyce Elmore, a national committee of 100 was created to raise a goal of $3 million for the Carnegie Chair. The Philadelphia subcommittee presented a $10,000 check to the University in December, 1994 (Fig. 2–8, left to right: Dolores Brewer; Betty Martin-Blount; chairperson Cynthia Flynn Capers; Rita Sellers; Dorothy L. Powell; Gloria McNeal; Mabel Morris). The purpose is to sustain scholarly work, especially large-scale minority health care research activities.

Two other nursing programs at historically black universities have endowed chairs—Tuskegee University, named in honor of Dr. Mary Harper, an alumna and outstanding nurse researcher, and Prairie View University. In 1993, the Board of Directors of Houston Endowment,

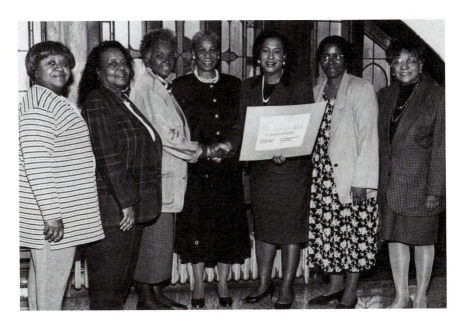

Figure 2–8   Check for Carnegie Chair presented to Howard University Dean Powell. (third from right).

Inc. authorized a grant of $750,000 to Prairie View A&M University to be maintained as a permanent endowment toward the Minority Health Research Chair at the College of Nursing. The $750,000 is matched with funds from the Texas A&M University system which will bring the College of Nursing Chair to a total of $1.5 million. The Chair will permit the College of Nursing to expand its services to the community, actively engage in research, and continue to grow as a college within Prairie View University.

Associate Degree

The President's Commission on Higher Education's recommendation that all American youth be given tuition-free education stimulated the growth of community and junior colleges in the United States (Brick, 1963).

Associate degree programs, based primarily in community colleges, are the latest type of basic nursing education. This type of program was launched in 1952, and the first nurses were graduated in 1954 after two years of education, with a combination of general and nursing education, including clinical experience, developed in accordance with college policy and the regulations of the state licensing authority. Graduates are prepared to give care to patients as beginning staff nurses, and to cooperate and share responsibility for their patients' welfare with other members of the nursing and health staff (Report of the Surgeon General's Consultant Group on Nursing, 1963).

A unique feature of associate degree education in nursing is that "it was the first program to be developed through research, rather than as the result of an historical accident" (Montag, 1980, p. 248). The Division of Nursing Education at Teachers College, Columbia University, New York initiated and sponsored the Cooperative Research Project in Junior and Community College Education for Nursing under the direction of Mildred Montag as the first major research undertaking of the Institute of Research and Service in Nursing Education at Teachers College. When the project was launched, there was less acceptance than today of the idea that education for nursing should be part of the nation's system of higher education, as recommended by Brown (1948).

The project's study and experimentation extended over five years and involved the cooperation of seven junior and community colleges and one hospital, located in six states. One of the colleges that participated was the Norfolk State University, a black institution, which entered the project in 1955 (Fig. 2–9). Beginning with these eight programs, the movement has

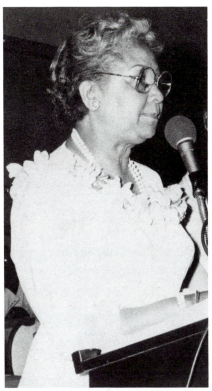

Figure 2–9 Dr. Hazle Blakeney, first chairman of the associate degree nursing program at the Norfolk State University.

spread so that in 1994, there were 848 programs located in all 50 states, the District of Columbia, Puerto Rico, the Virgin Islands, and Guam. More black students are enrolled in the associate degree program than in any other type. Were it not for the associate degree programs in community colleges, with low cost to the student and flexible standards in terms of age, marital status, and race, many qualified black students would be lost to the field of nursing. Then, too, those junior colleges located in black communities tend to have a high black enrollment in all areas of study.

In addition to the associate degree program at the Norfolk State University (established in 1955), eight associate degree programs were developed at historically black colleges and universities between 1963 and 1980: Alcorn State University, Natchez, Mississippi, 1963; Mississippi Valley College, which existed from 1964 to 1979; Kentucky State University, 1967; Bluefield State College, West Virginia, 1967; Lincoln University, Missouri, 1970; Bishop State Community College, Mobile, Alabama, in 1976; Tennessee State University, Nashville, 1980; and Oakwood College, Huntsville, Alabama, in 1987 (Table 2–2).

POST-BASIC PROGRAMS

As mentioned earlier, advanced education for registered nurses did not begin until 1899 at Teachers College, Columbia University, New York. Shortly thereafter, other universities, mostly in the North, began offering post-basic courses for nurses. A few black nurses completed these courses, commonly referred to as "postgraduate" education. However, black nurses in the South had no such opportunity. To meet this need, several programs were established especially for blacks. Two special courses in public health nursing and three in nurse-midwifery are discussed in this section, followed by a discussion of the five master's degree programs at historically black institutions.

Public Health Nursing

In 1936, the U.S. Public Health Service, in cooperation with the Medical College of Virginia in Richmond, established a program in public health nursing for black registered nurses at St. Philip Hospital, the black division of the College with Lillian Bischoff (white) as director (Fig. 2–10). Title VI of the Social Security Act provided scholarship aid with students being selected from 18 cooperating states. The program also attracted black nurses from other countries. The class of 1945, for example, had two foreign students: Mary Little from Liberia, West Africa, and Bernice Carnegie

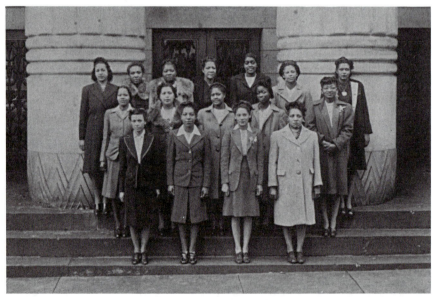

Figure 2–10   The 1943 graduating class, Public Health Nursing Program, St. Philip Hospital School of Nursing, Richmond, VA. Top row, left to right: Elizabeth Tyler, Savannah Sickles, Louise Blowe, Pansy McFadden Hicks, Ernestine Hill, Mary Cox, Veneley Narcisse. Second row, left to right: Thelma Abercrombie, Christine Haith, Lillian Carter Thompson, Sadie Ezelle, Nema Newell. First row, left to right: Lillian Henry, Ione Taylor Carey, Margaret Gilbert, Mozie Lee Thomas. (Courtesy Archives, Medical College of Virginia)

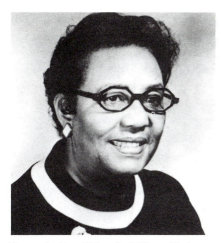

Figure 2–11   Helen S. Miller, Chairperson, North Carolina Central University, Durham when the generic program was established.

Redmon from Toronto, Ontario, Canada, who had completed her basic program the year before at St. Philip.

The program, approved by the National Organization for Public Health Nursing, which evaluated programs in public health nursing, was at first one-year long, including field experience and leading to a certificate. Before the program was discontinued in 1956, the curriculum had changed so that a bachelor's degree in nursing education, with a major in public health nursing, was offered. Academic courses were taken at Virginia Union University, a black institution in Richmond, but the degree was conferred by the Medical College of Virginia. In its 20 years of existence, 57 black nurses were graduated with qualifications for better positions, higher salaries, and the incentive for further education.

Because black registered nurses were denied admission to the public health nursing program at the University of North Carolina at Chapel Hill, a program for black nurses in this specialty leading to a certificate was established in 1946 at North Carolina College (renamed North Carolina Central University) in Durham, with Mary Mills as the first chairperson. Until black faculty could be found, faculty from the University of North Carolina at Chapel Hill conducted classes at the black school. Upon recommendation of the National League for Nursing during an accreditation visit in 1958, and under the leadership of Chairman Helen S. Miller (Fig. 2–11), the program was expanded to permit students to earn a bachelor's degree in public health nursing, while continuing with the program leading to a certificate. By this time, the program at St. Philip in public health nursing had closed, leaving North Carolina College the only school in the South offering public health nursing for black registered nurses. Its enrollment, therefore, consisted of more out-of-state students than those from the State of North Carolina. In 1969, North Carolina College discontinued its specialty program in public health nursing and began offering a generic program for high school graduates and registered nurses leading to a bachelor of science in nursing.

Midwifery

In many countries, midwifery is either a part of the basic nursing curriculum or a postgraduate course for those nurses who wish to become certified in this specialty. Formal training for nurse-midwives in this country did not begin until the early 1930s, with the establishment of the first school at the Maternity Center Association in New York. Need for such a school was recognized when the U.S. Children's Bureau found from its survey that there were at least 45,000 untrained midwives ("grannies") functioning and highlighted the appalling infant mortality rates—124 per 1,000 live births—and the terribly high maternal mortality rates, most coming under the classification of "preventable" (Hogan 1975).

In the South, maternal and infant mortality rates were far higher than for the nation as a whole; many needless deaths occurred, particularly in rural districts among families of sharecroppers—both black and white. Concern about the high infant mortality rates in the rural South led to the beginning of another nurse-midwifery school, this one for black nurses at Tuskegee, Alabama. The first aim of the project was to prepare black nurses in midwifery and then to reduce the number of rural deaths through improved and expanded maternity care and study.

As a demonstration project under the auspices of the Macon County Health Department, the U.S. Children's Bureau, the Julius Rosenwald Fund, Tuskegee University, and the Alabama Department of Health, the Tuskegee Nurse-Midwifery School opened September 15, 1941, with three students: Helen S. Pennington, Salina L. Johnson, and Fannye M. Prentice, who were graduated March 1942. The program was adapted from the curriculum of the Maternity Center Association (MCA) and organized by Margaret Thomas, a member of MCA staff. From 1945 until the school closed, one of its graduates, Claudia Durham (Fig. 2–12), directed the program. After the program was established at Tuskegee, it is reported that black nurses who applied for admission to MCA for training in midwifery were directed to Tuskegee, which had been established for blacks. The Association has since had black nurses on its staff. The first to be employed (in 1948) was Dorothy Doyle Harrison, a graduate of Mercy Hospital School of Nursing in Philadelphia.

The course at Tuskegee, for graduates of accredited schools of nursing, was six months long. One-third of the time was spent in theoretical instruction conducted by obstetricians, nurse-midwives, and other specialists. Students were given practical learning experiences in clinics and homes. Each student was required to manage under supervision at least 20

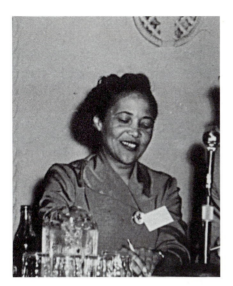

Figure 2–12   Claudia Durham, last Director, Tuskegee Nurse-Midwifery School.

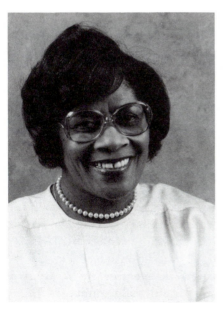

Figure 2–13   Pearline Gilpin, first Director, Nurse-Midwifery Program, Meharry Medical College, Nashville, TN.

to 30 deliveries and might assist the obstetrician with abnormal deliveries in the hospital. Standing orders were used as approved by consultants from the state health department and the county medical society (Thomas, 1942). When the school was established, the maternal mortality rate in Macon County was 8.5 per 1,000 live births. In its second year, the service was responsible for the delivery of one-third of all the mothers in the county, with a mortality rate of zero. The fetal death rate was 45.9 per 1,000 live births before the opening of the school; by the end of the second year of the demonstration, it was 14 per 1,000 for women under the care of the nurse-midwives (Maternity Center Association, 1955). Twenty-five black nurse midwives had been graduated from the Tuskegee program when it closed in 1946.

A second nurse-midwifery school for black nurses was established in 1942 in connection with Flint-Goodridge Hospital and Dillard University in New Orleans. Etta Mae Forte Miller, a native of Tuskegee in Alabama and a certified nurse-midwife from Maternity Center Association, helped to implement the program at Flint-Goodridge Hospital (Carter, 1982). This six-month course was also financed by the U.S. Children's Bureau. After one year, the school closed, having graduated only two black nurse-midwives, who subsequently were employed by the Departments of Health in Louisiana and Mississippi.

The third nurse-midwifery program was conducted at Meharry Medical College in Nashville, Tennessee from 1973 to 1982, under the leadership of Pearline D. Gilpin (Fig. 2–13), a nurse from Jamaica, West Indies, who had studied midwifery in England and held a master's degree in Nursing Administration from New York University. During its lifetime, Meharry's program, which was accredited by the American College of Nurse Midwives, had graduated 52 nurse-midwives.

The renaissance of nurse midwifery in the 1970s, coupled with women's rights movement and increasing interest in non-hospital deliveries, spurred research interest into alternative modes of service as well as continued research into the normal low-risk pregnancy and delivery (Gortner & Nahm, 1977).

Master's Degree Education

Since 1931, when the first black nurse, Estelle Massey Riddle Osborne, with a scholarship from the Rosenwald Fund, earned a master's degree in nursing at Teachers College, Columbia University, New York, many black nurses have earned master's degrees, receiving their education at historically white universities.

Today, master's degree nursing programs exist at five historically black institutions. The first one was established at Hampton University School of Nursing in Hampton, Virginia, followed by Howard University College of Nursing in Washington, DC, Albany State College in Georgia, Bowie State University in Maryland, and Southern University in Baton Rouge, Louisiana. Meharry Medical College Department of Nursing Education in Nashville, Tennessee, established a master's program in 1982, but closed it in June 1985.

Hampton University has had a basic baccalaureate nursing program since the first students were admitted in 1944, the first in the State of Virginia, initiated by Mary Elizabeth Lancaster Carnegie. It was established as a result of the wartime need for nurses for military and civilian service and for black nurses prepared for leadership positions (Lancaster, 1945). In 1976, under the leadership of Fostine G. Riddick Roach (Fig. 2–14), dean of the school at that time, the master's degree program was started, with major courses of study in community health and community mental health nursing. The program has expanded and now includes three specialty areas and two graduate head nurse-practitioner programs. The first master's degree from the program was bestowed in 1978 on Terry Williams

Dagrosa of Chesapeake, Virginia, who majored in community health nursing with a functional specialization in education. Her thesis was entitled "Correlation among Personality Traits Which May Facilitate Effective Relief of Chronic Pain by the Transcutaneous Nervous Stimulation Method."

Under the leadership of its first Dean, Dr. Anna B. Coles, (Fig. 2–15), the College of Nursing at Howard University in Washington, DC, has had a baccalaureate nursing program since 1969. This replaced the diploma program at Freedmen's Hospital, which, between 1894 and 1973, had graduated 1,700 nurses. In 1980, the Board of Trustees of Howard University approved the establishment of a graduate program leading to the degree of master of science in nursing. At first, the program had three major areas of concentration—gerontologic nursing, adult health nursing, and family nursing in the urban community. Later, nursing administration and mental health nursing were added to the curriculum as majors.

The graduate program in nursing at Albany State College, Albany, Georgia, under the direction of Dr. Lucille B. Wilson, was approved by the Board of Regents in August 1988 and admitted its first students that fall. The master's program offers options for two clinical majors: community health nursing and maternal-child health nursing. In conjunction with the

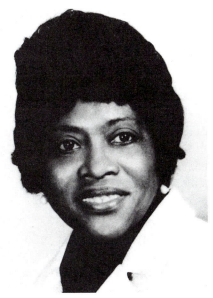

Figure 2–14 Fostine G. Riddick Roach, Dean, School of Nursing, Hampton Institute, when master's program was initiated.

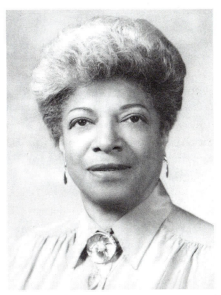

Figure 2–15 Dr. Anna B. Coles, Dean, College of Nursing, Howard University when master's program was established.

development of specialized competencies in one of these two clinical fields, the student may select preparation for a functional career as an administrator or as a clinical specialist.

The master's degree program in nursing at Bowie State University in Bowie, Maryland, was begun in 1989 under the direction of Dr. Joyce Bowles. The focus is on advanced clinical practice in adult health with emphasis on gerontology and role tracks of nursing administration and nursing education.

Southern University, Baton Rouge, Louisiana, under the leadership of Dr. Janet Rami, Dean of the School of Nursing, embarked on a master of science degree program in family health nursing in 1992—a two-year program that prepares graduates to assume leadership roles as administrators, clinical specialists, or educators in nursing. A master's program in rural health nursing is in the planning stage at Alcorn State University, Natchez, Mississippi.

Today, nurses engaged in advanced practice—nurse practitioners (NPs), clinical nurse specialists (CNs), certified nurse-midwives (CNMs), and certified registered nurse anesthetists (CRNAs)—are being prepared at the master's level and hold the title, "Advanced Practice Nurses (APNs)." In addition, nurses holding teaching and administrative positions in nursing programs at institutions of higher education are expected to have earned a master's degree in nursing.

SUMMARY

Before and after schools of nursing especially for blacks were established, a few black women entered and completed programs at predominantly white schools, the first being Mary Mahoney, who was graduated from the New England Hospital for Women and Children in 1879. The first diploma program established for blacks was at Spelman College in Atlanta, Georgia in 1886, followed by nearly 100 others before the last one at Grady Hospital closed in 1982.

Six years after the University of Cincinnati established the first baccalaureate program in the country in 1916, one was established at a black school, Howard University, but survived only three years—1922 to 1925. Currently (1994) there are 637 baccalaureate programs in the United States, 136 of which are for RNs only. Of the total, 23 are located at historically black colleges and universities, and all report mixed racial faculty and students.

Associate degree nursing education, the latest type of generic program, began in 1952 as an experimental project. One black school, Norfolk State University, participated in the project. Of the 848 associate degree nursing programs, six are located at historically black institutions.

In the 1930s and 1940s, public health and midwifery programs for registered nurses were established at historically black institutions: St. Philip in Richmond and North Carolina College at Durham in the area of public health nursing; and Tuskegee Institute in Alabama, Flint-Goodridge Hospital/Dillard University in New Orleans, and Meharry Medical College in Nashville, Tennessee in the area of nurse-midwifery.

Ongoing master's degree programs in nursing are at five black colleges and universities; Hampton University in Virginia; Howard University in Washington, DC; Albany State College in Georgia; Bowie State University in Maryland; and Southern University, Baton Rouge, Louisiana. Another is being planned at Alcorn State University in Mississippi. A master's program at Meharry Medical College in Nashville, Tennessee, existed from 1982 to 1985.

REFERENCES

American Nurses Association. (1965). First position on education for nursing. *American Journal of Nursing, 65,* 106–111.

Annual Report for 1878: New England Hospital for Women and Children, Boston.

Brick, M. (1963). *Forum and focus for the junior college movement.* New York: Teachers College Press.

Brown, E. L. (1948). *Nursing for the future.* New York: Russell Sage Foundation.

Carnegie, M. E. (1948). Nurse training becomes nursing education at Florida A&M College. *Journal of Negro Ed, 17,* 200–204.

Carter, A. J. (1982). Profiles of black registered nurses, *ANA Council on Intercultural Nursing Newsletter, 2,* 2–3.

Chayer, M. E. (1954). Mary Eliza Mahoney. *American Journal of Nursing, 54,* 429–431.

Davis, B. (1976). *The origins and growth of three nursing programs at Howard University, 1893–1973.* Unpublished doctoral Dissertation, Teachers College, Columbia University, New York.

Davis, B. L., Daniel, E. D., & Sloan, P. E. (1993). Research notes. *Association of Black Nursing Faculty Journal, 4,* 105.

Dyson, W. (1921). *The Founding of Howard University.* Washington, DC: Howard University Press.

Educational facilities for colored nurses (1925). *Trained Nurse and Hospital Review, 74,* 259–262.

Gage, N. D., & Haupt, A. D. (1932). Some observations on negro nursing in the south. *Public Health Nurse, 24,* 674–680.

Gortner, S., & Nahm, H. (1977). An overview of nursing research in the United States. *Nursing Research, 26,* 10–33.

Francis, G. (1967). A minority of one. *Nursing Outlook, 15,* 36–38.

Grippando, G. M. (1983). *Nursing Perspectives and Issues.* Albany, NY: Delmar, 93–95.

Hogan, A. (1975). A tribute to the pioneers. *Journal of Nurse Midwife, 20,* 6–11.

Jamieson, E. M., & Sewall, M. (1944). *Trends in nursing history, 2.* Philadelphia: Saunders.

Jones, J. (1981). *Bad blood, The Tuskegee syphilis experiment.* New York: Free Press.

Kessel, F. (1989). Black foundations: Meeting vital needs, *Crisis, 96,* 14–18.

Lancaster (Carnegie), M. E. (1945). How a collegiate nursing program developed in a negro college. *American Journal of Nursing, 45,* 119.

Maternity Center Association. (1955). *Twenty years of nurse-midwifery, 1933–1953.* A Report. New York.

Montag, M. (1980). Associate degree education in perspective, *Nursing Outlook, 28,* 248–250.

Mossell, N. F. (1908). *The work of the Afro-American woman* (2nd ed.) Philadelphia: George S. Ferguson.

Newell, H. (1951). *The history of the National Nursing Council.* New York: The Council.

Peck, E. S., & Pride, M. W. (1982). *Nurses in times: Developments in nursing education 1898–1981.* Berea College, Berea, Kentucky: Applachian Fund.

Peck, E. S., & Smith, E. A. (1982). *Berea's first 125 years.* Lexington: University Press of Kentucky.

Personnel Data Cards. (1898). Spanish-American War. Washington, DC: National Archives.

Report of the Surgeon General's Consultant Group on Nursing. (1963). *Toward quality in nursing: Needs and goals.* Washington, DC: USHEW.

Roberts, M. (1954). *American nursing: History and interpretation.* New York: Macmillan.

Spelman Messenger. (1908, March). Atlanta: Spelman College.

Spelman Messenger. (1914, February). Atlanta: Spelman College.

Staupers, M. K. (1961). *No time for prejudice.* New York: Macmillan.

Thomas, M. W. (1942). Social priority No. 1, mothers and babies. *Public Health Nursing, 34,* 442–445.

West, R. M. (1931). *History of nursing in Pennsylvania.* Harrisburg: Pennsylvania Nurses Association.

West, M., & Hawkins, C. (1950). *Nursing schools at the midcentury.* New York: National Committee for the Improvement of Nursing Services.

Chapter
3

~

From Dreams to Achievements

Prior to World War II, the only effort on a national scale to recruit blacks into the nursing profession was made by the National Association of Colored Graduate Nurses (NACGN), which had this as one of its objectives. During World War II, a mechanism was set into motion by the federal government to procure additional nursing personnel by financing basic nursing education. This was done through the Cadet Nurse Corps program in which many black nursing schools and students participated.

When the war was over and the Cadet Nurse Corps was terminated, again the only national recruitment program for black nursing students was conducted by NACGN. After NACGN dissolved in January, 1951, there was a noticeable decline in the number of black students being admitted to and graduated from nursing programs. The closing of a number of all-black schools, where the vast majority of black students had been enrolled, was a major factor influencing the decline. In the 1950s and 1960s, 15 black schools closed (Carnegie, 1964). There was a noticeable decrease in the registered black nurse population during these years as the number of would-be admissions to the closed black schools was not absorbed by the existing white schools. In fact, in 1969, while blacks made up the largest minority group in the United States (more than 11%), the percentage of blacks graduating from schools of nursing leading to registered nurse licensure was only 3.2 percent. This was also the time when integration efforts were stimulated by federal governmental prescriptions.

The Civil Rights Act of 1964, supreme court decision, and executive orders mandated the prohibition of racial segregation in institutions of higher education.

The Nurse Training Act of 1964 and its later revisions provided for special project monies to be expanded to increase the number of disadvantaged and minority students in schools of nursing. The Higher Education Act of 1965 greatly increased the availability of financial aid to low-income students and provided funds to institutions for special admission and support programs for minority students. These federal acts also stimulated state and local governmental prescriptions for racial integration. In addition, help came from the private sector.

In this chapter, five special projects are discussed—two privately funded and three federally funded. The Sealantic Project for the Disadvantaged received support from the Sealantic Fund which had been established in 1938 by John D. Rockefeller, Jr. The Faculty and Community Enhancement Project (FACE) is funded by the W. K. Kellogg Foundation. The Cadet Nurse Corps and the Breakthrough to Nursing Project of the National Student Nurses' Association were federally funded. The Ethnic/Minority Fellowship Project administered by the American Nurses' Association is still funded by the federal government.

CADET NURSE CORPS

The creation of the Cadet Nurse Corps played a significant role in procuring nursing personnel during World War II. In 1940, the United States began preparing for the possibility of war. In July of that year, the National Nursing Council on Defense was organized by six national organizations—the American Nurses' Association, the National League of Nursing Education, the Association of Collegiate Schools of Nursing, the National Organization for Public Health Nursing, the American Red Cross Nursing Service, and the National Association of Colored Graduate Nurses—as a means of working with problems that might arise in connection with nursing in national defense. One of the main purposes of the Council was to serve as a coordinating agency for the participating organizations. It began at once to recruit students and classify graduate nurses as to their availability for military service (Deloughery, 1977).

In the summer of 1941, the U.S. Congress was induced by Frances Payne Bolton, Congresswoman from Ohio, to appropriate $1,250,000 for nursing education, and in 1942, $3,500,000. Known as the first Bolton Bill, it provided for (1) refresher courses for graduate nurses, (2) assistance to schools of nursing so that they could increase their enrollments, (3) postgraduate courses, (4) preparation for instructors and other personnel, and (5) training in midwifery and other specialties (Goodnow, 1948).

In 1942, the National Council on Defense became the National Nursing Council for War Service (NNCWS). To increase the number of nurses for military service and at the same time ensure that civilians were cared for, the Council planned refresher courses for graduate nurses, pooled teaching staffs, helped to arrange for more centralized schools, and advised on all nursing activities (Goodnow, 1948).

The National Nursing Council for War Service also focused on untapped sources of nursing service—blacks, men, and practical nurses. NACGN worked closely with the Council and, in the early days of the war, inquiries about black nurses and opportunities for blacks in schools of nursing were referred by the Council to NACGN. NACGN's small staff and limited budget, however, could not carry this increased load. With financial aid from the General Education Board (GEB) of the Rockefeller Foundation, the Council elected to set up a black unit on an experimental basis and appointed a black nurse, Estelle Massey Riddle Osborne, to direct it with the title of consultant. The preliminary work was so promising that GEB funds were supplemented by the W.K. Kellogg Foundation and the U.S. Public Health Service (USPHS) and a second black consultant, Alma Vessells John, was employed and the unit was soon integrated into the general program.

The special functions of the two black consultants of NNCWS were (1) to compile data relative to the status and problems of black nurses and (2) to stimulate the progress of black nurses through further integration in the major professional nursing organizations (Roberts, 1954). These two consultants set into motion a series of institutes for nursing school directors, hospital administrators, members of governing boards, and officials responsible for the operation of schools of nursing in black colleges and universities. One very important conference of black college presidents and administrative deans was held at Dillard University in New Orleans in 1944 to develop ways of utilizing educational resources more fully for the preparation of black nurses (Riddle & Nelson, 1945).

In 1943, Congresswoman Frances Payne Bolton put through Congress a second bill, which became Public Law 74, Seventy-Eighth Congress, establishing the U.S. Cadet Nurse Corps under the administration of the USPHS. This had been carefully planned by the National Nursing Council for War Service, aiming to increase as rapidly as possible the number of nurses in the country. The bill passed both houses without a dissenting vote. Lucile Petry Leone was appointed director of the Division of Nurse

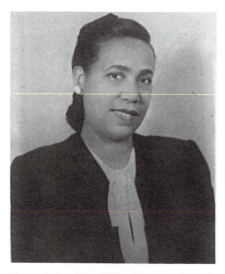

Figure 3–1 Rita Miller Dargan, Consultant, Cadet Nurse Corps.

Education of the USPHS to administer the Cadet Nurse Corps program. Included on her staff was a black nurse, Rita Miller Dargan (Fig. 3–1), as a consultant on a part-time basis, on leave from Dillard University in New Orleans where she chaired the Division of Nursing. Dargan's responsibilities were to assist black schools in applying for participation in the Cadet Nurse Corps program, to help black schools qualify for the Corps, and to facilitate inclusion of more black students in the program.

A committee on Recruitment of Nursing students, of which the author was a member, was estab-

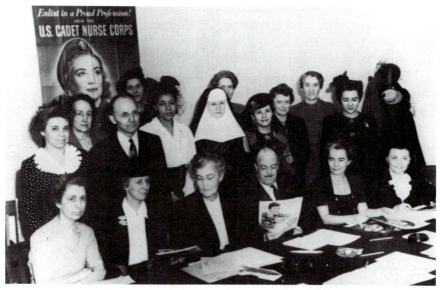

Figure 3–2 First Meeting of the National Nursing Council for War Service Committee on Recruitment of Student Nurses. Seated (left to right) Mrs. E. B. Wickendon, Mildred Reese, Edith H. Smith (chairman), Dr. Donald Smelzer (Vice-Chairman), Lucile Petry (Leone), Mrs. Eben J. Carey. Standing (left to right) Leah Blaisdell, Lucille Reynolds, Dr. Walter C. Ellis. Florence Meyers, Mary Elizabeth Lancaster (Carnegie), Sister Charles Marie, Katherine Faville, Mrs. Mary Anita Perez, Mildred Tuttle, M. Cordella Cowan, Jean Henderson. (Courtesy National Library of Medicine)

lished by the National Nursing Council for War Service, holding its first meeting February 24, 1944 (Fig. 3–2). A cooperative campaign by nurses, hospital administrators, educators, and civic leaders to meet the year's quota of 65,000 new students was mapped out.

Federal funds provided for maintenance of the students in the Cadet Nurse Corps during the first nine months, tuition and fees throughout the program, and necessary expansion of educational and residential facilities. Each student was provided school uniforms, the U.S. Cadet Nurse Corps outdoor uniform, and a stipend of $15 a month for the pre-cadet period and $20 a month for the junior cadet period—15 or 20 months. If up to six months were required before the student was eligible to take licensure examinations, during the Senior Cadet period, the using agency—home or other civilian or governmental hospital or health service—paid the cadet a minimum of $30 a month and maintenance. The student participant agreed to remain in essential civilian or military nursing service for the duration of the war, a pledge later determined not legally binding. For their senior experience, cadets served not only in their home hospitals, but also in hospitals of the Army, Navy, Veterans Administration, Public Health Service, and Indian Affairs plus other civilian hospitals and public health agencies. "Some 22 Negro cadets had served in six Army hospitals by the end of 1945" (Maxwell, 1976) (Fig. 3–3).

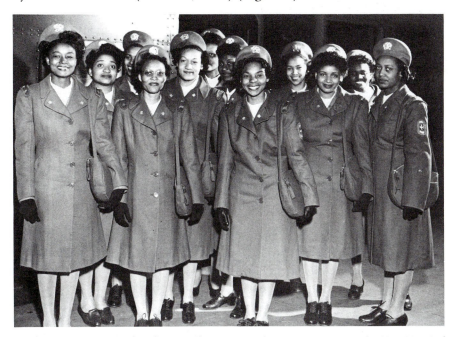

Figure 3–3   Senior cadets from Tuskegee Institute en route to Boston City Hospital to gain senior experiences, March, 1945.

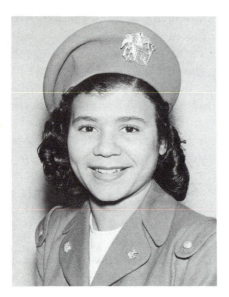

Figure 3–4 Orieanna Collins Syphax, recruiter for Cadet Nurse Corps.

It was deemed expedient and economical to strengthen the instructional staff and facilities of existing civilian schools of nursing. Although the establishment of the Cadet Nurse Corps was a defense measure, a precedent had been established—schools of nursing were given recognition as essential agencies in the protection of the nation's health (Shields, 1981). During the 1940s, the Corps recruited 169,000 of the nation's 179,000 nursing students (Kalisch, 1988) and of the 1,300 schools of nursing, 1,125 participated (U.S. Public Health Service, 1950).

In cooperation with the Cadet Nurse Corps, the National Nursing Council for War Service selected nurses with collegiate backgrounds to visit about 600 junior and senior colleges. Two black nurses, Orieanna Collins Syphax (Fig. 3–4) and Pauline Battle Butler "visited 82 [black] campuses and talked with thousands of black women students about the leadership positions awaiting the college-prepared nurse and about the free education offered through membership in the Cadet Nurse Corps" (Kalisch & Kalisch, 1978, p. 561).

The Cadet Nurse Corps proved beneficial to many black students, who otherwise might not have had a nursing education. When the war started in 1941, only 14 historically white schools had ever admitted blacks (Staupers, 1961). By the end of the war in 1945, 21 black schools had participated in the Cadet Nurse Corps as did 38 schools with integrated classes, training a total of 3,000 black nurses (Mullan, 1989).

The Cadet Nurse Corps, composed of student trainees, was not a branch of the armed forces or the civilian personnel force of the U.S. government. The corps pledge was a statement of good intentions, rather than a legal contract. Many of the 169,000 students recruited, however, did serve in the military.

After the war, in recognition of their contribution, faculty who had taught cadets, including the author, received a certificate signed by Surgeon General Thomas Parran. The certificate read, "This nation will always be indebted to the instructors in schools of nursing who prepared the largest classes of student nurses in history for military and essential civilian nursing . . . As an instructor your influence will be reflected in each of the young women to whom you have imparted your skill, knowledge, and wisdom. Through them you have cared for hundreds of patients. You have produced the graduate nurses of tomorrow who will be a vital factor in the public health of our country and of the world."

The training and experience of the cadets did not constitute federal service, and therefore, no veterans benefits accrued. In 1984, however, Beth Bohannon, a former cadet, started a major campaign to initiate national legislation that would credit time spent in the Cadet Nurse Corps during World War II toward Civil Service retirement (Larson, 1987).

On June 4, 1985, Congressman Jim Slattery of Kansas introduced a bill (H.R. 2663) in the House of Representatives. This bill, as originally written, mandated civil service status for all cadet nurses who served at least two years in the Corps. The House Bill met with much resistance from the Office of Personnel Management, the Budget Office, and members of the Reagan Administration who were concerned about the budgetary impact of the bill. Reluctantly, the bill was amended so that it applied only to registered nurses who were employed by the federal government on the date of enactment and who had at least two years of cadet service. The bill (P.L. 99-638) as amended was passed by the House and Senate and signed by President Reagan on November 10, 1986 ". . . to credit time spent in the Cadet Nurse Corps during World War II as creditable service for civil service retirement . . ." (CIS Annual Legislative History of US Public Laws, 1986, p. 725). In 1993, Congressman Slattery introduced another bill which would give benefits to all nurses who had been in the Cadet Nurse Corps.

The year, 1993, marked the fiftieth anniversary of the founding of the Cadet Nurse Corps and was celebrated in different ways. On June 15, the U.S. Public Health Service commemorated the signing of the Nurse Training Act which created the Corps with a reception in Washington, DC. Another tribute was made during the month of March by Sigma Theta Tau International, the honor society of nursing, via its television series, *Nursing Approach*—a monthly program by, for, and about nurses. Two of the interviewees on the television program were Lucile Petry Leone, Director of the Cadet Nurse Corps, and Mary Elizabeth Carnegie who had served on the National Recruitment Committee during the life of the Corps.

The Cadet Nurse Corps sparked a new beginning in nursing education in this country. Nursing schools became more independent; curricula were evaluated and restructured; thousands of nurses received post-graduate education; and hundreds of new facilities were built or upgraded. By the time the program officially ended in 1948, a precedent had been established— schools of nursing and the nurses they graduated were recognized as essential to protecting the nation's health (Bender, 1989).

On Friday, May 13, 1994, a golden anniversary celebration was held at the National Institutes of Health, Bethesda, Maryland, to honor the beginning of the Cadet Nurse Corps in 1943. The celebration included a conference with renowned speakers, a luncheon, and a dinner gala. The conference explored the historical significance and modern legacy of the Cadet Nurse Corps. Its plenary sessions focused on the future of nursing in health care reform, innovations in nursing practice, telemedicine advances, and health legislation.

BREAKTHROUGH

The National Student Nurses' Association (NSNA) is the only national organization for students in nursing. Its purpose is to aid in the development of the individual student and to urge students of nursing, as future health professionals, to be aware of and to contribute to improving the health care of all people.

In 1963, NSNA became actively involved in recruiting members of minority groups for schools of nursing. Recruitment of minorities continues to be a priority for the Association. "Breakthrough to Nursing" was first developed on the local level; it is now a project of national scope. From 1965 to 1970, the project was maintained solely by nursing students who volunteered their time. Funding came from local philanthropy and NSNA.

In June, 1971, the first contract of $100,000 from the Division of Nursing, U.S. Department of Health, Education, and Welfare enabled NSNA to employ a program director (Fig. 3–5) and staff to assist students to organize Breakthrough volunteer recruitment programs through local and state constituent student nurses associations; to establish five selected target areas for intensive effort as test project sites; and to develop program plans to identify strategies to recruit students from minority groups to enroll in nursing programs.

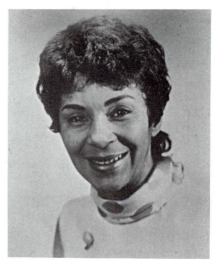

Figure 3–5   Alberta "Kit" Barnes, Project Director, NSNA Breakthrough Project, 1974–1977.

Although the money stabilized Breakthrough activities in the five selected target areas—Los Angeles, California; Phoenix, Arizona; Denver,
Colorado; Columbus, Ohio; and Charlotte, North Carolina—it was not
sufficient to mount a nationwide program. By the end of the contract period, over 600 potential candidates for nursing had been reached through
Breakthrough efforts, and there had been enough statistical data collected
to justify the need for the expansion of the project.

In June, 1974, NSNA obtained a three-year grant from the Division of
Nursing to initiate and maintain 40 local target areas where career opportunities for minority group students were available. During the first year
of the grant, approximately 500 NSNA members of various racial backgrounds worked on the Breakthrough project as recruiters in the target
areas. This was an average of about 20 percent more than had worked at
Breakthrough target areas the preceding year. Thirty-six students from
various minority groups were recruited and accepted into schools of nursing by the end of the first year.

During the 1975–1976 year of the grant, approximately 1,000 NSNA
members were involved in recruiting in the 40 target areas. By June,
1976, 86 more candidates had been recruited and were admitted to nursing programs, and 286 prospective applicants were targeted for the year
1976–1977.

The basic approach to the Breakthrough Project has been the establishment of one-to-one relationships with prospective candidates. When a
candidate expresses interest in pursuing the study of nursing, the person is
invited to meet with the local
Breakthrough Committee. The
Committee, composed of faculty
associates and students, determines
the type of assistance needed by the
candidate and also helps in finding
ways of providing it. Some students
need encouragement only, while
others may need assistance in fill-
ing out admission applications, in
making financial plans, or in determining high school course requirements (Fig. 3–6).

Through the persistent efforts of
the student volunteers and faculty
associates, the Breakthrough project has achieved the following:

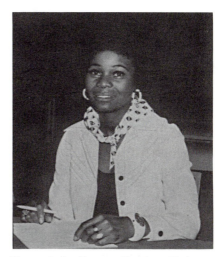

Figure 3–6   Frances Knight, Chairman,
NSNA Breakthrough Project, 1975–1976.

1. Encouraged schools of nursing to be more responsive to needs of minority-group students

2. Kept national nursing organizations aware of their responsibilities to
   minority-group [persons] in and out of nursing, and established good
   working relationships with these organizations

3. Established, through local campaigns and the mass media, good working relations with secondary schools, guidance counselors, and schools
   of nursing

4. Developed recruitment materials geared specifically to minority-
   group recruitment

5. Developed leadership ability and skill in intergroup relations among
   minority-and-nonminority-group student nurses

6. Obtained national and local scholarship funds for minority-group
   students

More than 50,000 pieces of literature about Breakthrough have been
distributed in junior and senior high schools, community centers,
churches, and neighborhood organizations. The effect of the literature
distribution is not known; however, the NSNA office receives thousands
of inquiries from prospective candidates who do not reside in the target
areas. In one week, over 3,000 inquiries were received at the NSNA office
from persons in the New York Metropolitan area following an NBC Television Network broadcast in which Dr. Frank Field, Science Editor,
filmed a recruitment session in the Manhattan/Bronx area and interviewed two Breakthrough student recruiters.

NSNA believes acceptance of and respect for minorities have increased
markedly over the last few years. Three of eight members of the NSNA
Board of Directors elected in 1976 were black. It is reasonable to assume
that without Breakthrough this would not have happened. And, as McGee
said, "The Breakthrough to Nursing Project . . . is forging a leadership
position in changing the image of the registered nurse as a 'white female
in a starched white uniform' as student nurses expand and increase their
local projects recruiting in minority communities all over the country"
(Breakthrough, 1972, p. 11).

Breakthrough has had an impact on schools, students, and the nursing
profession as the volunteer student recruiters have impressed administrative heads of nursing programs with the seriousness of purpose and
support of the project's goals. Hundreds of students, faculty, and practicing nurses are now more aware of the need to bring more people from

minority groups into the mainstream of American nursing. Students who are involved in Breakthrough realize that recruitment alone is insufficient and that efforts must also be directed toward helping students complete the program so that they will become licensed practitioners. Efforts to reduce attrition rates through a planned tutoring-advocacy-counseling program is also a part of the project.

Breakthrough continues to be one of the major avenues by which all nursing students can work in a unified way to ultimately improve the quality of nursing care given to diverse cultural groups, thus making nursing a more visible and attractive profession (Carnegie, 1988; Barnes, 1992).

SEALANTIC

Since the early part of this century, the Rockefeller Foundation has acted on the fundamental belief that trained intelligence can and does promote human welfare, and has been for many years deeply engaged in working with a number of outstanding universities and colleges in the United States to create new opportunities for students from deprived backgrounds (Schickel, 1965). In keeping with the Rockefeller Foundation's long-standing interest in helping the disadvantaged in the United States and other countries and its interest in helping to meet the health needs of the people, the Sealantic Fund was established in 1938 by John D. Rockefeller, Jr. Sealantic had funded several programs in nursing: the pilot project for the establishment of associate degree programs, the National League for Nursing Career program to recruit more students, and conferences for faculties of associate degree programs. In 1965, the fund began sponsoring a program in nursing education for the disadvantaged.

The purposes of the Sealantic project for the Disadvantaged in Nursing were (1) to assist selected schools of nursing to reach out for black and other disadvantaged youth and engage in educational and social action needed to prepare them for entering and completing programs in nursing and (2) to experiment with different ways of increasing the number of blacks and disadvantaged youth who enter nursing, with the expectation that many other schools, with or without financial assistance, would be stimulated to focus attention on this significant source of nurse power and on the expansion of educational opportunities for these youth.

In 1966, ten nursing programs participated in the Sealantic Project: Opening the Doors Wider in Nursing (ODWIN), Roxbury, Massachusetts; Cornell University-New York Hospital, New York; Goshen College, Indiana; Hunter College, New York; Loyola University, Chicago;

Spalding College, Louisville, Kentucky; University of Arizona, Tucson; University of Cincinnati, Ohio; University of Portland, Oregon, and Wagner College, Staten Island, New York. ODWIN, an outgrowth of a project sponsored and conducted by the Alumnae Association of Boston University School of Nursing to assist persons from minority and low income groups to enter and complete a program in nursing, became independently incorporated.

The initial grants awarded for all projects were two years. While all projects had the same goal of helping disadvantaged young people prepare for a career in nursing, each project identified different strategies for the attainment of the goal. Common elements in all programs included recruitment, academic remediation, counseling, cultural enrichment, and financial assistance.

An advisory committee, composed of nurse educators, representatives from the federal government, the National Urban League, national nursing organizations, and the Rockefeller Foundation formulated the criteria for participation in the Sealantic Project. The schools selected were required (1) to offer a baccalaureate program that was accredited by the National League for Nursing; (2) to admit freshmen directly from high school, or to admit students as sophomore or juniors; (3) to offer intensive counseling and special instruction, if needed, to students in the first or first two years of study in other colleges on the same campus; (4) to be desegregated and not admit a predominant number of blacks; (5) to be located in a community where a considerable number of blacks or other minority candidates were available; and (6) to have a dean and instructional staff who were known to possess interest in the purpose of the program.

On the basis of these criteria and the geographic spread, 58 baccalaureate nursing programs were selected and invited by letter to submit proposals to Sealantic that would include an estimate of funds needed. The schools were also informed of the availability of consultation services by the advisory committee through site visits. (The consultants who made the site visits were Lucile Petry Leone, Mary Elizabeth Carnegie, and Lillian Bischoff.) Twenty-four of the schools contacted indicated an interest, and visits were made. Nine schools submitted proposals, of which seven were approved for funding in 1966, with three additional programs funded later, bringing the number of participating programs to ten.

Since there were no forms for preparing the proposals, there was no uniformity among the proposals. All of the schools requested funds, however, for project directors, summer and Saturday school instructors, counselors, tutors, scholarships, and stipends for students. In all instances, universities contributed physical facilities, educational resources, and financial aid to enrolled Sealantic students. The budgets approved by Sealantic for individual schools ranged from $17,600 to $59,866. Four programs received $25,000; three received less than $25,000, and three received more than $25,000.

The project directors (Fig. 3–7), six of whom were nurses, were responsible for identifying potential candidates for nursing among the disadvantaged junior and senior high school students with identifiable potential and interest; preparing students for admission to nursing programs; maintaining the students' interest in nursing as a career; increasing the motivation of students to undertake and successfully complete the program; providing the students with an opportunity to pursue nursing as a career; working with high school counselors in providing information on nursing and in selecting promising students for nursing; expanding and maintaining enrollment of disadvantaged students; helping students to qualify for admission to nursing school; providing an opportunity for students to identify with nursing; raising the level of the intellectual and vocational aspiration of students; assisting students with financial aid; providing information about nursing to counselors; preparing students to function within the nursing career; and creating an awareness within the school and the university of the needs of the disadvantaged (Kibrick, 1970).

In addition, the project directors visited the families of the students to help them understand nursing, the Sealantic Project, and opportunities

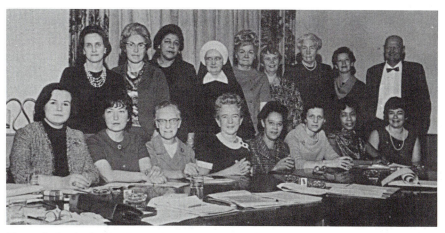

Figure 3–7   Sealantic Project Directors meet in Washington, DC, March 1967. Front row, left to right: Susan Dudas, Alice Cicerich, Orpah B. Mosemann, Lucile P. Leone, Anita Smith, Mary Malone, Doris B. Clement, Jean Scheinfeldt. Second row, left to right: Virginia Kettling, Vernia Jane Huffman, Mary Elizabeth Carnegie, Sister Agnes Miriam, Fannie L. Gardner, Doris Schwartz, Katharine Faville, Daphne A. Rolfe, Rhodes Arnold.

available in nursing. They also worked with community groups such as the Urban League and conducted field trips to hospitals, clinics, and public health agencies to sustain the students' interest in nursing and raise the level of their educational and professional aspirations. The project directors were also responsible for arranging culturally and socially enriching experiences. To provide further guidance, seven projects also had advisory committees composed of people in the community representing high school faculty and public service agencies. Members of these advisory committees represented various racial and ethnic groups in the community.

Recruitment plans and procedures varied. Six schools recruited specifically for baccalaureate programs, and four recruited for all types of nursing education programs; however, most efforts were aimed at high school students who had been identified by their counselors or teachers as having the interest in and potential for succeeding in nursing.

All projects conducted a prenursing program throughout the academic year, which included Saturday activities, and all but one had a summer program ranging from six to ten weeks. All the projects gave continued support to students, including financial aid and counseling, after admission to a nursing program. The summer programs included academic subjects and cultural enrichment activities, and several schools provided housing on campus. For those students who would ordinarily have to work, the Sealantic grants provided modest stipends. The amount varied from $30 to $40 per week.

The goals of the Sealantic Project were twofold: successful admission and completion of the program through graduation. After admission to a nursing school, the Sealantic students were given continuing counseling and guidance, academic assistance by volunteers who were often other students, and financial assistance by Sealantic in the form of scholarships for tuition and living expenses.

A study conducted in 1971 compared the Sealantic students who had had specialized counseling with a similar group of students in the National League for Nursing Career-Pattern Study who had had no such help (Carnegie, 1974). Findings of the study revealed that the dropout rate of the Sealantic students, who had been provided with special assistance, was 28.1 percent in contrast to those in the Career-Pattern group, who had a dropout rate of 48.4 percent. This finding alone supported the conclusion that the Sealantic Project was well worth the effort and money contributed, and resulted in adding more baccalaureate graduates to the population of black nurses. Although the Sealantic Project was in the 1960s, it is still being used by universities as a model.

ANA MINORITY FELLOWSHIP PROGRAMS

Doctoral education in nursing is relatively young; the first doctor of nursing science program was established in 1960 at Boston University. For years, however, nurses had been (and still are) pursuing doctoral studies in other disciplines to prepare them not only for leadership roles in service and education but also to conduct research in order to improve the quality of patient care. The first known nurse to hold a doctorate was Edith Bryan, who earned a Ph.D in psychology in 1927 from Johns Hopkins University, Baltimore, Maryland.

One of the main objectives of the American Nurses' Foundation (ANF), the research arm of the American Nurses' Association (ANA), is the encouragement of nursing research. To help meet this objective, ANF compiled a directory of nurses with doctoral degrees and published the first listing in the September-October 1969 issue of *Nursing Research,* with supplements in 1970, 1971, and 1972.

In 1973, the Foundation's directory, which included 1,019 nurses with doctorates in 19 countries, was presented in a separate publication entitled *International Directory of Nurses with Doctoral Degrees.* This directory included data such as educational preparation, country of residence, area of doctoral study, and subject of dissertation. A unique feature of the directory was the identification of minorities. Such identification was made with the permission of the persons involved. The data about minorities revealed that of the 964 nurse doctorates reporting in the United States, 41 (4.2%) were black, and three of these were men. Twenty-six (63%) of the 41 black nurses had acquired their basic nursing education at 13 historically black schools of nursing: Lincoln School for Nurses in New York and Freedmen's in Washington, DC—five each; Meharry in Nashville—three; Dillard University in New Orleans, Harlem Hospital in New York, and Florida A&M University in Tallahassee—two each; and Good Samaritan Hospital in Charlotte, North Carolina, Lincoln in Durham, Tuskegee in Alabama, St. Philip in Richmond, Mercy in Philadelphia, Hampton University in Virginia, and Kansas City General in Missouri—one each. Two of the 26 had earned doctorates in medicine.

In 1980, the ANA published a *Directory of Nurses with Doctoral Degrees.* This publication was funded by a grant from the Division of Nursing. Of the 1,964 respondents to a mailed questionnaire, 57 were identifiable as black, although race was not reported. However, 22 of these had appeared in ANF's 1973 directory, which did include data concerning race. Although the 1980 directory does not give the name of the nurse's basic program, of the 35 new black entries, 16, or nearly half, were known to have received their basic education at historically black schools: Freedmen's in Washington, DC, Florida A&M University, Harlem, Dillard University, Lincoln in New York, Homer G. Phillips in St. Louis, North Carolina A&T State University, and Tuskegee University. The two directories (1973 and 1980) presented a total listing of 76 black nurses with doctoral degrees. Of the questionnaires mailed in 1983 by ANA to 4,500 nurses, 3,650 elicited responses, which appear in the 1984 directory. Again, race was not included; however, 77 (2.1%) of the nurses were identifiable as black, 24 of whom were new entries. Although ANA has not issued a directory since 1984, the National Sample Survey of Registered Nurses indicates that in 1992 there were 11,304 nurses with doctoral degrees (4,261 in nursing and 7,043 in related fields) who have maintained their license in nursing (National Sample Survey, 1992). Of this number, between 300 and 400, or 3 percent, are black.

Based on the data in ANF's directory, an editorial which appeared in the November-December, 1973 issue of *Nursing Research,* entitled "ANF Directory Identifies Minorities with Doctorates," drew attention to the small number of minorities with earned doctorates (Carnegie, 1973). Two years earlier, 1971, the Center for Minority Group Mental Health Programs, a major component of the National Institute of Mental Health, Department of Health, Education, and Welfare, was established. According to Harper (1977), the idea of minority representation within NIMH began to ferment in the early 1960s, but did not succeed through its three initial attempts until black psychiatrists met with the Director, Dr. Bertram Brown, expressing the desire for an organized unit to basically serve four minority groups: American Indians, Asian-Americans, Spanish Speaking/Spanish surnamed, and blacks.

Following four national conferences with each of the ethnic groups, priorities in the areas of manpower, research, education and training were identified. Due to the lack of manpower, especially, it was decided to fund five fellowship programs to be administered by the following professional organizations: the American Psychological Association, the American Sociological Association, the American Nurses' Association, the American Psychiatric Association, and the Council on Social Work Education. These programs were to increase the number and quality of competent minority researchers, with the aim to enhance the professional minority manpower, and to provide scientific data through research to improve mental health and nursing care to ethnic minority consumers. In essence, the programs would supply researchers who could direct research and identify priorities by indigenous groups.

Because ANA was concerned about research in the area of ethnic minorities and the small number of doctorally prepared minorities to conduct such research, in 1974 it submitted a proposal to NIMH for a grant to help minority nurses earn doctorates. The grant of nearly $1 million was approved, and ANA received the funds in July of that year. This provided for a project director—Dr. Ruth Gordon (Fig. 3–8) was the first project director—secretarial services, and an advisory committee that included representatives of the racial minority categories and two white nurses. (The original advisory committee members were Hazle W. Blakeney, Mary Elizabeth Carnegie, Effie Poy Yew Chow, Signe Cooper, Herlinda Q. Jackson, Carmen D. Janosov, Myra E. Levine, Martha Primeaux, Gloria Smith, and Ethelrine Shaw-Nickerson.) The advisory committee was selected by the ANA Task Force on Affirmative Action and the ANA Board of Directors.

The purpose of the 1974 grant was to support candidates in behavioral and social science doctoral studies who had engaged in or who had demonstrated an interest in conducting research relating to the racial/cultural influences on mental health care delivery systems in ethnic minority communities. The objectives of this first ANA research grant were (1) to increase the quantity and quality of ethnic/racial minority nurse researchers and (2) to provide scientific data derived from research on ethnic/minority clientele as a basis for quality mental health and nursing service delivery. Since the first fellowships were given, the Registered Nurse Fellowship Program (RNFP) has changed its focus to center on the behavioral sciences only, as a result of the policies of the Reagan Administration, which dictated fewer research and training monies going to the social sciences.

The second grant to ANA was received in 1977 for the Clinical Fellowship Program (CFP) for Ethnic/Racial Minorities so that nurses could pursue doctoral studies in the area of psychiatric and mental health nursing. (Members of the

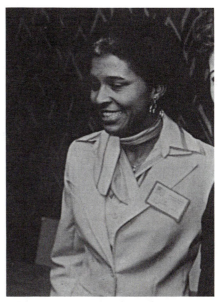

Figure 3–8   Dr. Ruth Gordon, first Project Director, ANA Minority Fellowship Program, 1974.

CFP Advisory Committee were Bette Evans, chairperson, Rosalie Jackson, Don Matheson, Helen Nakagawa, Oliver Osborne, and Janie Wilson.) The CFP prepares nurses to provide, supervise, and consult in the delivery of psychiatric and mental health nursing, particularly to ethnic and racial minority groups. Also in 1977, Dr. Hattie Bessent (Fig. 3–9) joined the project as its second director, bringing with her a vast amount of experience in administration, teaching, research, and consultation.

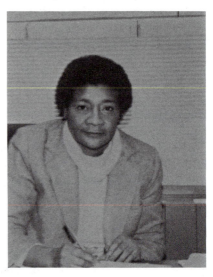

Figure 3–9   Dr. Hattie Bessent, ANA Minority Fellowship Programs, 1977–1992.

The rationale for the need for these minority nurse fellowship programs can be better understood in light of the mission of the Center for Studies of Minority Group Mental Health of NIMH, which is the funding agency. The Center's primary function is to improve the quality and quantity of research, manpower, and services to minority groups by funding supplemental technical assistance and developmental and enabling assistance. The Center's goal is to impact the health care delivery system for ethnic/racial minority groups through its programs and collaborative efforts with other federal, state, and local agency programs, regional and national consumer and professional programs, and private health and funding sources. Thus, although the two fellowship programs differ in the type of mental health disciplines being supported for doctoral study, both programs have a common objective—to improve the delivery of mental health care to ethnic/racial minority persons by increasing the pool of minority nurse researchers, educators, and administrators. The Fellows have been enrolled in nearly 50 universities throughout the country since the first fellowships were awarded in 1975. As of December 31, 1994, more than 200 Fellows have earned their doctorates, 95 percent of whom have been black. A number of ANA Fellows have pursued post-doctoral education, the first of whom was Cynthia Flynn Capers (Diploma, Freedmen's Hospital School of Nursing, Washington, DC; Ph.D., University of Pennsylvania, Philadelphia) (Fig. 3–10), who studied at the University of Pennsylvania in the area of coping of African-American families with low birth-weight babies.

As part of the minority fellowship program, a legislative internship (Fig. 3–11) existed from 1977 to 1990. It provided the Fellows with an opportunity to observe and participate in the legislative process at the national level, with particular emphasis on the enactment process of legislation dealing with healthcare policy, the nursing profession, and mental health and illness issues. The rationale for this was that the Fellows would benefit from having this kind of experience in public policy formation, and an internship would provide them with firsthand knowledge of the steps involved in having a bill introduced and its evolution into law. This political expertise helps the Fellows, as leaders in

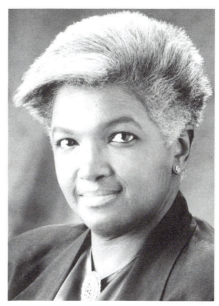

Figure 3–10   Dr. Cynthia Flynn Capers, first ANA Fellow to pursue post-doctoral education.

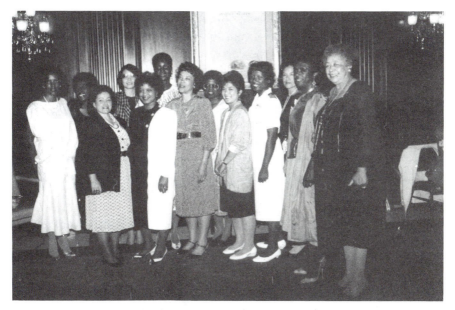

Figure 3–11   ANA Minority Legislative Interns, past and present (1989) with Dr. M. Elizabeth Carnegie (far right).

the health-care profession, make an impact in the legislative arena. As of 1990, 37 percent of the Fellows had interned in the offices of congressional lawmakers and committees, federal health regulatory agencies, and centers for research and development and policy studies. Placement of Fellows as interns in congressional offices and in federal health regulatory agencies is a means of monitoring and influencing federal legislative and administrative policies and their implementation as they affect the characteristics and numbers of nurses and the scope of their practice and accountability.

In addition to administering the project for ethnic/racial minorities funded by NIMH, the staff has been responsible for administering the Clara Lockwood Fund, the ANA Baccalaureate Scholarship Fund, the Allstate Foundation Fund, and the W.K. Kellogg Foundation project on leadership training. The Clara Lockwood Fund was originally established to assist in the education of American Indian nurses. In December 1983, however, the ANA Board of Directors approved the use of interest from the fund to help finance graduate education for all ethnic minority nurses.

The ANA House of Delegates at successive conventions passed two resolutions sponsored by the Commission on Human Rights. The 1978 resolution called for ANA to create a scholarship fund to support baccalaureate education for registered nurses, with the criteria for reflecting "national priorities for increasing access to nursing care" in medically underserved areas. The 1980 resolution proposed specific actions to increase informational, legislative, and financial support for minority students in basic and graduate nursing education programs, in response to the proposed changes in educational requirements for entry into practice. In their December 1983 meeting, the ANA Board of Directors committed $50,000 for five years toward the establishment of this fund, which was geared toward ethnic minorities, but not limited to them. In the five years that the program was in existence, 40 nurses completed bachelor's degrees.

From 1985 to 1989, the Allstate Foundation had financed education for American Indian/Alaska Native descent nurses through the Indian Nurses Association. When this association dissolved in 1985 because of financial difficulties, the ANA Minority Fellowship Program (MFP) assumed the administrative responsibility for the scholarship fund. Until the funds were depleted, 22 American Indian nurses received assistance and completed the bachelor's or the associate degree in nursing.

Also in 1983 with the strong conviction that a post-doctoral leadership training program was needed for the ANA Fellows, discussions toward this end were held between the MFP staff and officials of the W.K. Kellogg Foundation for possible funding. The preliminary proposal was submitted which would involve alumnae from all five minority fellowship programs—psychology, psychiatry, sociology, social work, and nursing. In 1986, a 3-year grant was secured from the Kellogg Foundation to provide postdoctoral leadership and management training in mental health and to improve the Fellows' contributions to the clients they serve. The thrust of the program recognized that our society . . . is in the process of change in terms of its perspectives in leadership roles and opportunities for women. The challenge was to design a program of excellence that would assist ethnic minority women in maintaining themselves in this environment of social change and in coping with those extra burdens placed on them because of the long history of society-imposed limitations (Bessent, 1989). A second three-year grant was made in 1989, which terminated in 1991.

The Kellogg program trained participants in a series of workshops that covered a wide range of administrative and communication skills. Faculty were selected from such prestigious sources as the Harvard School of Business and included America's leading women administrators. In the six years of the Kellogg program's existence, a total of 120 women of color participated. They included directors of university counseling centers, administrators, social and behavioral practitioners, and university faculty members. Most were interested in moving toward leadership roles in their academic, medical, and social service institutions where they could improve the status of their race and sex (Bessent, 1989).

Another innovative idea that Bessent had which came to fruition in 1988 was the establishment of an annual awards luncheon or dinner at ANA conventions, in collaboration with the Cabinet on Human Rights, to honor outstanding women of color—blacks, Hispanics, Asians, and American Indians. They were not limited to nursing, but to those women who had made a significant contribution to public service in the Armed Services, health management, public health, history, research, administration, education, social service, and public law.

In December, 1992, Dr. Bessent retired from the position of Project Director, having been praised by Hawaii Senator Daniel Inouye in the July 21, 1987 issue of the *Congressional Record* for providing more than $3 million to aid minority

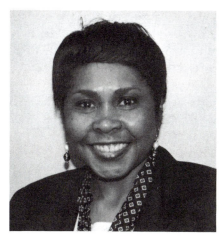

Figure 3–12   Dr. Carla J. Serlin, Director, ANA Minority Fellowship Programs, 1992.

nurses earn doctoral degrees and for operating Capitol Hill's nurse internship program. The Fellows paid tribute to her on June 22, 1992, at a special program at the ANA convention in Las Vegas, Nevada, titled, "The Role of Minority Nurses in Research, Education, and Practice." The ANA Board of Directors also voted to name a Minority Reading Room at its headquarters in honor of Dr. Bessent.

Dr. Bessent was succeeded by Dr. Carla Serlin (A.A., Bronx Community College; Ph.D., University of Colorado, Denver), January, 1992 (Fig. 3–12).

FACULTY AND COMMUNITY ENHANCEMENT PROJECT

Another project funded by the W.K. Kellogg Foundation was launched in 1992, with Dr. Hattie Bessent as its director. Project FACE (Faculty and Community Enhancement), of Florida A&M University, is designed to enhance scholarly productivity, skills in the transmission of knowledge, and service to the community. Participants are students enrolled in nursing and allied health programs at historically black colleges and universities (see Table 2–2, Chapter 2). These students now have access to more intimate mentoring from university faculty members than was possible in the past. Eighty-eight persons were initially selected to participate in Project FACE–two faculty and two students from each of the 22 historically black colleges and universities. In 1993, the project added the nursing program at the College of the U.S. Virgin Islands, bringing the total participants to 92.

The participating institutions serve as host or co-host for the nine workshops planned for the four years of the project (Fig. 3–13). The first workshop was held at Florida A&M University where the grant is housed. The workshops are designed so that at least two of the presentations at each one accommodates a large audience, composed of all faculty from the host and co-host institutions.

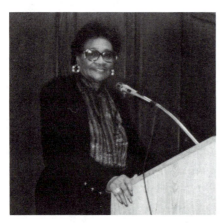

Figure 3–13   Dr. Hattie Bessent, Director, Project FACE, addresses participants at conference, Washington, DC, February, 1994.

Within the faculty teams, one faculty participant is expected to complete a proposal for funding and one to complete an article for journal publication. Both faculty members direct the student members of the team in the development and implementation of a community service project. Work with the faculty is individualized, depending on the need of the faculty member. Consultative visits, calls, and written feedback on work in progress are provided by Project FACE core faculty, composed of experts in nursing education, administration, and research.

SUMMARY

During World War II, the federal government financed basic nursing education through the Cadet Nurse Corps in an effort to procure more nurses to help meet military and civilian needs. Nearly 3,000 black students benefited from this program and received a nursing education.

To increase the number of blacks entering and successfully completing a basic program in nursing, in the 1960s and 1970s, special projects were established, two of which have been reported in this chapter: Breakthrough to Nursing and the Sealantic Project.

To increase the number of doctorally prepared minority nurses, including blacks, the Fellowship Program of the American Nurses' Association has been described. This project, which began in 1974, has been responsible for more than 200 minority nurses earning the highest academic credential—the doctorate, 95 percent of whom were black.

To support schools of nursing at historically black colleges and universities, a project was also funded by the W.K. Kellogg Foundation titled Faculty and Community Enhancement (FACE).

REFERENCES

Barnes, K. (1992). Breakthrough to nursing's early years. *Imprint, 39,* 103–109.

Bender, C. (1989). *Nurses in PHS celebrate proud history, dedication, service, commitment.* Washington, DC: U.S. Department of Health and Human Services, Public Health Service.

Bessent, H. (1983). *Future nurse researchers, Vol. II,* Kansas City American Nurses' Association.

Bessent, H. (1987). *Nursing researchers: Selected abstracts, Vol. II,* Kansas City: American Nurses' Association.

Bessent, H. (1989). Postdoctoral leadership training for women of color, *Journal of Professional Nursing, 5,* 279–82.

Breakthrough to nursing (1972). *Imprint, 4,* 11.

Breakthrough to nursing (1976). A proposal submitted by the National Student Nurses' Association to the Division of Nursing.

Carnegie, M. E. (1964). Are Negro schools of nursing needed today? *Nursing Outlook, 12,* 52–56.

Carnegie, M. E. (1973). ANF directory identifies minorities with doctoral degrees (editorial). *Nursing Research, 22,* 483.

Carnegie, M. E. (1974). Disadvantaged students in RN Programs. *National League for Nursing.*

Carnegie, M. E. (1988). Breakthrough to nursing: Twenty-five years of involvement. *Image, 35,* 55–59.

CIS Annual Legislative History of U.S. Public Laws (1986). Bethesda: Congressional Information Service.

Deloughery, G. L. (1977). *History and Trends in Professional Nursing, 8th ed.* St. Louis: C.V. Mosby.

Goodnow, M. (1948). *Nursing history, (8th ed.).* Philadelphia: Saunders.

Harper, M. S. (1977). The origin of the minority fellowship programs. *Fellowship.* Spring, 1977, 4.

Kalisch, P. A. (1988). Why not launch a new cadet nurse corps? *American Journal of Nursing, 88,* 316–317.

Kalisch, P. A., & Kalisch, B. (1978). *The Advance of American Nursing.* Boston: Little, Brown & Co.

Kibrick, A. (1970). A report of the Sealantic Project concerned with recruiting the disadvantaged in schools of nursing. New York: Sealantic Fund (unpublished).

Larson, D. V. (1987). Cadet nurses seek help from KNSA. *The Kansas Nurse, 5,* 14–15.

Maxwell, P. E. (1976). *History of the Army Nurse Corps 1775-1948.* Washington, DC: U.S. Army Center of Military History (unpublished), 92.

Mullan, F. (1989). *Plagues and politics: The story of the United States Public Health Service.* Philadelphia: Basic Books.

National Sample Survey of RNs (1992). Bureau of Health Professions, Division of Nursing, Department of Health and Human Services.

Riddle (Osborne) E., & Nelson, J. (1945). The negro nurse looks toward tomorrow. *American Journal of Nursing, 45,* 627–630.

Roberts, M. M. (1954). *American nursing: History and interpretation.* New York: Macmillan.

Schickel, R. (1965). *Equal opportunities for all.* New York: Rockefeller Foundation, Spring.

Shields, E. A. (1981). Highlights in the history of the Army Nurse Corps. Washington, DC: U.S. Government Printing Office.

Staupers, M. K. (1951). Story of the National Association of Colored Graduate Nurses, *American Journal of Nursing, 51,* 222–223.

Staupers, M. K. (1961). *No time for prejudice.* New York: Macmillan.

U.S. Public Health Service (1950). The United States Cadet Nurse Corps and other Federal Nurse Training Programs, 1943-1948. Washington, DC: Government Printing Office.

Chapter

4

~

Struggle for Recognition

This chapter discusses the involvement of black nurses in organizations that have been significant in their history. It begins with the National League for Nursing because its forerunner, the American Society of Superintendents of Training Schools for nurses in the United States and Canada, established in 1893, was the first nursing organization that was national in scope. This is followed by 25 others that have or have had black nurses in top leadership positions—elected or appointed.

THE NATIONAL LEAGUE FOR NURSING

At the Congress of Hospital and Dispensaries at the World's Fair in Chicago in 1893, held to celebrate the 400th anniversary of the "discovery" of America, the nursing section provided occasion for the first meeting of nurses on the North American continent. By that time, many schools of nursing had been established in the United States and Canada to train nurses. Concerned about the lack of educational standards for these existing schools, the directors, or superintendents of nurses who were attending the fair, created the American Society of Superintendents of Training Schools for Nurses in the United States and Canada for the purpose of exchanging ideas and establishing high educational standards. The work of the Society concentrated on (1) higher minimum entrance requirements to attract top students into nursing, (2) improvement of living and working conditions (for students), and (3) increased opportunities for postgraduate and specialized training. The Society was also concerned about the need for laws to protect the public from poorly trained nurses (Flanagan, 1976). Although there were a few trained black nurses in the country when the Society was formed, there was no indication of black involvement at the initial meeting.

In 1912, the Canadian nurses discontinued their membership in favor of establishing their own national organization, and so the name of the Society was changed to the National League of Nursing Education (NLNE), and membership was open on an individual basis to those nurses engaged in administration and education in schools of nursing.

As the result of an indepth study of the structure of the major national nursing organizations, NLNE, along with the Association of Collegiate Schools of Nursing and the National Organization for Public Health Nursing, and several national committees merged in 1952, becoming the National League for Nursing (NLN). The primary purpose of NLNE was to further the best interests of the nursing profession by establishing and maintaining a "universal" standard of training (*First Annual Report of the American Society,* 1897).

NLN's primary function is to work with health-care agencies, of which nursing services are a basic component, with educational institutions and with communities to improve health-care services, and to provide nursing education programs needed by society through services in accreditation, consultation, testing, continuing education, research, publications including videotapes, and through lobbying efforts on behalf of nursing and consumers of nursing.

Black nurses had participated in the National League of Nursing Education on all levels—national, state, and local—presenting scientific papers at conventions, and the like. As early as 1934, Estelle Massey Osborne read a paper at a general session of the fortieth annual convention in Washington, DC, entitled "The Negro Nurse Student." At its last convention in Atlantic City in 1952, Mary Elizabeth Carnegie participated in the symposium on curriculum. The papers by both these black nurses were published in the *American Journal of Nursing* (Massey, 1934; Carnegie, 1952).

When the structure was changed in 1912 from an organization of administrators, NLNE admitted to membership those who served in any teaching capacity in a school of nursing, directors in public health work, members of state boards of nurses examiners, and others actively concerned with education. For many years, however, black nurses in southern states were denied membership in NLNE because membership in their state nurses' association was a prerequisite. By virtue of their being denied membership in the state constituents of ANA, they were barred from NLNE membership. In 1942, NLNE set a precedent for individual membership by a change in its bylaws. This change was particularly significant because it broke the barriers related to race. Black nurses were also represented on committees related to areas such as curriculum, vocational guidance, postwar planning, educational policies in wartime, and the National Committee on Nursing School Libraries.

From its inception in 1952, NLN has had black representation on the Board of Directors, and it has continued to involve blacks on its boards, councils, committees, and professional staff. Willie Mae Johnson Jones (Diploma, Tuskegee University School of Nursing, Tuskegee, Alabama; B.S., New York University), a black nurse on the staff of the Community Nursing Services of Montclair, New Jersey, was elected on the first Board of Directors in 1952. She retired in 1974 as educational supervisor and died in 1982. While Lillian Harvey was on the board (1957 to 1961), she was a board-appointed advisor to the National Student Nurses' Association. Currently (1994) on the Board is Georgie C. Labadie (Fig. 4–1), having been elected in 1993. Labadie (B.S., Florida A&M University School of Nursing; Ed.D., Teachers College, Columbia University, New York) is Professor, School of Nursing, University of Miami, Florida.

In 1954, Estelle Massey Osborne joined NLN staff as Associate General Director for Administration and served in this capacity until her retirement in 1966. Many other blacks have held executive positions at NLN among whom were Eleanor Lynch, Test Construction Unit; Claudia Durham, Consultant, Maternal-Child Health project; Dr. Edith Ramsey Johnson, Dr. Betty Martin Blount, and Sylvia Edge, Council of Associate Degree Programs; Dr. Alma Yearwood Dixon, Director of Consultation; Dr. Ruth Johnson, Director of Council Affairs, Council of Baccalaureate and Higher Degree Programs (Fig. 4–2); Dr. Ngozi O. Nkongho, Program Evaluator; and Julia Kelly Jackson, director, Commonwealth-Funded Fellowship Program. Under

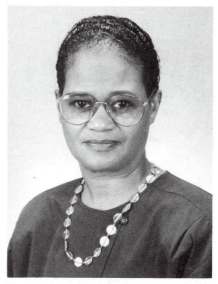

Figure 4–1 Dr. Georgie C. Labadie, elected to the NLN Board of Directors, 1993.

Jackson's direction, the fellowship program helped nurses with outstanding ability obtain advanced educational preparation. During its existence, from 1955 to 1963, 195 scholarships were given, 162 of which were for post-masters study.

NLN currently (1994) has two black nurses on its professional staff—Romaine Martin-Semeah and Ena Bailey. Martin-Semeah, who also holds a law degree, is Interim President and Chief Operating Officer of the Community Health Accreditation Program (CHAP). Bailey serves as CHAP's Senior Vice-President for Accreditation.

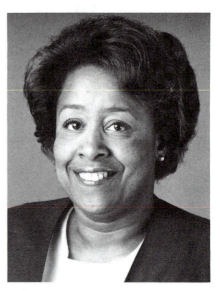

Figure 4–2   Dr. Ruth Johnson, former Director of Council Affairs, NLN Department of Baccalaureate & Higher Degree Programs, 1989–1994.

At each biennial convention, NLN presents awards to outstanding persons for various achievements. In 1973, Mabel K. Staupers, first executive director and last president, National Association of Colored Graduate Nurses, received the Linda Richards Award for her pioneering efforts to promote blacks in nursing. In 1975, Lillian Stokes (Fig. 4–3), faculty of Indiana University School of Nursing, Indianapolis, was the recipient of the Lucile Petry Leone Award for innovative teaching methods. Stokes is currently pursuing the doctoral degree as a Fellow of the ANA Minority Fellowship Program, and was profiled at the Indianapolis Children's Museum as one of the "Black Achievers in Science." In 1985, Vernice Ferguson received the Jean Mac Vicar Outstanding Nurse Executive Award and in 1987, the Marine Midland Bank/Margaret Heckler Award of $10,000 went to Carolyn Cuello, a black student at

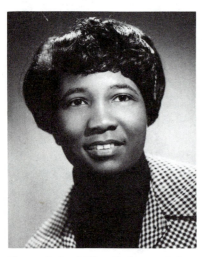

Figure 4–3   Lillian Stokes, recipient, Lucile Petry Leone Award, 1975.

North Carolina A&T State University School of Nursing, Greensboro, for excellence in writing. In 1993, the Mary Adelaide Nutting Award went to Dr. Gloria R. Smith, coordinator and Program Director of Health Programming, W.K. Kellogg Foundation, in recognition of outstanding leadership and achievement in nursing education and nursing service of national significance (Fig. 4–4). Smith's prior positions include Dean, Wayne State University College of Nursing, Detroit, and Director, Michigan Department of Public Health. Most recently, she has been especially acclaimed for her devotion to problems of the poor and disenfranchised and for

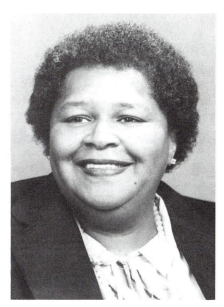

Figure 4–4　Dr. Gloria Smith, recipient, Nutting Award, 1993.

international leadership with special focus on nursing and health care in Southern Africa.

In 1953, NLN issued a statement on civil rights, "All activities of NLN shall include all groups regardless of race, color, religion, and sex." This statement was reviewed in 1964 by the Executive Committee of the Board which expressed its conviction that the principles inherent in the statement had been practiced and the statement should not be changed or amplified. The League vowed to continue its past policy of nondiscrimination in employment practices and all other activities. Since 1991, NLN has had a special committee on racial, ethnic, and cultural diversity and as of 1993 all appointed committees reflect its policy of inclusion.

In 1990, NLN produced a videotape, edited by Ellen Baer, entitled *Nursing in America: A History of Social Reform,* which includes black nurse leaders. In addition, NLN Press has published a 1991 historical calendar, compiled by Mary Elizabeth Carnegie, saluting the 23 baccalaureate and higher degree nursing programs at historically black colleges and universities (see Chapter 2 for a listing of these schools). In 1993, NLN produced a videotape titled, *A Conversation with Elizabeth Carnegie*—a recap of her 50 years of professional and personal experiences in nursing; and *Critical Thinking: Lessons from Tuskegee,* a commentary of the tragic syphilis experiment.

THE AMERICAN NURSES' ASSOCIATION

As schools of nursing developed, graduates of these schools formed alumnae associations not only for social and professional purposes but also for promoting their own schools (Flanagan, 1976). The graduates of Bellevue Hospital Training School were first to organize, in 1889, followed by the Illinois Training School in 1891, Massachusetts General and Johns Hopkins in 1892, and St. Louis Protestant Hospital in 1895 (Seymer, 1933; Christ, 1957). In addition to social and professional purposes, many of these organizations had the more serious intention of providing both moral support and financial assistance to their members in time of need. The service feature of the St. Louis Protestant Hospital Alumnae, for example, provided for "pecuniary assistance in time of illness, or death among its members" (Christ, 1957, p. 103). Such a provision was a common function of American secret societies originating during the eighteenth and nineteenth centuries, many of which, even today, still offer their members mutual assistance in the form of burial insurance, life insurance, endowment plans, and so on (Gist, 1940).

In 1896, with the support of the American Society of Superintendents of Training Schools for Nurses in the United States and Canada, representatives of nurse alumnae societies formed a national association to embrace the general betterment of the profession. The name chosen for the new organization was The Nurses' Associated Alumnae of the United States and Canada. For legal reasons that involved matters of incorporation, the Canadian members withdrew from the Association in 1911. That year the name was changed to the American Nurses' Association (ANA).

Today, the ANA is the national professional organization of registered nurses, comprising 53 constituent state and territorial associations in the 50 states, the District of Columbia, Guam, and the Virgin Islands, and over 900 district associations. The association establishes the standards of nursing practice, education, and service, and promotes the professional and educational advancement of nurses, and the general welfare of nurses, to the end that all people may have better nursing care. These purposes are unrestricted by consideration of nationality, race, creed, color, or gender (*This is ANA*, 1975).

From its founding in 1896, the ANA has always offered membership to all qualified professional nurses regardless of race, color, creed, or national origin, and before 1916, all nurses joined ANA through their alumnae associations. This reorganization set up the state association as the basic unit of membership. Because of segregation laws at that time, black nurses in 16 southern states and the District of Columbia were denied membership on the state level, thereby precluding their membership in ANA. Black nurse membership in ANA was one problem upon which the NACGN, which had been established in 1908, spent most of its time and efforts. The first major step taken by the ANA House of Delegates in 1942 toward this end was the authorization of the Committee on Constitution and By-laws to consider some type of membership for those black nurses who were barred from membership in a state association because of race. With ANA's encouragement, a few southern states that year dropped their color bars and admitted black nurses—Delaware was first, followed by Florida and Maryland (Staupers, 1951). It was a simple procedure to admit blacks to membership in Florida: The word "white" was merely deleted from the bylaws. However, this was not the total solution. It took years before black nurses participated fully in the Florida Nurses' Association.

The 1942 action was followed in 1946 by the adoption of a plank in the ANA 1946–1948 platform, which read: "Removal, as rapidly as possible, of barriers that prevent the full employment and professional development of nurses belonging to minority racial groups." At the 1946 convention, there was vigorous debate on this issue—pro and con—with some nurses from the southern states voicing their strong objections to black member-ship. Georgia delegates were particularly vocal and almost vehement in their protests, with one delegate referring to black nurses as "our darkies." The house immediately voted that this be stricken from the record. The house was reminded by the president, Katharine Densford Dreves, that the barring of professionally qualified black nurses from membership in a state or district association was clearly against the nondiscriminatory policies of the ANA. After the convention, Tennessee dropped its color bar. In 1947, a subcommittee of a joint committee of ANA and NACGN, chaired by Anna Heisler of the U.S. Public Health Service, was set up to study and plan ways in which ANA could absorb the functions of NACGN should the latter vote to dissolve. In a letter to Rita Miller dated July 1, 1949, Linnie Laird, Secretary, American Nurses' Association, wrote "You have been appointed by the President and Board of Directors of ANA as a member of the Special Committee to study the functions of the NACGN as they relate to comparable areas within the ANA program."

In 1948, the ANA House of Delegates inaugurated the Individual Membership Program, which offered direct membership and benefits in ANA to those qualified nurses who were not accepted by a state or district association. To implement the program, Elizabeth Ann Edwards was ap-pointed assistant executive secretary. She was the first black to hold a po-sition as an executive on the staff of ANA. Edwards, a Harlem Hospital School of Nursing in New York graduate with a master's degree from

Teacher's College, Columbia University, New York, had served as secretary of Health and Housing, Urban League of Greater New York. She had also been an instructor in psychiatric nursing at Bellevue Hospital, New York, and director of student personnel and guidance at Harlem Hospital School of Nursing.

Also in 1948, the first black nurse, Estelle Massey Osborne (Fig. 4–5), was elected to the Board of Directors for a four-year term, having been nominated by the State of Oregon. Osborne brought with her to the ANA Board not only professional knowledge and experience, but also experience as former president of NACGN. In 1949, the board selected her to represent ANA as one of its delegates to the International Congress of Nurses in Stockholm, Sweden.

At NACGN's final convention in 1949 in Louisville, Kentucky, the report of the ANA Special Committee to Study the Functions of NACGN as they related to Comparable Areas Within the ANA Program was unanimously approved. In essence, ANA had agreed to absorb the functions of NACGN should the membership vote to dissolve. Votes to accept the report of the ANA committee and to dissolve NACGN were taken in Louisville, and the wheels were set in motion immediately for legal dissolution, which would take a couple of years to accomplish.

At the final NACGN Convention (1949), a panel of presidents of state associations of Colored Graduate Nurses, of which the author was one, in those southern states that had accepted black nurse membership to the

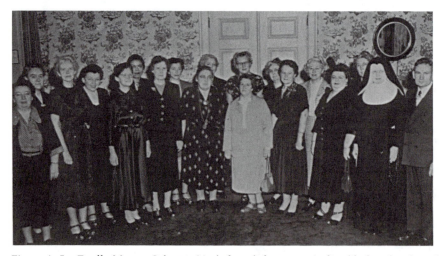

Figure 4–5   Estelle Massey Osborne (sixth from left, top row), first black to be elected to ANA Board. (Courtesy AJN Co.)

formerly all-white associations described the different problems. A common problem was finding meeting places that would accommodate both races. In 1948, the Board of the Florida State Nurses Association (FSNA) first gave courtesy membership without voice or vote to Grace Higgs, president of the Florida State Association of Colored Graduate Nurses, followed by Mary Elizabeth Carnegie. However, at the 1949 meeting of FSNA, the President of the FACGN, Mary Elizabeth Carnegie (Fig. 4–6), was placed on the ballot and elected to the Board of FSNA for a one-year term and reelected the following year for a three-year term. Florida was the first state to elect a black to its state nursing association board of directors.

At the 1950 convention of ANA, a Code for Professional Nurses, embracing 17 principles, was adopted. The preface states:

> Service to mankind is the primary function of nurses and the reason for the existence of the nursing profession. Need for nursing service is universal. Professional nursing service is therefore unrestricted by consideration of nationality, race, creed, or color.

The code had been prepared by a committee after receiving suggestions from some 5,000 persons, chiefly nurses, representing a cross section of the profession (Roberts, 1954). Adoption of such a code had significance in that a democratic philosophy was expressed.

The platform adopted by the ANA House of Delegates in 1950 carried a clear statement of the association's policy in Plank 14, which emphasized

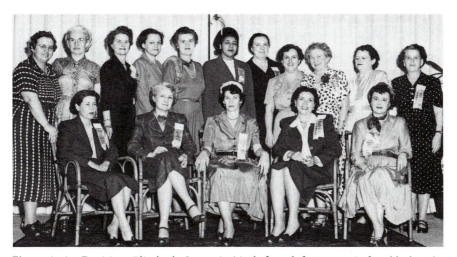

Figure 4–6   Dr. Mary Elizabeth Carnegie (sixth from left, top row), first black to be elected to Board of a state association (Florida), 1949.

"full participation of minority groups in association activities," and the elimination of "discrimination in job opportunities, salaries, and other working conditions." As a follow-up of this unprecedented action, the House of Delegates further approved a resolution urging that biracial committees be set up in district and state associations to implement programs of education and interpretation in their respective areas to promote sound development of intergroup relations, a program that had been inaugurated by ANA in 1950. The ANA's Intergroup Relations Committee was charged with the responsibility of seeing that these policies were carried out (Staupers, 1951). Serving on the Committee was Rita Miller Dargan, chair, Division of Nursing, Dillard University. In her letter of appointment to the Committee dated October 15, 1952, Agnes Ohlson, Secretary of ANA, referred to its function as "To consider problems in relation to the promotion of participation by nurses of the minority groups in the affairs of the professional nursing organization. Currently, the major problem of the Committee is to effect the absorption of the functions of the NACGN into the ANA program."

In 1951, Elouise Collier Duncan (Fig. 4–7), who was the first black nurse to graduate from Yale University School of Nursing, New Haven, Connecticut, was appointed to ANA's executive staff to work across the board; her responsibilities in the area of Constitution and Bylaws were not race-related. She remained in this position until 1953, when she resigned to marry the Honorable Henry B. Duncan, Secretary of Public Works and Utilities, Liberia, West Africa. She has since represented nursing in numerous capacities: president of the Liberian Nurses Association, member of the Board of Directors of the International Council of Nurses, and adviser to the Liberian delegation to the 19th General Assembly of the United Nations.

In 1951, NACGN dissolved its organization, largely through the patient and persistent effort of its leaders who worked for many years for the integration of black nurses into the profession. Mabel K. Staupers was president of the NACGN at the time of its dissolution. Upon acceptance of the statement of the formal dissolution of NACGN,

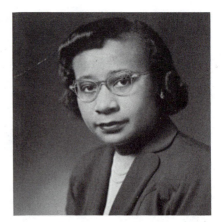

Figure 4–7   Elouise Collier Duncan, first black appointed to ANA staff to work "across the board."

Elizabeth K. Porter, President of ANA, pledged the assumption by ANA of NACGN functions. NACGN then began to make preparations for the final hours. At NACGN's testimonial dinner, January 26, 1951, certificates of honor were distributed to organizations and individuals who had been involved in its mission. ANA's certificate read: "For the recognition of the problems . . . [of] Negro nurses and the resulting action of the House of Delegates in 1946, in voting to make membership available to all American nurses, regardless of color, and the substantial interest in encouraging the removal of all restrictive barriers on the district and state levels."

From 1936 to 1951, NACGN presented the Mary Mahoney Award to persons for their contributions to the profession in the area of intergroup relations. At the convention in 1952, ANA awarded its first Mary Mahoney Medal to Marguerette Creth Jackson, public health nurse and longtime nurse leader in Harlem, who led the fight for the integration of the Henry Street Visiting Nurse Service. The Mary Mahoney Award is still given by ANA (Fig. 4–8). It is awarded to a person, or group of persons regardless of race, who, in addition to making a significant contribution to nursing generally, has been outstandingly instrumental in achieving the opening and advancement of opportunities in nursing on the same basis to members of all races, creeds, colors, and national origins.

Because of the concerted efforts of nurses and aided by ANA, the state associations gradually accepted the nondiscriminatory principles, and by

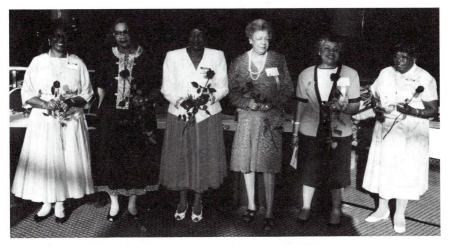

Figure 4–8 Mary Mahoney Medal recipients attending 1990 ANA convention, Boston. Left to right: Dr. Ethelrine Shaw-Nickerson, 1990; Dr. Hattie Bessent, 1988; Verdelle Bellamy, 1984; Dr. Mary Elizabeth Carnegie, 1980; Vernice Ferguson, 1970; Mary Mills, 1972. (Courtesy American Nurses Association)

1953, all states except one (Georgia) admitted all professionally qualified nurses to membership. At the 1960 biennial convention of ANA in Miami Beach, the House of Delegates considered the question of whether Georgia, which had not complied with the ANA nondiscriminatory principle of membership, should continue to be accepted as a constituent. After much discussion, the House accepted a resolution stating that "The state association be further encouraged in its efforts to provide membership for all qualified professional nurses, so that by at least the time of the next biennium, all states will accept all professional nurses as members." Georgia finally dropped its color bar in 1961; but one district in Louisiana (New Orleans) held out until 1964.

Although the ANA bylaws for many years had included a nondiscriminatory principle as one of the association's functions, in 1962 this principle was more appropriately placed within the statement of purposes of the organization. The statement (Section 2 of ANA Bylaws) now reads as follows:

> The purpose of the American Nurses' Association shall be to foster high standards of nursing practice, promote the professional and educational advancement of nurses, and promote the welfare of nurses to the end that all people may have better nursing care. The purposes shall be unrestricted by consideration of nationality, race, creed, or color.

The platform of ANA states that the association will "encourage all members, unrestricted by consideration of nationality, race, creed, or color, to participate fully in association activities and to work for full access to employment and education opportunities for nurses."

In 1964, through one of the membership memos, members were encouraged to recruit nurses from minority groups and to involve them in the work of the state and district associations. In addition, that year, the Economic Security Unit reviewed the Minimum Employment Standards of SNA sections. Wherever the Standards did not include provisions against discrimination in employment, omission was called to the attention of the SNA.

For nearly 20 years, from 1952, the year that Estelle Osborne, the first black elected to the ANA Board, completed her four-year term, until 1970, when Fay Wilson (Fig. 4–9), was elected to the board, there was no black representation on the board. This lack of representation on the policy-making level concerned the black membership. It was pointed out to the house of delegates at the 1972 convention that the only function of NACGN that ANA had assumed responsibility for was the awarding of the Mary Mahoney Medal.

Despite the perceived inaction on behalf of state and local constituents, the ANA House of Delegates, at the 1972 convention, did pass an affirmative action resolution calling for a task force to develop and implement a program to correct inequities. The resolution had been drafted by the Commission on Nursing Research, of which two black nurses were members: Dr. Lauranne Sams and Dr. Mary Harper. It was resolved that the ANA honor its commitment by taking immediate steps to establish an Affirmative Action Program at the national level, which would include the appointment of a task force to develop and implement such a pro-

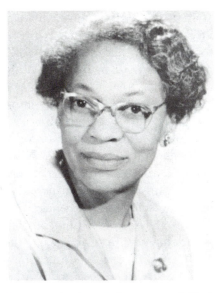

Figure 4–9 Fay Wilson, second black elected to ANA Board, 1970.

gram, to appoint a qualified black nurse to the ANA staff to work with the task force in developing and implementing the program, and to actively seek greater numbers of minority-group members in elected, appointed, and staff positions within ANA and urge states and districts to do likewise.

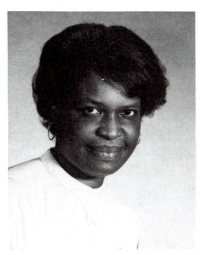

Figure 4–10 Dr. Ethelrine Shaw-Nickerson, first Chair, ANA Affirmative Action Task Force, 1972.

It was also resolved that ANA encourage and promote affirmative action programs on the state and local levels; and that an ombudsman be appointed to the ANA staff (*ANA Proceedings,* 1972). At the same convention, the house of delegates adopted a comprehensive resolution on the Universal Declaration of Human Rights. This placed the organization on record in support of specific issues on human rights and race relations; for example, employment opportunities, education, and implementation of the 1965 Civil Rights Act.

An Affirmative Action Task Force was established in 1972 and was chaired by Ethelrine Shaw-Nickerson

(Fig. 4–10), a black nurse who had just been elected to the office of third vice-president. Other members of the task force were Teresa Bello (California), Gean Mathwig (New York), Janice E. Ruffin (Connecticut), Lauranne Sams (Alabama), Betty Williams (California), and Rosemary Wood (Oklahoma), Irene Minor was appointed staff coordinator.

This action marked the beginning of a new commitment by the majority group nurses to the minority membership. The House of Delegates also provided for the position of ombudsman to evaluate involvement of minorities in leadership roles within the organization, and to treat complaints received from applicants or members that they had been discriminated against in participating in ANA because of nationality, race, creed, life-style, color, age, or gender.

Through the establishment of the affirmative action program, ANA joined a widespread movement that had grown dramatically during the 1960s. Affirmative action programs exist today within industry, government agencies, educational institutions, hospitals, and trade, professional, and community organizations (Minor & Shaw, 1973). During 1975, the Affirmative Action Task Force held two regional conferences that focused on improving nursing care and health-care delivery for ethnic/minority consumers and on promoting affirmative action programs in nursing (Flanagan, 1976).

In 1974, Barbara Nichols, a black nurse who had been president of the Wisconsin Nurses' Association, was elected to the ANA Board and served until 1978, when she became president. The year 1974 is significant because that was when ANA received a million dollar grant from the National Institute of Mental Health, designed to increase the quality and quantity of ethnic/racial minority nurse researchers with doctorates (see Chapter 3).

As a result of house of delegates' action establishing the Task Force on Affirmative Action, the need to establish a broader permanent unit focusing on human rights became evident, and a Commission on Human Rights was established in 1976. It was chaired for two terms by Ethelrine Shaw-Nickerson, prime mover in the development of ANA's Affirmative Action program. The first item in Article 8 of the 1976 bylaws states: The Commission (retitled Cabinet) on Human Rights "shall establish the scope of the Association's responsibility for addressing and responding to the equal opportunity and human rights concerns of nurses and health care recipients, with the major focus on ethnic people of color."

Looking at the Cabinet in terms of its scope and long-range goals, Shaw-Nickerson pointed out that although the focus is on ethnic people of color at the present time, she expected that eventually "programming will be broadened to encompass many significant human rights issues." Marian Whiteside (Fig. 4–11), chairperson from 1980 to 1982, added that "the Cabinet's primary focus is to protect the rights of nurses and patients, particularly those who are racial and ethnic minorities." Whiteside also viewed the Cabinet as needing to be sensitive to the sociopolitical issues that affect the inalienable rights of people around the world. The Cabinet has, since 1976, been influential in having the vast majority of the states change their bylaws to incorporate provisions for a formal mechanism for human rights.

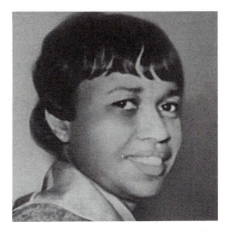

Figure 4–11 Marian Davis Whiteside, Chair, ANA Cabinet on Human Rights, 1980–1982.

In 1977, the Commission on Human Rights honored, with a luncheon in New York, the surviving leaders of NACGN. Present were Mabel K. Staupers, Estelle Osborne, Mabel Northcross, Marguerette Jackson, Alma John, Leota Brown, and Verdelle Bellamy. At the 1978 ANA Convention, the Commission on Human Rights initiated an award to a constituent association or structural unit that had evidenced the most growth in programming and policies reflecting affirmative action efforts and human rights concerns.

Under the jurisdiction of the Cabinet on Human Rights is a Council on Intercultural Nursing, composed of interested members. The Council's purpose is to improve the quality of nursing care by being responsive to cultural and ethnic variances among consumers. One function of the Council is to promote the inclusion of cultural diversity in the curriculum of nursing programs throughout the country.

In 1984, the Council on Intercultural Nursing was renamed the Council on Cultural Diversity in Nursing Practice. Its new purpose—to improve nursing practice based on the inclusion of cultural conditions, values, beliefs, and attitudes of our society, health-care consumers, and practitioners of nursing—takes into account the need to change with our society as the character of that society changes.

At the 1976 convention in Atlantic City, as part of the country's bicentennial celebration, ANA paid tribute to 15 pioneers in nursing and named them as the first members of ANA's Hall of Fame. These women, all deceased, were recognized for their crusades and reforms in health care through the significant contributions they had made in nursing practice, education, service, and research, at least 20 years before the time of selection. Three of the 15 nurses were black: Mary Eliza Mahoney, Martha M. Franklin, and Adah B. Thoms. Mary Mahoney (1845–1926), America's first black professional nurse, was known for her outstanding personal career and her contributions to local and national professional organizations. Martha Franklin (1870–1968) founded the NACGN in 1908 to promote the standards and welfare of black nurses and to break down racial discrimination in the profession. Adah B. Thoms (1879–1943) worked for acceptance of black nurses as members of the American Red Cross and for equal rights in the U.S. Army Nurse Corps. She also wrote the first account of black nurses, *Pathfinders,* published in 1929. For seven years, Thoms was president of NACGN and received the first Mary Mahoney Medal in 1936. Estelle Massey Osborne (1901–1981), another black nurse, was one of the 13 new members inducted into the Hall of Fame at the 1984 ANA convention.

In 1978, for the first time in the history of the ANA, a black nurse, Barbara Nichols (Fig. 4–12), a member of the board of directors for four years, was on the ballot running for president. Nichols ran against two white candidates, Marion Murphy and Laura Simms, and won the election. At the 1980 convention in Houston, Texas, Nichols was elected to a second two-year term. In balloting by the 773-member house of delegates, she received 452 votes; Jean Steel, a white nurse from Boston, who was nominated from the floor, received 282 votes.

During her four years in office as president of ANA (1978–1982), Nichols spent much of her time traveling to represent ANA, addressing hundreds of meetings of state nurses associations, meeting with officials of other health organizations and government officials, traveling to Nairobi, Kenya, and Geneva, Switzerland, for conferences of the International Council of Nurses, and walking the picket line with nurses in Ashtabula, Ohio. In answer to the question by the

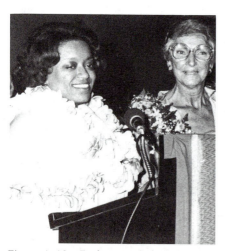

Figure 4–12 Barbara Nichols (left), first black President of ANA and Anne Zimmerman.

American Nurse, "What do you consider to be your greatest achievements as president," Nichols said:

> I consider the following to be developments that I have helped to influence: movement toward baccalaureate education as the basis of professional nursing practice; legitimizing the professional association's right to represent registered nurses for collective bargaining; and strengthening the interaction with the American Hospital Association, the Joint Commission on Accreditation of Hospitals, the American Medical Association, the National Council of State Boards of Nursing, and the Federation of Specialty Nursing Organizations. (ANA Presidency, 1982)

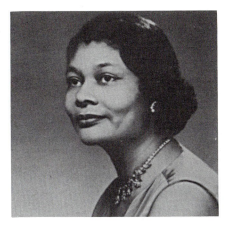

Figure 4–13   Dr. Lillian Harvey, 1982 recipient of Mahoney Award.

In 1986 at the convention, Nichols was the recipient of the ANA Honorary Recognition Award.

At the 1982 ANA convention, presided over by Barbara Nichols, Lillian Harvey (Lincoln School for Nurses, New York; Ed.D., Teachers College, Columbia University, New York; Fig. 4–13). Dean Emerita, Tuskegee University School of Nursing in Alabama, was the 29th recipient of the Mary Mahoney Award. Because her experiences were typical of many of the Mahoney Awardees, presented here is the full text of Lillian Harvey's citation (Dr. Harvey died in October, 1994):

> Her life is a profile of dynamic leadership, an example of service dedicated to advancing opportunities for thousands of black young people to enter nursing and to become successful practitioners. Dr. Harvey arrived in Tuskegee, Alabama, as a young woman in 1944, becoming the first dean of the School of Nursing at Tuskegee University. Upon her arrival at Tuskegee, Lillian met 75 students who were enrolled in a three-year diploma program. While engaging in activities to assure their successful completion of the program in which they were enrolled, she also embarked upon activities necessary for the establishment of the first baccalaureate program in the state of Alabama, which began in 1948.
> Lillian was instrumental in advancing opportunities for black nurses to enter the Army Nurse Corps during World War II. She maintained a program at Tuskegee University that prepared black nurses for military service.

Our Mary Mahoney Award recipient has been an active participant in community and nursing activities at all levels: local, state, and national. She used her talents to work through established organizations for the purpose of contributing to and advancing causes of the nursing profession. She is a former member of the Nursing Advisory Committee of the American National Red Cross and the Kellogg Foundation, and was a member of the Board of Directors of the National League for Nursing. She is a former member of the Board of Directors of the American Journal of Nursing Company and a former secretary of the Educational Administrators, Consultants, and Teachers Section of the American Nurses' Association and of the Alabama Nurses' Association. She has held committee membership in the Alabama State Nurses' Association and in the Alabama League for Nursing.

While it was necessary to work within the segregated system that was mandated by law in the deep South, Lillian worked endlessly toward breaking these barriers and promoting an open system. Some of her efforts may seem diminished because of the passing of time, and changes that have occurred over time. The impact of some of her actions, however, cannot be measured by time. For example, during the early years of her career, she singularly undertook the task of desegregating the Alabama Nurses' Association by attending its meetings. This required an 80-mile round-trip drive from Tuskegee to Montgomery. Although she had to sit in a separate section of the room, she spoke for the needs of black nurses and nursing students without hesitation. It took courage to bear humiliation. Moreover, going into white communities in southern cities was an actual physical threat that most black people chose not to chance.

That the baccalaureate program, which Lillian started in 1948, remains an active, viable, accredited offering that admits students without regard to race, sex, or national origin, is the strongest statement necessary for demonstrating the current and perpetual nature of her work.

Dr. Lillian Harvey is an example of a truly authentic nursing leader who knew how to face and tackle problems no matter how difficult, always maintaining belief in the ability to attain that which countless others would have viewed as unattainable.

Dr. Lillian Harvey is an example for us all. As Phillips Brooks said, if every person were such as you and every life like yours, this earth would be God's paradise. (Summary of Proceedings, 1982, p. 16–17)

Another event that had genuine meaning for black nurses at the 1982 ANA convention was the address by the President of the International Council of Nurses, Eunice Muringo Kiereini, a black nurse from Kenya, East Africa, who had been elected at the 17th quadrennial International Congress of Nursing—the first black to hold that office.

When elected to the presidency of the American Nurses' Association, Barbara Nichols (Massachusetts General Hospital School of Nursing, Boston; M.S., University of Wisconsin-Madison) was director of inservice education for all employees at St. Mary's Hospital, Madison, Wisconsin. Among her many honors, Nichols has had three honorary doctoral degrees bestowed upon her: one from the University of Wisconsin at Milwaukee, one from Rhode Island College, Providence, and one from Lowell University, Massachusetts. She was one of eight women to receive the 1984 Outstanding Women of Color Award, sponsored by the National Institute for Women of Color. Established in 1981, the purpose of the award is "to enhance the strength of diversity and to promote educational and economic equity for women of color." Nichols joins a celebrated group of recipients: Coretta Scott King, the civil rights activist, Connie Chung, television news reporter, and Patricia Roberts Harris, former Secretary, U.S. Department of Health and Human Services.

On July 29, 1984, at its convention in Montreal, Quebec, Canada, the National Medical Association, an organization of black physicians in the United States, presented to Nichols a Scroll of Merit,

> . . . in recognition of her distinguished leadership and service as secretary of the Department of Regulation and Licensure for the State of Wisconsin, and her unique contribution as teacher, nurse, and scholar in the field of health care and human services.

In June 1985, Barbara Nichols was elected ICN North America Area Member of the Board. She had been member-at-large of ICN Board since 1981.

In working toward the objectives set forth in ANA's platform, which would place greater emphasis on legislative activities, in 1951, the association opened the Division of Governmental Affairs office in Washington, DC. Staff are responsible for the review of congressional and state bills affecting nurses, nursing, and health care; preparation and distribution of informative materials on legislation, legislative problems, and the government relations program of ANA; and preparation of congressional testimony reflecting nurses' interests and concerns (Flanagan, 1976). From 1984 to 1986, Retired Brigadier General Hazel Johnson-Brown served as Director of the Washington office.

In 1983, a black nurse, Donna Rae Richardson (Fig. 4–14), who also holds a law degree, was added to the staff of the Washington office as Senior Staff Specialist/Lobbyist. She became Director of Congressional and Agency Relations in 1989 and became Director of Governmental Affairs in

1992. Richardson worked with the Clinton Administration, Congress, and organized nursing on the national campaign for health care reform. During that time, Richardson was appointed to the Montgomery County (MD) Commission for Women by the County Executive. She was elected its president for 1993–1994—the first nurse to serve on the Commission and the first African-American woman to serve as president of the Commission.

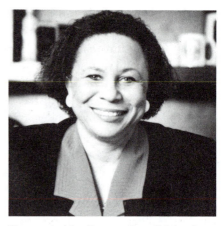

Figure 4–14   Donna Rae Richardson, nurse and lawyer, ANA Senior Staff Specialist/Lobbyist.

Richardson (Akron City Hospital School of Nursing, Akron, Ohio; J.D., Howard University, Washington, DC) represents the ANA's position and policy statements on nursing and health issues to federal agencies, Congress, the executive branch, and constituent forums. She assists in the development and implementation of legislative strategy, prepares ANA testimony and witnesses for public presentations, and acts as liaison with state nurses' associations and regional congressional delegates. Eunice Turner, another black nurse, is senior staff policy analyst for Practice, Economics, and Policy.

In a memorandum to the Executive Director, dated July 12, 1990, Richardson referred to specific initiatives and activities undertaken by the Governmental Affairs Division on issues related to ethics and human rights. Among these were lobbying for the Civil Rights Act Reauthorization (passed in 1989) and Civil Rights Restoration Act (1990); pushing for examination of federal pay classification systems to determine if wage discrimination is based on gender or race; and lobbying for the Minority Health Professions bill which has intended to increase the numbers of minority health professionals as well as access to care for minorities. In addition, ANA participates in a number of coalition activities which support human rights and ethics positions. She also worked with an internal staff task force on the report of the Cultural Diversity Task Force addressed by the House of Delegates in 1994.

In 1973, an ad hoc committee of the ANA Board of Directors met to consider the establishment of a political action arm for ANA. Representatives from states with political action committees served as resources to the Board. As an outcome of the meeting, the ANA Board accepted the following recommendations: (1) that ANA establish a carefully structured nonpartisan political action unit to be voluntary, unincorporated non-profit organization of nurses and others. The committee (PAC) will function in areas of political activity not open to ANA and will be independent but work in a close cooperative relationship with state and local nursing political action units; (2) the Bylaws for the unit would provide for up to 50 percent of the Board of Trustees to be named by the ANA Board of Directors; and (3) the ANA would provide budget to support the political action unit.

The purposes of the Political Action Committee (PAC) are to educate nurses and others on the relevant political issues; assist nurses and others in organizing for effective action in the political arena and in carrying out civic responsibilities; and to raise funds and make contributions to candidates for public office who have demonstrated or indicated supportive positions on the issues of importance to nurses and health care.

In 1986, ANA-PAC became the official name of ANA's political action committee. Currently (1994), two black nurses are serving on its board of trustees: Jean Marshall (NJ) (Fig. 4–15) and Gwendolyn Johnson (DC) (Fig. 4–16), treasurer. Both have served as elected president of their state nurses' associations. In 1992, Marshall was the recipient of the ANA Distinguished Membership Award in recognition of her outstanding leadership, participation in, and contributions to the American Nurses' Association.

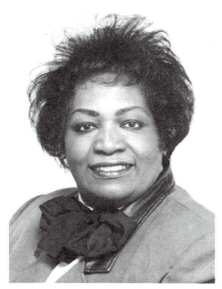

Figure 4–15 Jean Marshall, Board of Trustees, Political Action Committee.

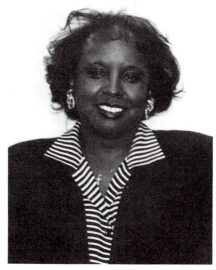

Figure 4–16 Gwendolyn Johnson, Treasurer, Political Action Committee.

Because so many national nursing organizations had developed since the major ones were restructured in 1952, the American Nurses' Association deemed it timely to reexamine organizational arrangements. To that end, in 1982, ANA appointed the Commission on Organizational Assessment and Renewal (COAR). The goal of COAR was to strengthen ANA on behalf of its members, the nursing profession, and the American people through study of its structure, function, membership base, and interorganizational relationships.

The Commission proposed a number of recommendations, which resulted in the disbanding of ANA cabinets, including the Cabinet on Human Rights, called for the strands of ethics, human rights, nursing education, and nursing research to be recognized as part of the work of all ANA units.

The House further directed that the Board appoint an ad hoc committee to determine what mechanism should be developed to address human rights and ethics issues. The committee, chaired by Dr. Beverly Malone (Fig. 4–17), proposed that a Center for Ethics and Human Rights be established. The proposal was adopted by the Board in December of 1989 and a program director was appointed in 1990, charged with the responsibility of insuring that ethics and human rights are considered in all activities of ANA, including its strategic plan, its labor relations, governmental and practice programs. The center makes ANA's efforts and resources more available to nurses across the country. At its April 1991 meeting, the ANA Board of Directors appointed an Advisory Board to the Center for Ethics and Human Rights, which held its first meeting September of that year. Three of the seven members were black: Dr. Cynthia Capers (Pennsylvania), Gwendolyn Johnson (District of Columbia), and Karen D. Bankston (Ohio).

The 1982 ANA bylaws revision created the Nursing Organization Liaison Forum (NOLF) in an attempt to permit ANA to collaborate with representatives from the growing number of other national nursing organizations—general and specialty. In its operating guidelines adopted by ANA

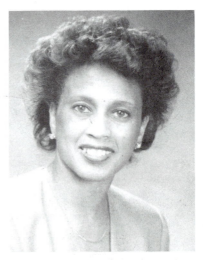

Figure 4–17 Dr. Beverly Malone, ANA Board and Chair, Committee on the proposed Center for Ethics and Human Rights.

Board of Directors in 1984, NOLF has two purposes: (1) to provide within the formal structure of ANA a forum for discussion between national nursing organizations and ANA regarding questions of professional policy and national health policy issues of mutual concern; and (2) to promote concerted action by national nursing organizations on professional policy and national health policy issues, as participating organizations deem appropriate (*The Evolution of Nursing Professional Organizations,* 1987). In 1987, NOLF listed 41 participating organizations of which two were black: Chi Eta Phi Sorority and the National Black Nurses' Association. When the Association of Black Nursing Faculty in Higher Education was organized, it, too, became a member of NOLF. The forum then included 47 national nursing organizations and 12 ANA Councils.

On May 10, 1994, in celebration of National Nurses Week, ANA and the American Organization of Nurse Executives paid tribute in Washington, DC to the nurses in Congress and the Executive Branch, including President Clinton who addressed the group. Among those honored was the Honorable Eddie Bernice Johnson (Diploma, St. Mary's College of the University of Notre Dame; MPA, Southern Methodist University, Dallas, Texas) (Fig. 4–18), a black from Texas who is the first nurse to be elected to the U.S. Congress. Before going to the House of Representatives, she had been a State Senator in Texas.

As has been pointed out, blacks have had representation on the board

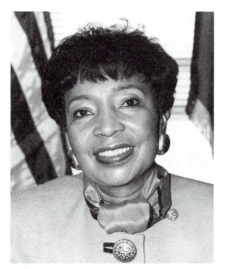

Figure 4–18 The Honorable Eddie Bernice Johnson, first nurse to be elected to U.S. Congress, 1992.

and staff of ANA since 1948, but not consecutively on the board until 1970. From 1978 to 1982, there was an elected black president, and today, 1994, there are elected and appointed black officials, such as Carrie Houser James, President of South Carolina Nurses Association, who was elected chair of ANA Constituent Assembly of Presidents of State Nurses Associations. Blacks are also represented on ANA's professional staff.

ANA is the only full-service professional organization representing the nation's 2,239,816 registered nurses through its 53 constituent associations. ANA advances the nursing profession by fostering high standards of nursing practice, promoting economic and general welfare of nurses in the workplace, projecting a positive and realistic view of nursing, and lobbying the Congress and regulatory agencies on health care issues affecting nurses and the public. ANA-affiliated organizations include the American Nurses Foundation, the American Academy of Nursing, and the American Nurses Credentialing Center.

Since 1948, when the first black nurse, Estelle Massey Osborne, was elected to the board of directors, a few other black nurses have served on the board, including Fay Wilson, Ethelrine Shaw-Nickerson, Barbara Nichols (who later became president), Juanita Fleming, Beverly Malone, Gwendolyn Johnson, and Mary Long. Elected to the ANA Board of Directors at the 1994 ANA convention in San Antonio, Texas, was Verlia Brown (New York). Also at the convention, four black nurses were recipients of awards: Dorothy Ramsey, Bernardine Lacey, Juanita Fleming, and Jessie M. Colin. Ramsey (Diploma, Jewish Hospital and Medical Center School of Nursing, Brooklyn, NY; Ed.D., Teachers College, Columbia University, NY) (Fig. 4–19), professor at Adelphi University, Garden City, NY, received the Mary Mahoney Award. Dr. Ramsey, an advocate for nursing, has spent a lifetime promoting mentoring programs that include recruiting students of color, retaining them through graduation, and assisting to assure their success in the professional arena. (See Appendix C for past Mary Mahoney Award recipients.)

Lacey (Diploma, Mississippi Baptist Hospital School of Nursing, Jackson; Ed.D., Teachers College, Columbia University, NY) (Fig. 4–20), received the Pearl McIver Award for her work with the homeless and the establishment of health services for the homeless in Washington, DC.

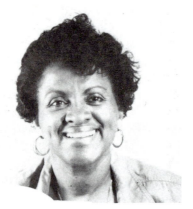

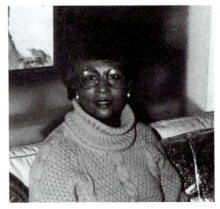

Figure 4–19 Dr. Dorothy Ramsey, 1994 Mahoney Medal recipient.

Figure 4–20 Dr. Bernardine Lacey, 1994 recipient, McIver Award.

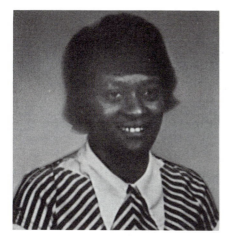

Figure 4–21 Dr. Juanita Fleming, 1994 recipient, Distinguished Membership Award.

Fleming, (B.S., Hampton University School of Nursing, Hampton, VA; Ph.D. Catholic University of America, Washington, DC) (Fig. 4–21), professor and special assistant to the President for Academic Affairs at the University of Kentucky, Lexington, was chosen to be the recipient of the ANA Distinguished Membership Award in recognition of her professional association involvement and her commitment to the improvement and availability of the health care services for the people. Dr. Fleming serves on a number of federal, state, and civic organizations. In 1992, Jean Marshall (NJ) received this award.

Colin, received the Shirley Titus Award in recognition of her contributions to the economic and general welfare program.

INTERNATIONAL COUNCIL OF NURSES

In January, 1899, the International Council of Women held its meeting in London. At the suggestion of one of its members, Ethel Bedford Fenwick, a British nurse, the Council held a one-day program on trained nursing. At this meeting, Fenwick, editor of the *British Journal of Nursing,* conceived the idea for developing an international organization of professional nurses which would be a nongovernmental, voluntary federation of national nurses associations. The next month, after the meeting of the International Council of Women adjourned, Fenwick proposed her idea at a meeting of the Matron's Council of Great Britain and Ireland to which nurses from several other countries attended as invited guests. The idea was accepted and a committee was appointed to work out an organizational plan (Bridges, 1967). This was to become the first international organization in the health field.

Although the date of the founding of the International Council of Nurses (ICN) is recorded in the history books as 1899, the organization was not officially organized until the provisional committee, representing nine countries, met in London in 1900 and adopted a constitution. Ethel

Fenwick of England was elected president; Mary Agnes Snively of Canada, treasurer; and Lavinia Dock of the United States, secretary. Congresses were planned for the participation of individual members from the member associations. The first executive meeting and Congress was held in Buffalo, New York in 1901; the next in Berlin, Germany in 1904. By 1910, ten national organizations were members.

The preamble to the original constitution of the International Council of Nurses stated the purpose of the council as follows: "We, nurses of all nations, sincerely believing that the best good of one profession will be advanced by greater unity of thought, sympathy, and purpose, do hereby band ourselves in a confederation of workers to further the efficient care of the sick, and to secure the honor and the interests of the Nursing Profession" (Breay & Fenwick, 1931). Article 2 of the current constitution states that "The ICN is a federation of national nurses' associations . . . and has functions unrestricted by consideration of nationality, race, creed, color, politics, gender, life style, or social station" (ICN Constitution, 1993).

ICN has a council of national representatives, a board of directors, one standing committee on professional services, expert panels, and a secretariat. Its member organizations number 111 and represent over 1.3 million nurses from all over the world, including those from more than 30 African and Caribbean countries.

According to the criteria for membership, "Within a country, one national nurses' association or federation of nurses, or where neither of these exists, a separate nurses section or chapter of a national association composed of other health workers, may become a member of ICN provided that: its constitution, regulations or rules define objectives which are not in conflict with Article 2 (see above)." Its purpose must be in harmony with ICN's stated purpose: to provide a medium through which national nurses' associations share their common interests working together to develop the contribution of nursing to the promotion of the health of all people and the care of the sick. The association must be controlled by nurses, gaining its authority from its members and speak on nursing matters and it is the most representative of nurses in the country. The term, "nurse," is defined by ICN, for membership purposes only, as "a person who has completed a program of basic nursing education and is qualified and authorized in her/his country to practice nursing" (ICN Constitution, 1993).

The activities of ICN are carried out from headquarters, located in Geneva, Switzerland. Every two years, the Council of National Representatives meet, and every four years ICN holds a Congress in a different country for international communication and fellowship. These are mostly program sessions with a general theme and there are simultaneous translations of speeches in English, French, and Spanish. Attendance at the last Congress held in Madrid, Spain, 1993 was about 8,000 persons from 90 nations. The Congress is complex blend of pomp and circumstance, international nursing business and politics, and provides many educational opportunities.

In 1978, ICN heeded the call of the World Health Organization to strive for "Health for All by the Year 2000." Since then ICN has been dedicated to the primary health care approach, and to helping nurses act out their new roles. Programs have been undertaken to assist in shifting the emphasis in education and to show the national nursing associations how to change national regulations to allow nurses to fulfill their expanded responsibilities (Kim, 1993).

In 1988, the Carnegie Corporation of New York granted $200,000 to ICN to help fund its "Regulation of Nursing" project in 10 African countries that were members or former members of the British Commonwealth. It was a three-year project to help nurses develop policies to regulate education and practice that will raise nursing effectiveness in primary health care, particularly in maternal and child health services. ICN introduced the project at an invitational workshop in Lusaka, Zambia, July 4–9, 1988.

Also in 1988, the ICN/Florence Nightingale International Foundation and the W.K. Kellogg Foundation held the first workshop to implement "The Regulation of Nurses" in Tobago with 28 participants from 14 countries, including Belize, Guyana, Lesotho, Botswana, Swaziland, and Zimbabwe.

In 1993, the International Council of Nurses Foundation (ICNF) received a $186,210 grant from the W.K. Kellogg Foundation to fund a project to improve nurses' contribution to primary health care practice through development of an international classification for nursing practice standards of quality and uniform data sets. According to the Chief Executive Officer of ICN, "the international classification for nursing practice will enhance more cost-effective delivery of quality nursing care and such a system will provide nursing with a common language that can be used across borders to describe and organize nursing data and thus provide nursing with a tool for use in practice, planning and management, policy development, teaching, and research" (ICNF Receives Funding, 1994).

Whereas ICN has had black nurses on its committees, board, council of national representatives, and staff, it was not until the quadrennium 1981–1985 that a black nurse from Kenya, East Africa, Eunice Muringo Kiereini, served as president (Fig. 4–22). In this quadrennium (1993–1997), the following black nurses are serving in elected positions: Yvonne Pilgrin (Trinidad & Tobago) is a member at large of the ICN Board; Sererā S.

Kupé (Botswana) and Eleane I. Hunte (Barbados) are area members of the Board. Dr. Kupé is serving a third term on the board, having been first elected in 1981 and again in 1989.

In 1994, Gebrehiwet Tesfami-cael, (B.S.N., University of Indi-ana, U.S.A.; Ph.D., University of Southampton, United Kingdom), a native of Eritrea, which had been a part of Ethiopia, joined the staff of ICN as nurse consultant. Equipped with a master's degree in commu-nity health from Liverpool Univer-sity School of Tropical Medicine

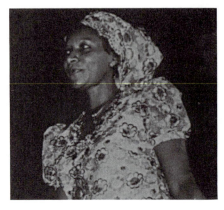

Figure 4–22   Eunice Muringo Kierini of Kenya, East Africa, President of Inter-national Council of Nurses, 1981–1985. (Courtesy ANA)

and a doctorate in health education and health promotion from the Uni-versity of Southhampton U.K., his main areas of responsibility include primary health care, community health, substance abuse, and HIV/AIDS.

ICN has been awarding competitive fellowships for post-basic, bac-calaureate, master's, and doctoral study to members of its national associ-ations since 1970. Established at ICN's 14th quadrennial Congress in Montreal, Canada in 1969 and supported by the Minnesota Mining and Manufacturing Company (3M), the fellowship competition has attracted hundreds of nominees (Marshall-Burnett, 1985). Among the recipients of the ICN/3M fellowships have been 16 nurses from Black African and Caribbean countries: Trinidad and Tobago—1 (Fig. 4–23); Tanzania—1; Nigeria—1; Jamaica—3; St. Lucia—1; Botswana—2; Sierra Leone—1; Ethiopia—1; Ghana—3; Uganda—1; and Barbados—1. The award carries a monetary amount of $9,000 and the recipients attend the university of their choice.

In 1995, ICN will have completed a four-year historical project, an in-vestigation of the impact of organized nursing as countries around the world became industrialized, nationalized,

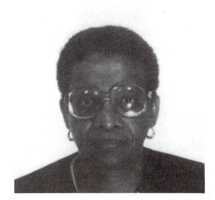

Figure 4–23   Dr. Jean Grayson of Trinidad & Tobago, first recipient of ICN/3M fellowship, 1989. (Courtesy ICN)

and radically reorganized through war and changing political and economic alignments. The role of ICN will have been examined from its founding and interrelated to the historical and international context in which it has operated through the years. Represented on the project consultant team, along with its director, Joan Lynaugh from the United States, is Dorothy Namate, a black nurse from Malawi, who is currently pursuing a doctoral degree at the University of Pennsylvania, Philadelphia (*The Thalamus,* 1993).

Black English-speaking Caribbean countries that have or have had membership in ICN are highlighted in Chapter 7; African countries in Chapter 8.

AMERICAN JOURNAL OF NURSING COMPANY

Upon the suggestion in 1895 of the American Society of Superintendents of Training Schools for Nurses that nurses needed a journal "managed, edited, and owned by the women of the profession," the Nurses' Associated Alumnae (forerunner of ANA) appointed a Committee on Periodicals, led by Mary E. P. Davis. The committee formed a joint stock company and sold shares to nurses only at $100 each. With this capital, plus 550 subscriptions pledged at $2 each, the nursing profession in 1900 launched its own magazine titled the *American Journal of Nursing* (Fondiller, 1990).

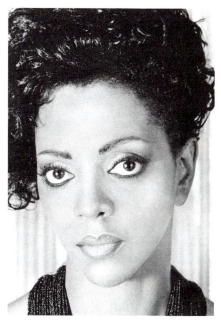

The Company conducts its business under the direction of a board of directors, but since ANA is the sole stockholder of the Company, the Journal Company board members are elected by the ANA Board of Directors. Since 1951, black nurses have been represented on the *American Journal of Nursing* Board of Directors, with Estelle M. Osborne being the first. Dr. Ora Strickland (Fig. 4–24), was on the board from 1980–1988, serving as chairperson from 1984 to 1986—two terms.

Figure 4–24   Dr. Ora Strickland, AJN Co. Board of Directors, 1980–1988.

Until 1952, the *American Journal of Nursing* was the Company's only publication, serving as the official organ of ANA and the National League of Nursing Education. Although there had been a few other magazines for nurses, e.g., *The Nightingale* and *Trained Nurse and Hospital Review,* the *Journal* was the first official professional nursing journal established in the United States.

In 1952, at the request of the Association of Collegiate Schools of Nursing, the Journal Company began publishing its second magazine, *Nursing Research,* devoted exclusively to research reporting in nursing. From 1953 to 1980, when the National League for Nursing (NLN) started publishing its own

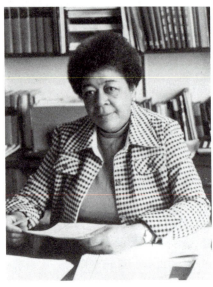

Figure 4–25 Dr. Mary Elizabeth Carnegie, Chief Editor, *Nursing Research,* 1973–1978.

journal, *Nursing and Health Care, Nursing Outlook* had been published by the Company as the official organ of NLN. In 1966, the company began publishing the *International Nursing Index; MCN, the Journal of Maternal Child Nursing* in 1975; *Geriatric Nursing* in 1980; and the *AJN Guide.* The Company also produces multimedia materials (books, other printed matter, audiocassettes, filmstrips, videocassettes, and films) through its Educational Services Division. In addition, the Company manages seminars, holds national professional conferences, and conducts other communications activities.

In July, 1953, Mary Elizabeth Carnegie was the first black nurse to join the American Journal of Nursing Company as Assistant Editor of the *American Journal of Nursing.* She moved to *Nursing Outlook* in 1956 as Associate Editor. In 1970, she became Senior Editor of *Nursing Outlook,* and in 1973, equipped with a doctoral degree, she was made Chief Editor of *Nursing Research* (Fig. 4–25), the position she held until her retirement from the American Journal of Nursing Company in 1978. At that time, the board, in the form of a resolution, commended her "for her illustrious record and meritorius service in the editing of its publications," and expressed "its gratitude . . . for her quarter of a century of contributions and accomplishments."

THE NATIONAL ASSOCIATION OF COLORED GRADUATE NURSES

Until the structure of the ANA changed in 1916, setting up the state association as the basic unit of membership, black nurses who were members of their nursing school alumnae associations could join ANA, and many of them did. Little was done to encourage their participation, however, nor was any concern shown for their special problems of segregation and discrimination (Staupers, 1961).

Scattered throughout the country, black nurses had little or no medium through which they might keep abreast of developments in nursing in general and little opportunity for useful action to advance the standards of nursing among black nurses. There was a unity of desire on the part of black nurses to organize, however, and, as a result, local groups began to form as early as 1900 in cities such as Norfolk, Washington, New York, and Chicago. It was not until 1908 that the first group of black graduate nurses came together for the purpose of considering plans for organizing a permanent national association to help improve their conditions. The title selected was the National Association of Colored Graduate Nurses (NACGN). (See Appendix B for a list of the NACGN Charter Members.)

The guiding light in the movement toward a national organization was

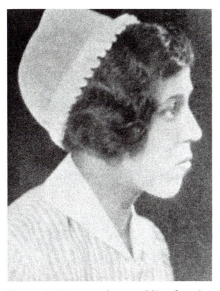

Martha M. Franklin (1870–1968) (Fig. 4–26) of Connecticut, a graduate of Women's Hospital in Philadelphia in 1897, the only black in her class. Because of her concern for the welfare of black nurses, she zealously studied their status as graduate nurses in America by writing hundreds of letters in her own hand to black nurses, superintendents of nursing schools, and nursing organizations. The survey took two years to complete. Finally, in 1908, she mailed 1,500 letters at her own expense to all the black nurses with whom she had been in contact, polling them on the advisability of a national gathering. Franklin, one of the first to campaign actively for racial equality in

Figure 4–26   Martha Franklin, founder, National Association of Colored Graduate Nurses, 1908.

nursing, was the catalyst for collective action by black nurses. Not only did she recognize that black nurses needed help to improve their professional status, but that they would have to initiate it themselves.

At the invitation of the Alumnae Association of Lincoln School for Nurses in New York City, under the leadership of Adah B. Thoms, 52 nurses attended the organizing 3-day meeting, which began on August 23, 1908, at St. Mark Methodist Church. They heard a statesmanlike report from Franklin, in which she outlined the manifold need for a national organization of their own. After much discussion, the group adopted the following purposes for the new organization: (1) to achieve higher professional standards; (2) to break down the discriminatory practices facing blacks in schools of nursing, in jobs, and in nursing organizations; and (3) to develop leadership among black nurses. By organizing, these women proclaimed to the entire profession that they had created an instrument through which they could oppose discrimination in the nursing field on all fronts. Franklin, the founder of the NACGN, was elected president and served two terms.

Lavinia Dock, nursing's premier historian and Lillian Wald, founder of the Henry Street Settlement House—both social activists, supported the formation of NACGN and hosted a reception at Henry Street for this new organization (Staupers, 1961). Dock went on record with her support, saying, "Negro nurses are held among the most valuable members, not only for good nursing, but for intelligent altruism" (Dock, 1912, p. 198).

Franklin seldom missed a national meeting of NACGN. Her last attendance was at the convention in Washington, DC, in 1921. Those attending were received at the White House by President Warren G. Harding. The membership presented the President and his wife with a large basket of American beauty roses and requested that NACGN be placed on record as an organization of 2,000 trained nurses ready for world service when needed.

In the early days of NACGN's existence, the work of the organization, which served as an instrument for the advancement of the black nurse, was done by volunteer members. Among the projects of these volunteers was a central registry, begun in 1918 and operating out of New York, to serve black nurses in every area of work and in every section of the country. This was an important program because at that time private and official registries, which had sprung up all over the United States, seldom accepted black registrants.

Along with the registry program, a campaign was instituted to focus attention on better opportunities for black nurses in leadership positions in hospitals, schools of nursing, and public health agencies. NACGN was not only concerned with the plight of the black nurse, but with the general improvement of conditions of all blacks. To this end, NACGN worked with other civic organizations, including those that focused on civil rights. Because of her experience in a number of professional and community organizations and because of the knowledge of the many facets of nursing, Mabel C. Northcross (Fig. 4–27) of St. Louis, Missouri, was elected president of the NACGN in 1930 and served four years. During her administration, she was responsible for several innovations, the most impor-

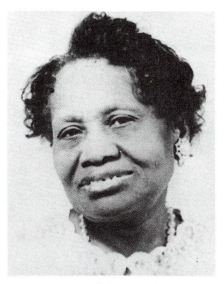

Figure 4–27   Mabel C. Northcross, President, NACGN, 1930–1934.

tant of which was the conduct of educational programs, called institutes, held during the national conventions as a form of postgraduate education to help increase the level of skills, knowledge, and job potential of members. The first institute was held during the national convention in 1932. Northcross was ahead of her time in terms of continuing education, a vital part of most conventions and meetings today.

To meet the continuing-education needs of black nurses, beginning in 1934 under the presidency of Estelle Massey Riddle Osborne and with the support of a grant from the General Education Board of the Rockefeller Foundation, NACGN instituted regional conferences as a vehicle through which black nurses could keep abreast of developments in the nursing profession. Participants in the first regional conference, held in New York City, included the executive secretaries of the three major national nursing organizations—the ANA, the National League of Nursing Education, and the National Organization for Public Health Nursing; officials of the Rosenwald Fund, the National Medical Association, and the National Health Circle for Colored People; directors of schools of nursing for black students; and the black press. At the time of this conference, America was feeling the effects of the Great Depression. There was great need for a program that would bring into clear focus the fact that black nurses not only needed jobs, but that these needs were aggravated by racial bias (Staupers, 1951).

The many projects, educational programs, consultation services, and day-to-day business of operating a national organization made it mandatory that NACGN establish headquarters with a paid staff. In 1934, through the generosity of the National Health Circle for Colored People, office space was shared and Mabel K. Staupers was employed as executive secretary—a position she held for 12 years. In 1936 with grants from the General Education Board and the Rosenwald Fund, NACGN acquired its own permanent office located in the same building with the three major national nursing organizations. As executive secretary, Staupers was responsible for collecting facts, advising the black nurse and translating her to the community, holding conferences, organizing state and local nursing associations, as well as strengthening those already in existence, and working closely with the national advisory council, biracial in composition, which was organized in 1938 as a means of developing greater interest in and support for the programs of NACGN. In short, the executive had the tremendous responsibility for developing greater unity in order to combat the policies and practices that were hampering the professional development of black nurses. Staupers was truly the ombudsman for the black nurse.

The year 1936 was also the year that NACGN established the annual Mary Mahoney Award in recognition of individual achievement in nursing, presenting it to Adah B. Thoms (Fig. 4–28), past president of NACGN and author of the first account of black nurses, *Pathfinders*. She was also recognized for her active single-handed campaign during 1917 and 1918 in opposing discrimination in the military against black nurses.

Another program of NACGN was to work for progressive health legislation, making its voice heard and its influence felt regarding health and nursing legislation, as well as other progressive legislation that would benefit all Americans. A major feat was NACGN's joining with other organizations to support the amendment to the Bolton Bill of 1943 for the creation of the Cadet Nurse Corps during World War II. This amendment ensured for students in black schools the privilege of joining the Corps. By the end of the war, over

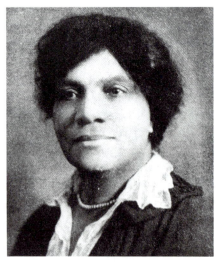

Figure 4–28   Adah B. Thoms, first recipient of Mary Mahoney Award, 1936.

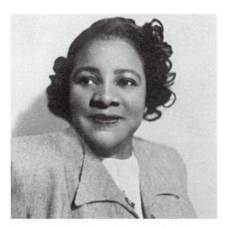

Figure 4–29   Alma Vessells John, Executive Director, NACGN, 1946–1951.

3,000 black students had participated in the Cadet Nurse Corps.

At the time of Pearl Harbor in 1941, NACGN was in the midst of leading a vigorous campaign to break down racial barriers in the Army and Navy. In 1941, the Army established a quota of 56 black nurses, and the Navy had flatly refused to admit them. Through the efforts of NACGN, the Army quota was abolished before the end of the war, and the Navy dropped its color bar in January, 1945. By the end of the war, over 500 black nurses had served in the Army and four in the Navy. NACGN's campaign, led by Mabel Staupers, stimulated wide public interest and support because discrimination was costing the lives of American fighting men (Staupers, 1951).

In 1946, for health reasons, Staupers (1890–1989) resigned as executive secretary of NACGN and Alma Vessells John (Fig. 4–29) was appointed to fill this position which she held until NACGN dissolved in 1951. John, a graduate of Harlem Hospital School of Nursing in New York with a bachelor's degree from New York University, had, since 1943, served on the staff of the National Nursing Council for War Service as assistant consultant. She brought to her position with NACGN firsthand knowledge of the problems of the black nurse in this country. She had worked closely with the consultant, Estelle Massey Osborne, to help integrate blacks into schools of nursing, as well as into the military nursing services. John died in New York in 1986.

Of all battles waged by NACGN, whose quest was to place the black nurse into the mainstream of professional nursing in America, the longest and hardest was with the ANA, the professional organization which nurses joined through their states. When the barriers were finally removed, the NACGN, at convention in Louisville, Kentucky in 1949, under the presidency of Alida Dailey (Fig. 4–30), voted itself out of existence. By that time, provisions had been made for black nurses to bypass those southern states that denied them membership and join the ANA directly as individual members.

At the 1949 convention, Staupers, who had been executive secretary from 1934 to 1946, agreed to serve as president of NACGN until the organization legally dissolved in 1951. The forward steps that had been made during NACGN's lifetime are not as important in themselves as in the development of capable leadership, broadened understanding on both sides, and determination to accept nothing less than full and equal opportunity for all nurses (Staupers, 1951).

On January 26, 1951, approximately 1,000 persons, including members of the boards of the three major national nursing organizations, representatives from government and private agencies, and many distinguished citizens, assembled at the Essex House in New York for the formal dissolution of NACGN, which had purposefully and successfully worked itself out of

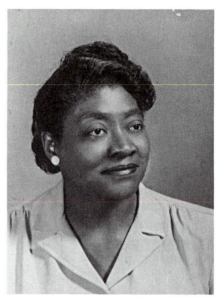

Figure 4–30 Alida Dailey, President of NACGN when vote was taken to dissolve the organization.

existence. This occasion was also used to present certificates of honor to 11 individuals and 21 organizations who had worked with and for black nurses.

As keynote speaker at the dinner, the Honorable Judge William H. Hastie, former Governor of the United States Virgin Islands and Judge of the First District Federal Court, said:

> The passing of an organization can be only somewhat less sad than the death of a human being, but in this case I rejoice, as I believe all of the guests here tonight do, that a splendid organization has accomplished its mission and then deliberately determined to release its membership to continue work under more comprehensive auspices. It is a grand thing that there is no longer need for a separate organization of Negro nurses . . . To me the meaning of this far transcends the nursing profession, its organization, and its internal policies. It points up something of great consequences which is happening to American life as well as the reaction of the Negro to the change . . . I can think of no incident which symbolizes the dynamics of constructive social evolution at its best more effectively or more dramatically than this gathering and its occasion.

Writing in a column in the *Chicago Defender,* after attending the testimonial dinner, Walter White, then executive secretary of the National Association for the Advancement of Colored People (NAACP), said:

> For the first time in my life I have enjoyed a funeral, instead of being lugubrious the obituaries were gay and congratulatory. The quite lively corpse handed out thank you scrolls to individuals and organizations which had held and cooperated with the late departed. Stripping off its sable shroud, the corpse promptly marched into a new life of greater usefulness . . . [through amalgamation with the American Nurses' Association].

While happy about the progress NACGN had made from 1908 to 1951, the nurse leaders in the movement for integration reflected seriously on the challenges still to be faced. They recognized that, although black nurses had taken a giant step forward in the fight for equality, there was still much that remained to be done. In presenting certificates of honor at the testimonial dinner, NACGN's past president, Estelle M. Osborne, had this to say:

> There are still the problems of segregated and inadequately supported nursing schools for Negroes, salary differentials on a racial basis, inequalities in job opportunity and advancement, racial inequalities in preliminary education, and frequently there is merely token or no representation of Negro nurses in the policy-making areas at the higher levels of participation. These and other problems constitute a considerable amount of unfinished business of democracy, as well as the unfinished business of NACGN. These problems [with dissolution of NACGN] automatically become a part of the unfinished business of the entire nursing profession.

So, 1951 marked the end of one era in the fight for equality for all nurses and the beginning of another. That is, to the public, it was the formal recognition of a giant step taken by the nursing profession to prove that its democratic principles are real and workable.

Because of her devotion to the nursing profession and to the advancement of black nurses, Mabel Staupers received many honors, none more deserved than the Mary Mahoney Award presented to her in 1947. Other awards have been the prestigious Spingarn Medal, black America's highest honor, from the National Association for the Advancement of Colored People for leadership in the movement to integrate black nurses as equals in the national professional nursing organization in 1951 (Fig. 4–31) (The

Spingarn Medal was established in 1914 by the late Joel E. Spingarn, chair, NAACP Board of Directors, to call attention to distinguished merit and achievement by Americans of African descent, and with that recognition to stimulate black youth to similar aspiration.); the Sojourner Truth Award, 1947; the National Urban League Team Work Award; the John V. Lindsay Citation, 1967, presented by the Mayor of New York City to an immigrant (Staupers was born in Barbados, British West Indies) who had become an outstanding American Citizen and leader; the Medgar Evers Human Rights Award, 1965; Howard University Alumni Award for distinguished achievement in the fields of nursing and community service, 1970; Caribbean American Intercultural Organization for outstanding contributions

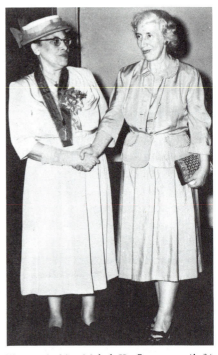

Figure 4–31   Mabel K. **Staupers** (left) presented NAACP Spingarn Medal by Lillian Smith, 1951.

to the field of nursing and civil rights, 1972; the Linda Richards Award for unique and pioneering contributions to nursing, given by the National League for Nursing, 1973.

In 1972, Staupers was invited to the ANA convention in Detroit to attend a reception given by ANA for Mary Mahoney Medal awardees. She declined the invitation because, as she explained, "The ANA has not completely acted upon the Resolution accepted from the NACGN in 1951 and therefore, I cannot in good conscience accept recognition from the ANA. The Board of Directors has not given full attention to the problem of minority nurses, but rather has shown mere tokenism" (Bourne, 1989, p. 37).

AMERICAN RED CROSS NURSING SERVICE

Aware of Florence Nightingale's work in the Crimea, Henri Dunant, a native of Switzerland, used his influence to establish national societies that would render aid to all combatants in time of war. Beginning in 1864,

National Red Cross societies were organized, but it was not until 1882 that one appeared in the United States (Jamieson & Sewall, 1944).

Upon her return from service with the Red Cross Society in Germany in the Franco-Prussian war of 1870, Clara Barton was determined to win her country's approval of this new type of neutral society. In 1882, the American Red Cross Society was founded, and Miss Barton became its first president, serving in this capacity until 1905 (Jamieson & Sewall, 1944).

Public health nursing was first proposed as a Red Cross program by Lillian Wald as early as 1908, and the American Red Cross Nursing Service was established in 1909, created by Jane Delano. The public health nursing component was financed mainly by Jacob H. Schiff, an officer of the New York branch of the Red Cross. Because the number of nurses employed was inadequate to meet the needs of the country, in 1912 the Red Cross organized its rural nursing service, known as the American Red Cross Town and Country Nursing Service. This was the first plan of a nationwide scope to supply trained nurses to rural districts. By 1913, the service was extended to towns having populations as large as 25,000. After 1918, the service was known as the American Red Cross Public Health Nursing Service.

Frances Reed Elliott Davis (Fig. 4–32), a graduate of Freedmen's Hospital School of Nursing in Washington, DC, was the first black nurse to be accepted in the American Red Cross Nursing Service in 1918. Her pin read "1-A"—"A" designating "Negro." Before being accepted by the Red Cross, Elliott was required to take a year's course at Teachers College, Columbia University, in New York. She was the first black nurse to take the course, which included conferences each week with Adelaide Nutting, the head of the Nursing Department. Elliott's practice work was at the Henry Street Visiting Nursing Service and the New York Board of Charities. Upon completing the course, she was assigned to work in Jackson, Tennessee, which had requested a black Red Cross nurse.

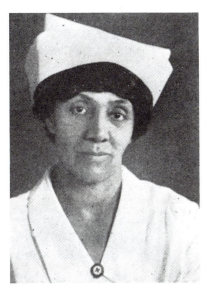

Figure 4–32 Frances Reed Elliott Davis, first black accepted by American Red Cross Nursing Service, 1918.

Sixty-four years after Davis received her Red Cross pin, Irmatrude

Grant (Fig. 4–33), a black nurse who had become chairperson of recruitment and enrollment, Nursing and Health Services, American Red Cross in greater New York, received the Ann Magnussen Award, the highest recognition given for outstanding volunteer nursing leadership in the American Red Cross. The award was made at the 1982 National Convention of the Red Cross in St. Louis, Missouri, and presented by Dr. Jerome Holland, a black man and former U.S. Ambassador to Sweden, who was National Chairman.

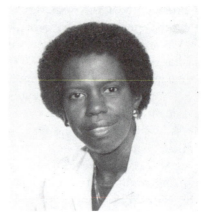

Figure 4–33   Irmatrude Grant, recipient of American Red Cross Ann Magnussen Award, 1982.

NATIONAL ORGANIZATION FOR PUBLIC HEALTH NURSING

By the turn of the century, public health nursing had been identified as a separate field, and the nurses in this specialty felt the need to form an organization that would meet their needs. As a result, in 1911, a joint committee was appointed by the ANA and the American Society of Superintendents of Training Schools for Nurses for the purpose of standardizing nurses' services outside the hospital. Lillian Wald, who had established the public health nursing service and the Henry Street Settlement to meet the needs of the poor in New York City's lower East Side, mostly immigrants whose port of entry to the United States was Ellis Island, New York, was appointed chairperson. In June 1912, at the meeting of the two established nursing organizations in Chicago, with invited representatives from 800 public health agencies, the National Organization for Public Health Nursing (NOPHN) was voted into existence with Lillian Wald as president.

Wald had also been one of the moving spirits in the establishment of the National Association for the Advancement of Colored People, which was formed to press for full citizenship rights for blacks and public understanding of their contribution to America's stability and progress. She was one of the "Committee of Forty" who in 1909 signed the call to conference on the hundredth anniversary of Abraham Lincoln's birthday the driving force in the establishment of NAACP several months later. On the eve of the conference, Wald hosted a reception for the group at her Henry Street Settlement House (Hughes, 1962).

As an association of nurses, laypersons, and education and service agencies, NOPHN grew out of a pressing need to provide a mechanism through which standards could be developed for public health nursing services operating under voluntary auspices with direction of lay boards (Fitzpatrick, 1975). During its lifetime of 40 years (it became part of National League for Nursing in 1952), black nurses were involved. Unlike the ANA, NOPHN was not confronted with any significant difficulties regarding membership of blacks. Members joined the national body directly, while members joined ANA through their state associations. NOPHN accepted black members if they met the usual eligibility requirements. Its purposes were to stimulate the general public and the visiting nurse associations to the extension and support of public health nursing service, to facilitate harmonious cooperation among the workers and supporters, to develop a standard of ethics and teaching, and also to act as a clearing house for information for those interested in such work.

After the Gage and Haupt survey of Black schools in the South, made under the auspices of NOPHN in 1932 (see Chapter 2), NOPHN became concerned about the poor quality of education for blacks in these southern schools, many of which made no provisions for public health nursing theory or practice in the curriculum, thus prohibiting their graduates' acceptance as nurse members of the organization. To help remedy this situation, NOPHN awarded public health nursing scholarships to black nurses. In addition, NOPHN members participated in conferences held to discuss the health of blacks, making the services of its Education Committee available for advice and consultation to black schools of nursing. After the Gage and Haupt tour, Estelle Riddle Osborne and Mabel Staupers were invited to join two important NOPHN committees. Osborne represented NACGN on the Education Committee and Staupers represented NACGN on the Committee on Organization and Administration.

Along with ANA and NLNE in 1940, NOPHN was represented on a special joint committee to work with the NACGN. An additional mechanism to work with black nurses was NOPHN's establishment of a Council on Negro Nursing to study the education and development of the black public health nurse. Its objective was to foster and enhance the complete integration of the Negro nurse in all phases of public health nursing so that they would receive all benefits and emoluments based on the effort and programs achieved in their work (Report of NOPHN Council on Negro Nursing, 1942).

The problems faced by black nurses continued to be of vital interest and concern to NOPHN, and it, probably more than any other nursing organization, took action to support and help NACGN.

In October 1993, Wald, the founder of NOPHN, was inducted into the National Women's Hall of Fame at Seneca Falls, New York, having been nominated by the Lucy Lincoln Drown Nursing History Society of the Massachusetts Nurses Association. This recognition was based on her having been an outstanding nurse and social activist during the early twentieth century—a dynamic force for social reform, creating widely adopted models of public health and social service programs. Because Wald died in 1949, the award was accepted by Dr. Nettie Birnbach, president of the New York State Nurses Association, for the American Nurses Association.

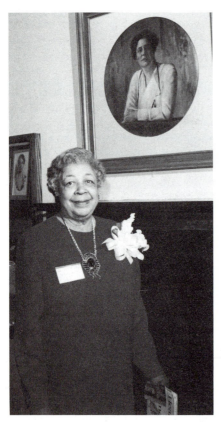

Figure 4–34   Dr. Mary Elizabeth Carnegie, recipient of Visiting Nurse Service of New York's Lillian D. Wald Spirit of Nursing Award, 1994.

On March 15, 1994 the Visiting Nurse Service of New York, an outgrowth of the Henry Street Visiting Nurse Service, as a closing event of its centennial year, hosted a Celebration of Nursing at the Ellis Island National Monument, which houses the Immigration Museum. Attending were more than 1,000 nurses representing all walks of nursing life. The grand highlight of the event was the presentation of the Agency's Lillian D. Wald Spirit of Nursing Award to seven nurses who were pioneers in the advancement and delivery of health care in the United States as practitioners, researchers, educators, authors, and administrators: Diane Carlson Evans, Claire M. Fagin, Loretta Ford, Ruth Lubic, Doris Schwartz, Jessie Scott, and Mary Elizabeth Carnegie, a black nurse. Carnegie (Fig. 4–34) was cited for not only pioneering baccalaureate education for nurses in two states—Virginia and Florida, but for four decades of leadership in the civil rights struggle for the integration of the black nurse into the mainstream of professional nursing, which included breaking down the barriers to membership of blacks in the southern states and the District of Columbia which, in turn, had denied them entry to the American Nurses Association.

AMERICAN PUBLIC HEALTH ASSOCIATION

The American Public Health Association (APHA) is the largest organization of public health professionals in the world, representing more than 50,000 members (including state affiliate members) from more than 70,000 public health occupations and offers 30 sections and special primary interest groups. The Association and its members have been influencing policies and setting priorities in public health since 1872. APHA brings together researchers, health service providers, administrators, teachers, and other health workers in a unique, multidisciplinary environment of professional exchange, study, and action.

APHA is concerned with a broad set of issues affecting personal and environmental health. In recent years, this has included topics such as state and federal funding for health programs, movement toward a national health program, air pollution control, promotion of water fluoridation, health care in jails and prisons, full funding for the World Health Organization, public health programs and policies related to AIDS, a smoke-free society by the year 2000, and professional education in public health.

The Association's programs are based on scientific study of health problems and service issues, utilizing the expertise and diverse resources of its members. Whether APHA is proposing solutions based on research, helping to set public health practice standards, or working closely with national and international health agencies to improve health worldwide, it continually strives to improve public health.

From 1988 to 1989, Iris R. Shannon, Ph.D., RN, FAAN,

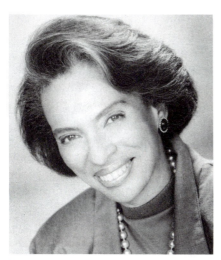

Figure 4–35 Dr. Iris Shannon, President, American Public Health Associate, 1988–1989.

Associate Professor, Community Health Nursing, Rush University, Chicago, Illinois, served as the elected president of APHA and presided at the 117th annual meeting in Chicago in 1989 with 8,700 in attendance (Fig. 4–35).

SIGMA THETA TAU INTERNATIONAL

Sigma Theta Tau International, honor society of Nursing, which was founded by six nursing students in 1922 at Indiana University, Indianapolis, is now the second largest nursing organization in the United States. As of January, 1994, there were 189,469 members and 322 chapters at 359 colleges and universities with accredited baccalaureate and higher degree programs in nursing, four of which are at historically black institutions: Hampton University in Virginia, Howard University in Washington, D.C., Prairie View A&M University, Houston, Texas, and North Carolina A&T State University in Greensboro.

The organization's mission encompasses recognizing superior achievement in nursing, facilitating leadership development, fostering high nursing standards, stimulating creative work, and strengthening the commitment to the ideals of the profession. Membership in Sigma Theta Tau International is a distinct honor conferred by active chapters on students demonstrating academic excellence and distinguished nursing leaders who demonstrate excellence and achievement in nursing practice, education, research, and administration.

The commitment of Sigma Theta Tau International to knowledge dissemination and utilization, and to resource development, human or otherwise, assists its members to improve the health care of people worldwide. The Society advances the scientific base of nursing practice and facilitates nursing leadership and scholarship. The organization furthers the use of nursing research in health care delivery and public policy.

Vernice D. Ferguson, a black nurse who, at that time, was Deputy Assistant Chief Medical Director for Nursing Programs, Department of Veterans Affairs, became the society's sixteenth president in 1985 (Fig. 4–36). She served for two years. In 1987, Mary Elizabeth Carnegie was nominated to receive a "Founders Award for Excellence in Leadership," one of Sigma Theta Tau's most prestigious awards recognizing nursing excellence and scholarship. In 1991, Carnegie was elected to the Board of Directors and reelected in 1993.

In 1989, Sigma Theta Tau International dedicated its elegant new International Center for Nursing Scholarship and the Virginia Henderson

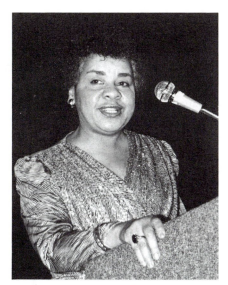

Figure 4–36   Vernice Ferguson, President, Sigma Theta Tau International, 1985–1987.

International Nursing Library on the Indiana University-Indianapolis campus. The 32,000-square foot facility serves as an international focal point for nursing research, continuing education, and other professional activities. It also houses Sigma Theta Tau's international headquarters. The state-of-the-art, electronic library offers quick, easy, on-line computer access to a unique information database featuring "fugitive," or unpublished nursing literature, and additional information valuable to nurse clinicians, educators, researchers, and entrepreneurs, as well as other health care professionals. November, 1993 marked the debut of its *Online Journal of Knowledge Synthesis for Nursing*. This electronic nursing periodical offers peer-reviewed articles and critiques of research literature. More than 16,000 nurses, 100 nursing groups, 75 foundations and corporations, 270 Sigma Theta Tau chapters, and friends of nursing contributed approximately $5 million to the center and library. Many black nurses who participate in Sigma Theta Tau's national activities and hold chapter offices throughout the country strongly supported the fund raising effort. The successful Campaign for the Center for Nursing Scholarship was the first national capital funds campaign ever conducted by a nursing organization.

Sigma Theta Tau's strong commitment to research is exemplified by its numerous scholarly publications, including *Image: Journal of Nursing Scholarship*; the *Directory of Nurse Researchers,* which lists and classifies the work of more than 3,600 nurse researchers; and periodic research monographs. The society underwrote the first known nursing research grant in 1936, and has since that time funded an impressive body of work through a series of small grants to hundreds of highly qualified nurse researchers. In 1989, it presented the first Baxter Foundation Episteme Award for breakthrough nursing research, which includes a $10,000 honorarium and original onyx sculpture. Local, national, and international theory, research, and writers' conferences and congresses are frequently sponsored by Sigma Theta Tau. Hundreds of thousands of nurses around the world have benefitted from those events and the society's other scholarly activities, including research conferences that have been held not only in the United States, but in Spain (twice) (Fig. 4–37), Egypt, Korea, Thailand, Israel, Scotland, and Australia (Fig. 4–38).

Sponsored by Mosby-Yearbook, Inc. and local cable television station managers and produced by Sigma Theta Tau and Samuel Merritt College's Studio Three Productions of Oakland, California, the television programs titled, *Nursing Approach* marked the first time in history that nurses have had their own television show, which was created by, for, and about nurses. It was launched in January 1993. The March 1993 program highlighted the fiftieth anniversary of the Cadet Nurse Corps and included interviews with Lucile Petry Leone, director of the Corps, and Mary Elizabeth Carnegie, member of the National Recruitment Committee. This particular program won second prize at the 1994 American Journal of Nursing Media Festival.

In 1991, Sigma Theta Tau initiated a leadership extern program designed to assist in preparing Sigma Theta Tau members for leadership roles in nursing. One of the four 1993–1995 externs is Bettye Davis-Lewis (B.S., Prairie View A&M University, Houston, Texas; Ed.D.,

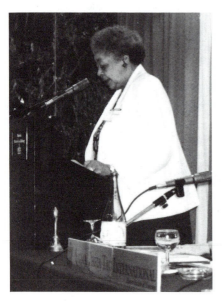

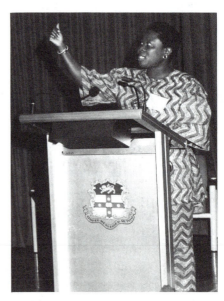

Figure 4–37   Dr. Mary Elizabeth Carnegie presenting a paper at Sigma Theta Tau International Research Conference, Madrid, Spain, 1993.

Figure 4–38   At the Australian Congress, Dr. Dora Carbonu, originally from Ghana, presented a paper based on her research conducted in Pakistan.

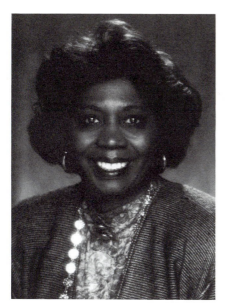

Figure 4–39   Dr. Bettye Davis-Lewis, Sigma Theta Tau International extern, 1993–1995.

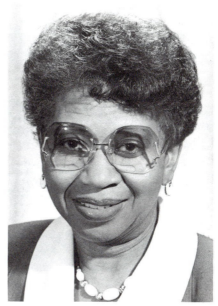

Figure 4–40   Dr. Juanita Hunter, Distinguished Lecturer Sigma Theta Tau.

Texas Southern University, Houston), chief executive officer and owner, Diversified Health Care Systems, Inc. (Fig. 4–39). She is gaining leadership skills in working with diverse populations.

In 1987, Sigma Theta Tau established a Distinguished Lecturer Program designed to foster its mission of promoting leadership and scholarship. Over 150 members have participated in this program over the past seven years. Nursing leaders agree to share their knowledge and expertise with other members. The program provides an excellent opportunity for chapters to use these resources to further implement the goals of Sigma Theta Tau at the local and regional levels. One of the lecturers is Dr. Juanita K. Hunter, Clinical Associate Professor, State University of New York at Buffalo (Fig. 4–40). Because of her experiences with a homeless project, her topic is in this area, which includes nursing care of the homeless.

CHI ETA PHI

Chi Eta Phi is a national sorority of registered professional nurses, founded at Freedmen's Hospital, Washington, DC, in 1932 by Aliene Carrington Ewell (Fig. 4–41), along with 11 other women—all Freedmen's

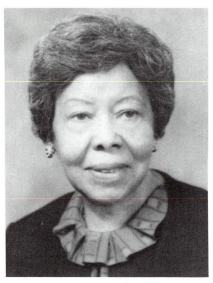

Figure 4–41   Aliene C. Ewell, Founder, Chi Eta Phi Sorority, 1932.

nurses. The organization was incorporated in 1934 under the laws of the District of Columbia.

Chi Eta Phi Sorority consists of more than 5,000 professional nurses and nursing students (predominantly black), representing many cultures and diverse ethnic backgrounds. It has 93 chapters—75 graduate and 23 active undergraduate—in 26 states, and the District of Columbia; Monrovia, Liberia, West Africa; and the U.S. Virgin Islands. Its purposes are to develop a corps of nursing leaders; encourage continuing education; conduct continuous recruitment for nursing and other health professions; stimulate close and friendly relationships among members; and develop working relationships with other professional groups.

Among the 65 Honorary members of Chi Eta Phi are five white nurses, including the late Lillian Carter ("Miss Lillian"), the mother of Jimmy Carter, the 39th president of the United States. (See Appendix E.) Its official publications are *The Glowing Lamp* and *JOCEPS, Journal of Chi Eta Phi,* published annually, which presents peer-reviewed scientific articles, as well as chapter news. The organization also supports civic and charitable efforts.

Except for the NACGN, there was little opportunity for black nurses to develop leadership skills in professional nursing organizations when Chi Eta Phi was organized in 1932. In the South, including the District of Columbia, black nurses were barred from membership in their state nurses' associations; in the North, even with open membership, there was little evidence of black nurses at that time having held office in the state and district constituents of the ANA, let alone on the national level.

For 20 years, between 1951 when NACGN was dissolved and 1971 when the National Black Nurses' Association came into existence, Chi Eta Phi was the only organization in which black nurses were given the opportunity to develop organizational leadership skills. Many of the black nurses who have occupied and are now occupying leadership roles in ANA and other organizations on all levels—national, regional, state, and local—

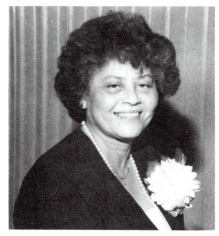

Figure 4–42   Catherine W. Binns, Supreme Baileus, Chi Eta Phi, elected 1993.

rose through the ranks of Chi Eta Phi, where they had held key offices. When Fay Wilson, for example, was elected to the board of directors of the ANA in 1970, she not only brought with her a history of experience in nursing service, education, administration, and consultation, but valuable experience from having served three terms as national president of Chi Eta Phi. Before her death in 1992, she had also served on the California Board of Nursing.

Others with leadership experience in Chi Eta Phi include Marguerette Creth Jackson, who had been first vice-president of the joint boards of the six national nursing organizations (ANA, NLNE, NOPHN, ACSN, AAIN, NACGN) to study the Structure; Fostine Riddick Roach, member of the Virginia State Board of Health and alumni representative on the Board of Trustees of Tuskegee University; Verdelle Bellamy, president of the Georgia State Board of Nursing; Helen Miller, who had been vice-president of the National League for Nursing and member of the Board of Nursing in North Carolina; and Mary Long, president of the Georgia Nurses' Association and board, American Nurses' Association. The current Supreme Basileus is Catherine Binns (Fig. 4–42), having been elected in 1993.

Beginning as an organization of black female nurses, Chi Eta Phi Sorority has become interracial and also accepts men as members. With a chapter in Africa and the Caribbean, this organization can also be classified as international in scope. In keeping with its goals of encouraging continuing education among its members and scholastic achievements, all chapters of Chi Eta Phi conduct continuing education workshops and award generous scholarships to worthy students in their communities to study nursing.

NATIONAL STUDENT NURSES' ASSOCIATION

When the National Student Nurses' Association (NSNA) organized in 1953, it was under the aegis of the ANA and NLN. Today NSNA is an autonomous, student-financed and student-run organization. According to its bylaws, its purpose is "to aid in the development of the individual student and to urge all students of nursing, as future health professionals, to be aware of and to contribute to improving the health of all people."

The functions of NSNA are related to its purpose and demonstrate the scope of its work: promoting community participation directed toward improved health care and related social issues; speaking for nursing students when and where this is indicated; influencing the development of recruitment of minorities into schools of nursing; and promoting collaborative relationships with the Ameri-

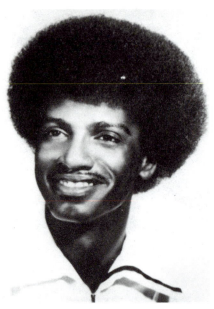

Figure 4–43   Cleo Doster (1931–1985) elected President NSNA, 1976.

can Nurses' Association, the National League for Nursing, the International Council of Nurses, and other nursing and related health organizations (National Student Nurses' Association Bylaws, 1972).

At the 1976 convention of NSNA, a black student, Cleo Doster (Fig. 4–43) from California, was elected president. After serving one term, he was made an honorary member of NSNA. Doster organized and chaired the Student Assembly at the ICN in Tokyo in 1977. He died November 25, 1985 at the age of 44. There is currently one black student serving on the NSNA Board of Directors as the Breakthrough to Nursing Director. NSNA's major and most successful project is its Breakthrough to Nursing (see Chapter 3).

NURSES' EDUCATIONAL FUNDS

Nurses' Educational Funds (NEF) was incorporated in 1954 as an extension of the Isabel Hampton Robb Memorial Fund, established in 1910, and the Isabel McIsaac Loan Fund, established in 1914. An independent, nonprofit organization, NEF grants and administers scholarships to registered nurses for masters and doctoral study. The corporation, with a chief executive officer, is governed by an interracial board consisting of members selected from nursing and business leaders. Current membership includes two black nurses—Dr. M. Elizabeth Carnegie, and Dr. Hattie Bessent. NEF is supported by contributions from the business community, foundations, nurses, and individuals interested in the advancement of nursing.

In addition to providing scholarships from interest on the endowment funds, NEF administers named grants. Although black nurses may win any of the awards, two of the named scholarships are designated for black nurses: The M. Elizabeth Carnegie Scholarship for doctoral study initiated in 1982 and the Estelle M. Osborne Memorial Scholarship for master's study initiated in 1983.

Between 1982 and 1994, the Carnegie scholarship for doctoral study has been awarded to Bobbie Jean Cotton, Virginia Polytechnic Institute and State University; Sadie Smalls, Althea Davis, and Marie Mosley, Teachers College, Columbia University, New York; Patricia McElvy, Marcia Wells, Harvard University, Cambridge, Massachusetts; Cynthia Archer-Gift, Wayne State University, Detroit, Michigan; Vicki Hines-Martin, University of Kentucky, Lexington; Kaye L. Claytor, Indiana University; Rosie Lee Calvin, Louisiana State University; Marva L. Price, University of North Carolina, Chapel Hill; and Brenda Owens, Texas Woman's University, Houston.

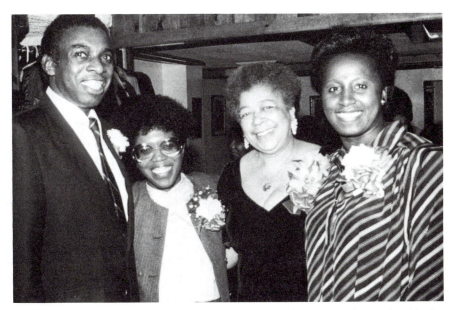

Figure 4–44   At NEF fund-raising reception, New York, 1983. Left to right: Charles Hargett, Dr. Barbara Holder, Dr. Mary Elizabeth Carnegie, Sadie Smalls.

Between 1983 and 1994, the Osborne scholarship for master's study has been awarded to: Vicki Hines-Martin, University of Cincinnati; Cheryl Williams Thompson, Columbia University, New York; Sandra Picot; Constance M. Dallas, St. Xavier College; Carol Gibson and Vickie C. Scott, Howard University, Washington, DC; Barbara H. McCall, Emory University, Atlanta, Georgia; Jacqueline B. Patton, Indiana University; Elizabeth A. Simms and Erna Josiah, University of California, San Francisco.

In the spirit of helping other black nurses earn doctorates, Sadie Smalls, a Carnegie Scholarship recipient, along with Charles Hargett and Barbara Holder, initiated an annual fund-raising activity (Fig. 4–44). Major annual donors to the Osborne Scholarship to help black nurses earn a master's degree are Chi Eta Phi Sorority and Freedmen's Hospital School of Nursing Alumni Association.

AMERICAN NURSES' FOUNDATION

The American Nurses' Foundation (ANF) was established by the American Nurses' Association in 1955 pursuant to action of the 1954 House of Delegates calling for a mechanism through which tax-exempt funds could flow in support of nursing programs, particularly those in nursing research. ANF's Nursing Research Grants Program supports research directed by registered nurses. It was created chiefly for beginning nurse researchers, but consideration is also given to experienced nurse researchers who are entering new fields of investigation.

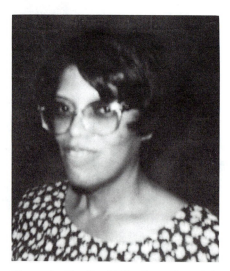

Several black nurses have received grants from ANF to support their research: Dr. Juanita Fleming's project in 1970–1971 was "Understanding Hospitalized Children Through Drawings"; Dr. Willa Doswell's research in 1979 was entitled "Physiology and Behavior: An Investigation of the Relation Between Race, Repression-Sensitization and Systolic Blood Pressure Response in Female Registered Nurses."

In 1992, Doswell (Fig. 4–45), was again funded by ANF, as the

Figure 4–45 Dr. Willa Doswell, recipient of ANA Research Grant, 1992.

Sterling Drug Company Scholar, to support her research on the physiological and behavioral effects of swaddling cocaine-exposed neonates. At the time of funding, Doswell was the associate director, Nursing Research and Quality Assurance, Health and Hospitals Corporation, New York City. She is now research assistant professor and associate director, Center for Nursing Research, University of Pittsburgh School of Nursing, Pittsburgh, PA. Among the 1992 ANF Research Scholars was Vicki P. Hines-Martin whose research focused on African-American Caregivers and the Chronic Mentally Ill.

In 1976, Evelyn K. Tomes, professor and chair of the Department of Nursing Education at Meharry Medical College in Nashville, Tennessee, received one of six grants from ANF to investigate the contributions of black nurses to health services and health education. Says Dr. Tomes:

> Black nurses are interested in being recognized for their contributions to the progress of nursing in this country. Throughout the development of the profession, there have been black women so concerned about the improvement of health services, and the involvement of black nurses in the profession that they have overcome many insurmountable odds to accomplish these goals. It is such contributions that need to be researched, highlighted, and incorporated into nursing history. Bringing these events into focus should provide a long overdue redress to this group of nurse pioneers, and also influence the future direction of professional nursing. (*Nursing Research Report,* 1976, p. 7)

The 29 grants awarded by ANF in 1990 marked the largest number of nurse researchers funded since its beginning in 1955. Funded recipients are titled scholars of the sponsoring corporation, organization, or individual. In 1987, Dr. Gloria Smith became the fourth recipient of the ANF Distinguished Scholar Award, and conducted a study titled, "Influencing Public Policy: Rethinking Public Health Nursing Practice Dilemmas."

ANF is directed by a nine-member board of trustees—all registered nurses. In 1985, Dr. Ethelrine Shaw-Nickerson became president—the first black—and served until 1989. Currently on the board of trustees as vice-president is Dr. Beverly Malone, North Carolina A&T University, Greensboro, and Verlie Brown, New York. Two other black nurses have played important leadership roles for ANF: Mary N. Long (Georgia) and Jean Marshall (New Jersey). Long chaired the Foundation's successful Nursing on the Move capital campaign (1990–1992) to enable headquarters' move from Kansas City to Washington, DC. Marshall chaired the first ANF special event (1993), a dinner to raise funds for immunization projects for underserved children in rural communities, featuring Children's Defense Fund President Marian Wright Edelman as guest speaker.

THE AMERICAN ASSOCIATION OF COLLEGES OF NURSING

Beginning in 1966, a group of deans and directors, concerned about making baccalaureate preparation for beginning professional nursing practice a reality, and who were also members of the National League for Nursing Department of Baccalaureate and Higher Degree Programs, held a series of meetings with NLN staff to explore the kind of organizational arrangement that could focus on significant issues through an effective forum, and then take the necessary actions (Fondiller, 1989).

In 1969, the deliberations of these early sessions culminated in the formation of an independent conference of deans of college and university schools of nursing. By 1972, the name of the group had become the American Association of Colleges of Nursing (AACN), which became incorporated in the District of Columbia in 1973. From the original 121-member institutions in 1969, AACN today represents 463 schools of nursing at public and private universities and four-year colleges nationwide.

The mission of AACN, with offices in Washington, DC, focuses on three main areas: to advance the quality of baccalaureate and graduate nursing education, promote nursing research, and provide for the development of academic leaders. AACN administers programs in education, research, government relations, publications, public affairs, and data base operations (Fondiller, 1989). In 1985, AACN began publishing its official organ, *The Journal of Professional Nursing*—a bimonthly.

From its inception, black deans have played an active role—holding office, serving on task forces, and the like. In 1988, Geraldene Felton, dean, University of Iowa College of Nursing, was elected president and served until 1990 (Fig. 4–46). Currently serving on the board of directors is Margie Johnson, dean, Tuskegee University School of Nursing. In addition, Dorothy Powell, dean of the College of Nursing at Howard University, continues to represent AACN on the U.S. Preventive Services Coordinating Committee. Brenda Cherry, dean, University of Massachusetts, Boston, College of Nursing, chairs the AACN Interest Group on Fostering Publication and Scholarly Effort.

The historically black schools that hold membership as of 1994 are: Tuskegee University, Alabama; University of Arkansas at Pine Bluff;

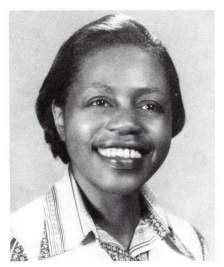

Figure 4–46 Dr. Geraldene Felton, President AACN, 1988–1990. (Courtesy AACN)

Howard University, Washington, DC; Florida A&M University, Tallahassee; Bowie State University, Maryland; Coppin State College, Baltimore, Maryland; Alcorn State University, Natchez, Mississippi; North Carolina A&T State University, Greensboro; Winston-Salem State University, North Carolina; Tennessee State University, Nashville; Prairie View A&M University, Texas; Hampton University, Hampton, Virginia; Norfolk State University, Norfolk, Virginia; North Carolina Central University, Durham, North Carolina; Southern University and A&M College, Baton Rouge, Louisiana; Albany State College, Albany, Georgia; and Dillard University, New Orleans, Louisiana. The predominantly black member schools are: Chicago State University, Chicago, Illinois; Medgar Evers College of CUNY, Brooklyn, New York; and the University of the District of Columbia, Washington, DC.

THE NATIONAL BLACK NURSES' ASSOCIATION

In 1970, the national convention of the American Nurses' Association was held in Miami, Florida, with approximately 200 black nurses in attendance. To learn more about those present, one black nurse from Indiana, Dr. Lauranne Sams (Fig. 4–47), called for a caucus to which over 150 black nurses responded. This was an initial attempt to develop a channel of communication among concerned black nurses. From the caucus, it was determined that they were concerned about and accountable to black people in a special way. The caucus also felt there was a need for them to articulate the health needs of the black community, as well as provide equal access to and mobility within the health care system.

Later, a small group of black nurses was called by Sams and met in the home of Dr. Mary Harper in Cleveland, Ohio. The primary purpose was to organize a black nurses association that would be an independent group. They also met to plan for a caucus at the ANA convention. Those present noted what many other black nurses had voiced: concern over the absence of black nurses in leadership positions in ANA (at that time, there had never been a black president or vice-president); limited opportunities for blacks to share in shaping ANA policies and priorities; persistent tokenism; limited recognition of the black nurse's contribution to nursing; no significant increase in the number of black registered nurses; no recognition of achievement in terms of awards, other than the Mary Mahoney Award honoring the first black trained nurse; limited appointments to committees and commissions, presentation of papers, and the like.

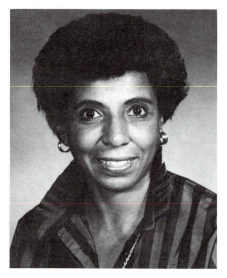

Figure 4–47   Dr. Lauranne Sams, first President, National Black Nurses Association.

In December 1971, the National Black Nurses' Association (NBNA) was formed with Sams as its first president. In 1972, NBNA was incorporated, with membership open to all registered nurses, licensed practical nurses, licensed vocational nurses, and student nurses. (See Appendix F for a list of Charter Members.)

The purpose and objectives of the NBNA are as follows:

1. Define and determine nursing care for black consumers for optimum quality of care by acting as their advocates.

2. Act as change agent in restructuring existing institutions and/or helping to establish institutions to suit (black nurses') needs.

3. Serve as the national body to influence legislation and policies that affect black people and work cooperatively and collaboratively with other health care workers to this end.

4. Conduct, analyze, and publish research to increase the body of knowledge about health needs of blacks.

5. Compile and maintain a National Directory of black nurses to assist with the dissemination of information regarding black nurses and nursing on a national level by the use of all media.

6. Set standards and guidelines for quality education of black nurses on all levels by providing consultation to nursing faculties and by monitoring for proper utilization and placement of black nurses.

7. Recruit, counsel, and assist black persons into the field.

8. Be the vehicle for unification of black nurses of varied age groups, educational levels, and geographic locations to insure continuity and flow of our common heritage.

9. Collaborate with other black groups to compile archives relevant to the historical, current, and future activities of black nurses.

10. Provide the impetus and means for black nurses to write and publish on an individual or collaborative basis. (Smith, 1975)

In addition to regular organization business, NBNA sponsors annual national institutes. The first one held in Cleveland, Ohio, in 1973 with the theme, "Emerging Roles for Black Nurses," focused national attention on the relationship between the health needs of the black consumer and the current practice of nursing. The purpose of this institute was to design and implement a program that would provide an opportunity for black nurses and other health-related workers to begin to explore systematically the health needs of the black consumer.

NBNA, with headquarters in Washington, DC, has 7,000 members in more than 51 chapters representing the 130,000 black nurses in the United States, 90,611 of whom are registered nurses (National Sample Survey of R.N.'s, 1992). With a special focus on minorities, the association recruits for nursing, serves as a job bank, functions as an information resource for federal agencies concerned with health care, monitors federal legislation, and provides health education seminars for nurses and allied health professionals. It is an active member of the Black Congress on Health Law, and Economics. NBNA's refereed journal, *Journal of*

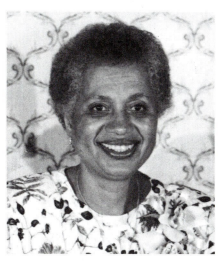

Figure 4–48 Dr. Hilda Richards, editor, *Journal of the NBA* and Chancellor, Indiana University Northwest, Gary.

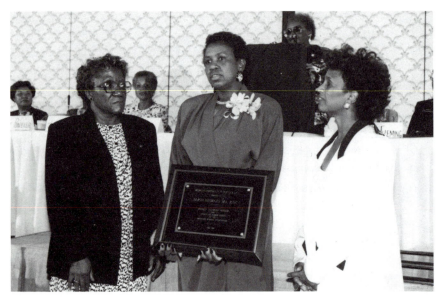

Figure 4–49   C. Alicia Georges (center), President, NBNA Foundation.

NBNA, is edited by Dr. Hilda Richards (Fig. 4–48), chancellor, Indiana University Northeast, Gary.

Beginning in 1986, at several ANA biennial conventions, the ANA Minority Fellowship Program and the ANA Cabinet on Human Rights presented awards to women of color who had made a contribution to public service. In 1990, C. Alicia Georges (Fig. 4–49), then president of NBNA, and Dr. Hilda Richards were among those so honored.

In 1991, under the leadership of its president, Dr. Linda Burnes–Bolton, the National Black Nurses Foundation was established to serve as an educational research and fund-raising arm of NBNA. The Foundation, with C. Alicia Georges as President, solicits support for the long-term activities of NBNA and support activities designed to encourage continuing education for nurses and promote nursing as a career. These activities include nurturing networking relations with historically black colleges and universities with nursing programs by helping to increase enrollment and offering mentoring to nursing students; recruiting, counseling, and assisting African-American persons interested in nursing to ensure a constant procession of persons of African-American heritage into the field; and conducting, analyzing, and publishing research to increase the body of knowledge about the health needs of African-Americans.

AMERICAN ASSOCIATION FOR THE HISTORY OF NURSING

Spearheaded by the late Teresa Christy, nurse historiographer, the International History of Nursing Society was founded in the Midwest in 1978. Because of problems with making the organization international in scope, in 1980 the name was changed to the American Association for the History of Nursing. From 1982 to 1984, M. Elizabeth Carnegie served as corresponding secretary.

Annual conferences, co-sponsored by the Association and a university upon invitation, have been held since 1984. In 1992, the annual conference was held in Canada with the Canadian Association for the History of Nursing. The conferences are designed to provide a forum for members to share their historical research. As of 1994, AAHN's membership totaled over 400, with representation from all 50 states and several foreign countries, including Australia, Canada, England, Finland, Germany, Italy, and Portugal.

The purposes of AAHN are to stimulate national and international interest in the history of nursing and promote collaboration among its supporters; encourage research in the history of nursing; promote the development of centers for the preservation and use of materials of historical importance to nursing; serve as a resource for information related to nursing history; and produce and distribute materials related to the history and heritage of the nursing profession.

Among the many presentations have been a few that focused on black nurses and their contributions; for example, Dr. Althea Davis' paper, based on her dissertation, paid tribute to three early "architects" of integration: Adah B. Thoms, Martha Franklin, and Mary Eliza Mahoney. Another by Janice Barnes Young described black nurses' experiences in the Cadet Nurse Corps. Another by Pegge L. Bell was on the "Influence of the Tuskegee School of Nurse Midwifery for Colored Nurses on the Health Status of Southern Blacks in the 1940s." Still another by Dr. Arlene Lowenstein, described "Racial Segregation in Nursing Education: The Lamar Experience."

At the 1990 conference, held at the University of Texas—Galveston, Darlene Clark Hine (Fig. 4–50), John Hannah Professor of History at Michigan State University, who has written five books and published 11 journal articles on the history of blacks, was the recipient of the coveted Lavinia Dock Award (Dock was America's first nurse historian). Dr. Hine's latest book is *Black Women in White: Racial Conflict and Cooperation in the*

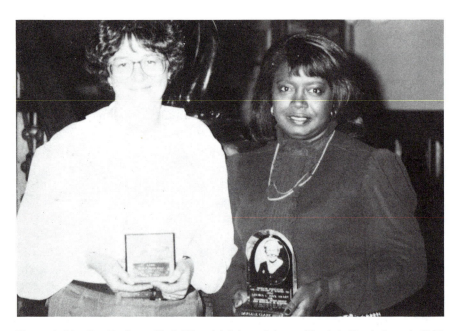

Figure 4–50   Dr. Darlene Clark Hine (right), recipient of Lavinia Dock Award, 1990. (Courtesy University of Texas Medical Branch at Galveston)

Nursing Profession, 1890–1950, published by Indiana University Press in 1989. According to the *Women's Review of Books,* "the book is full of poignant and sympathetic portraits of black nurses in their dedication and idealism, in their pain and anger . . . and in their deep concern for their community's health needs . . . ." At the 1993 conference, Marie Mosley presented a paper based on her doctoral dissertation, titled "The Development of Black Community Health Nursing in the Northeastern United States, 1906–1934: Contributions of Elizabeth Tyler and Edith Carter."

At the 1994 Conference in Chicago, Jeanette Waits of the University of Mississippi, presented a paper on a black nurse, "Eliza Parish Pillars: Pioneer Mississippi Public Health Nurse." (See Chapter 5 for a profile of Pillars.)

Since 1988, the American Association for the History of Nursing has been cooperating with the Museum of Nursing History in Philadelphia and the Center for the study of the History of Nursing at the University of Pennsylvania in holding an annual invitational Nursing History Conference at the historic Pennsylvania Hospital. The conference not only addresses important issues in the history of nursing such as the ethics of historical research, but also serves as a forum for the critique of historical research.

AAHN publishes the *Bulletin,* a quarterly newsletter, and an annual scholarly journal *Nursing History Review,* devoted to history of nursing and health care.

THE ASSOCIATION OF BLACK NURSING FACULTY IN HIGHER EDUCATION

In 1986, at the invitation of Sallie Tucker-Allen, a group of black nursing faculty from several universities in Illinois met to share experiences on how to best meet their professional needs and to determine how to best serve their constituencies (see Appendix G). The result was the founding of the Association of Black Nursing Faculty in Higher Education, Inc. (ABNF), with Dr. Tucker-Allen as its first president (Fig. 4–51).

Membership in ABNF consists of black registered nurses with an earned graduate degree in nursing who are teaching at an institution of higher education. Its functions are to: provide a center for communication among members; develop strategies for promulgating group concerns to other individuals, institutions, and communities; assist members in professional development; develop, initiate, and sponsor continuing education activities; encourage and support research efforts among members; support black consumer advocacy issues; act and speak on health-related issues of legislation, government programs, and community activities; and serve as a forum for the exchange of new ideas and research findings.

ABNF's first annual meeting was held in 1988 in Washington, DC. At this conference, awards of recognition were presented to two outstanding nurses—Dr. Hattie Bessent and Dr. Helen Grace; honorary membership was bestowed upon Dr. M. Elizabeth Carnegie. At its second annual meeting in August, 1989, in the Bahamas, Dr. Carnegie received the ABNF Lifetime

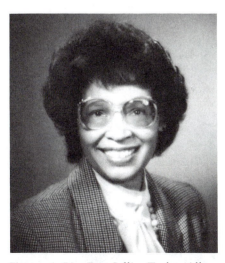

Figure 4–51 Dr. Sallie Tucker-Allen, Founder and first President, Association of Black Nursing Faculty.

Achievement Award in Education and Research. The current president (1994) is Dr. Ruth Johnson.

Like other professional nursing organizations, ABNF has an official journal which is refereed. ABNF is also a member of the American Nurses' Association Nursing Organizational Liaison Forum.

ASSOCIATION OF BLACK SEVENTH-DAY ADVENTIST NURSES

The Association of Black Adventist Nurses (ABAN) is a professional nursing organization targeting black Seventh-Day Adventist nurses. One of the primary goals is to unite this body of professionals for the purpose of promoting excellence in Christ-centered education and professional development. The objective which is holistic, addresses the physical, mental, and spiritual needs of individuals, families, and communities of African-American descent.

The organizational meeting was held on April 19, 1987 at Oakwood College in Huntsville, Alabama. The idea of establishing such an organization was conceived by Kathleen Woodfork Bradley (Fig. 4–52), who was voted ABAN's first president. She served in that capacity until 1993 when Donna Manier was voted her successor. Bradley was named President Emerita. ABAN is committed to its mission and meets annually at Oakwood College, where its literary materials are housed in the Archives of the Eva B. Dykes Library.

Since ABAN's inception, the organization has worked to meet the needs of its members by forming numerous local chapters, providing nursing scholarships and continuing education, networking, and fostering mentor-mentee relationships. It also addresses ethnic health care issues, health screening, and makes referrals.

At present, ABAN is a national organization extending across the

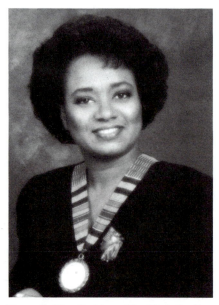

Figure 4–52   Kathleen Woodfork Bradley, Founder and first President, ABAN.

United States. There are established interests in the Caribbean, England, and the continent of Africa. Further development is planned for these areas and more.

THE AMERICAN ACADEMY OF NURSING

Within most professions is a body referred to as an academy, composed of a cadre of scholars who deal with issues that concern the profession and take positions in the name of the academy. Nursing, a young profession, has such an academy under the aegis of the professional association. The academy was established by the ANA Board of Directors in 1973. The board, acting on the criteria that had been established to recognized substantial achievement and contributions in nursing, designated 36 Charter Fellows, among whom were two blacks: Rhetaugh Dumas and Geraldene Felton. The Charter Fellows were chosen from more than 100 nominees and symbolize the high degree of commitment of today's nursing to providing high-quality care. Those selected for charter membership were highly expert clinical practitioners, academicians, administrators, and researchers.

The American Academy of Nursing is constituted to provide visionary leadership to the nursing profession and the public in shaping health policy and practice that epitomize the well-being of the American people. The Academy identifies emerging nursing and health care issues, promotes their scholarly exploration, challenges the status quo, and proposes creative solutions.

The mission of the Academy is framed within nursing's historic commitment to an ethos of caring and the responsible generation and application of science. The Academy facilitates the synthesis of scientific and philosophic knowledge as the basis for effective health care policy and practice. The Academy pursues its mission by facilitating scholarly debate on issues that are identified as significant to nursing and health care; evaluating and interpreting scientific and philosophic knowledge as a basis for proposing new directions in health care policy and practice; initiating studies to generate new knowledge relevant to health care; disseminating proposals for health policy and practice through publications, conferences, and other professional activities; and forming interactive linkages with other groups to recommend health care policy and practice to meet emerging health care needs (*American Academy of Nursing Mission Statement,* 1990). *Nursing Outlook,* published by Mosby-Yearbook, is the official journal of the American Academy of Nursing.

As of 1994, 1,050 nurses have been admitted to the Academy, 68, or 6 percent, of whom are black (see Appendix H). Seventy-five percent of the Fellows are doctorally prepared; the remainder are masters prepared. The Academy also has had three black elected presidents: Mary Elizabeth Carnegie, 1978–1979; Vernice Ferguson, 1981–1983; and Rhetaugh Dumas, 1987–1989.

At the 1992 Academy meeting in St. Louis, Missouri, Dr. Hattie Bessent was the recipient of the Academy's Distinguished Service Award "for having done more than any other single individual in this country to develop a pool of minority nurse scholars and researchers; and to prepare leaders in nursing to assume roles as practitioners and clinicians. Administered by ANA with funding from NIMH, she kept the program viable and vigorous for 15 years (she retired in 1992)." At that same meeting, M. Elizabeth Carnegie received a Media Award (see Preface to Third Edition).

The 1994 Media Award went to the series of articles submitted by Gloria J. McNeal, showcasing the Thomas Jefferson University Mobile Immunization Unit/ICARE project. McNeal is an assistant professor at The Thomas Jefferson University College of Allied Health Sciences, Department of Nursing, Philadelphia.

Also in 1994, the Academy instituted a new tradition by designating each year some Fellows as "Living Legends" to recognize the most stellar Fellows as role models and to provide an opportunity each year for newer Fellows to socialize with long-established Fellows, so various generations of leaders can become better acquainted with each other. Among the first honored was a black, M. Elizabeth Carnegie. Others so honored were: Myrtle Aydelotte, Ildaura Murillo-Rohde, Hildegarde Peplau, Jessie Scott, Faye Abdellah, and Harriet Werley. Lifetime fellowship status is bestowed upon the Legends.

Reference is made here to the two black Charter Fellows and the two black Honorary Fellows. See Appendix H for a complete listing of the black Fellows, with year of induction into the Academy.

Charter Fellows

Rhetaugh Dumas (Dillard University Division of Nursing, New Orleans, LA; Ph.D., Union Graduate School, Yellow Springs, Ohio) (Fig. 4–53), was chief of Psychiatric Nursing Education Branch, Division of Manpower and Training Programs, NIMH, when she was selected by the ANA Board of Directors for membership in the American Academy of Nursing as a Charter Fellow. She became Deputy Director of that Division in 1977. In 1979, she was promoted to deputy director, NIMH, Alcohol, Drug Abuse, and Mental Health Administration, Public Health Service,

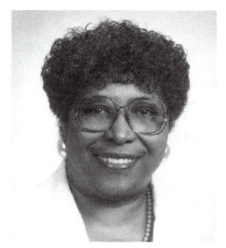

Figure 4–53 Dr. Rhetaugh Dumas, Charter Fellow, American Academy of Nursing, 1973.

U.S. Department of Health and Human Services. From 1981 to 1994, she was dean, University of Michigan School of Nursing, Ann Arbor. In her honor is the Rhetaugh G. Dumas Award for Student Excellence in Leadership at the School of Nursing to be given annually at commencement. She has also been awarded the Lucille Cole Professorship of Nursing, named after the first black faculty member in the School of Nursing.

In 1994, Dumas became vice provost for health affairs at the University of Michigan, with the responsibility for fostering cooperation among the various health units on campus, including the schools of Nursing, Public Health, Pharmacy, Dentistry, Medicine, and Social Work.

Prior to Dumas' appointment to federal posts beginning in 1972, her career had spanned teaching, clinical practice, administration, consultation, and research. She had served as chairperson of the Psychiatric Nursing Program at Yale University and Director of Nursing Service at the Connecticut Mental Health Center at Yale-New Haven Medical Center. In the area of research, she is credited with being the first nurse to conduct clinical experiments to evaluate nursing practice. In this connection, she was principal investigator of federally funded research projects. Robert C. Leonard, Ph.D., was her collaborator. Results of their studies on "The Effect of Nursing Care on Postoperative Vomiting" (1961) have been widely published and have stimulated many similar studies over the years. Dumas is the author of numerous publications.

Dumas is in constant demand, in this country and abroad, as a consultant to organizations and as a speaker at conventions and scientific meetings. In the spring of 1982, she was invited by the U.S. Department of Health and Human Services to travel with a team of nurses to Nigeria, West Africa, to consult with the Federal Ministry of Health on nursing and nursing education. In July, 1983, she participated in a Working Conference for the Examination of Group Behavior Within an Institution, sponsored by the Washington-Baltimore Center of the A. K. Rice Institute and the University of Maryland European Division for the 7th Medical Command, United States Army at Waldorf, Germany. In 1990, she gave the keynote address at the Fifth Southern African Network Conference, Gaborone, Botswana.

Five honorary doctorates have been bestowed on Dumas: Doctor of Public Service, University of Cincinnati; Doctor of Public Service, Simmons College, Boston; Doctor of Humane Letters, Yale University, and her alma mater, Dillard University; and Doctor of Humane Letters, University of San Diego, California. Her numerous awards includes Distinguished Alumnae Award from Yale University, which reads, "No catalogue of her personal and professional accomplishments does justice to the power of her person, the scope of her service, or the depths of the ways she has touched the lives of others." In 1985, she received the University of Michigan's First Annual Academic Women's Career Award. In 1986 and 1987, she served on the Advisory Committee to the Director of the National Institutes of Health.

Geraldene Felton (Mercy Hospital School of Nursing, Philadelphia, PA; Ed.D., New York University) (Fig. 4–54), was on loan from the Department of the Army in the position of associate professor, University of Hawaii School of nursing when she was named a Charter Fellow of the American Academy of Nursing. She had served as a nurse anesthetist and researcher in the Army Nurse Corps from 1949 to 1975 and had achieved the rank of Lieutenant Colonel after having served in Japan, Korea, and Germany. She had also been principal investigator on a Health, Education, and Welfare research project: "Rhythmic Correlates of Shift Work." Later she was a research nurse and deputy director, Walter Reed Army Institute of Research, Division of Nursing, Washington, DC.

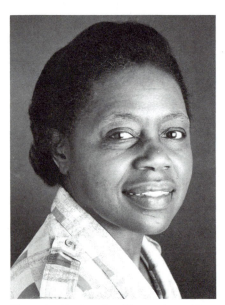

After 20 years of service with the U.S. Army Nurse Corps, and as professor and researcher, Felton retired and became professor and dean of nursing at Oakland University in Rochester, Michigan. In 1981, she assumed the position of professor and dean, College of Nursing, University of Iowa, Iowa City.

Figure 4–54   Dr. Geraldene Felton, Charter Fellow, AAN, 1973.

Felton has published widely in professional and refereed journals; has delivered innumerable papers at scientific meetings; is a member of Sigma Xi, Scientific Research Society of North America; has held office in major nursing organizations; and has served on the boards of the American Journal of Nursing Company and St. Joseph Mercy Hospital, Pontiac, Michigan. With her administrative responsibilities, she continues to be actively engaged in teaching, consultation, research, and scholarly publication. In 1984, she became the assistant editor for research for the *Journal of Professional Nursing,* the official publication of the AACN. She was chair, Iowa Academy of Science Nursing Section, 1984–1985; president elect, Association of Colleges of Nursing (AACN), 1986–1988; President, AACN, 1988–1990; chair, Nursing Research Study Section, National Science Institute of Health Division of Research Grants, 1987–1991; is serving a second four-year term as member, Special Medical Advisory Group, Department of Veterans Affairs, 1988–1996; is on the board of directors, North Central Association Commission on Institutions of Higher Education; and serves on the Pew Robert Wood Johnson National Advisory Committee on "Strengthening Hospital Nursing."

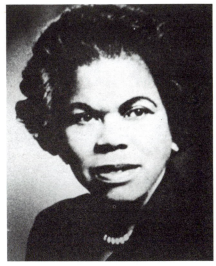

Figure 4–55   Estelle M. Osborne, Honorary Fellow, AAN, 1978.

Honorary Fellows

Estelle M. Osborne. (Fig. 4–55) was the first black nurse to be inducted into the American Academy of Nursing as an honorary Fellow (1978), and in 1984 she was inducted into the ANA Hall of Fame. The following is the complete text of the statement read in 1982 at the memorial service for deceased Fellows.

In Memoriam

Estelle Massey Riddle Osborne, honorary Fellow of the American Academy of Nursing, died December 12, 1981 in California at the age of 80 following a long illness.

During her distinguished career in nursing, Mrs. Osborne made lasting contributions to nursing in the areas of teaching; public health; educational administration, consultation, and research; publications; and public service in local and nationwide communities. Mrs. Osborne's teaching experience occurred on all levels—from elementary school in rural Texas prior to entering nursing, to high school in Kansas City, Missouri, to diploma programs at Lincoln and Harlem in New York, and to New York University Division of Nurse Education as assistant professor. Her first experience after graduating from nursing school was with the St. Louis Municipal Visiting Nurses. Upon earning the master degree in 1931 from Teachers College in New York, she served as educational director at Freedmen's Hospital School of Nursing in Washington, DC. At the invitation of the board of directors of the nursing program from which she was graduated, Mrs. Osborne became the first black director of nursing at Homer G. Phillips Hospital in St. Louis.

Realizing the odds against the black nurse in the areas of education, employment, and organized nursing, Mrs. Osborne joined forces with other members of the National Association of Colored Graduate Nurses (NACGN) to fight discrimination on all those fronts. Not only did she provide leadership as president for five years, striking hard for principles and convictions, but she was instrumental in securing financial support for NACGN from such sources as the Rosenwald Fund, the Rockefeller Foundation, and personal affluent friends among whom was Congresswoman Frances Payne Bolton of Ohio. Having been the recipient of two Julius Rosenwald fellowships to complete her bachelor's and master's degrees, Mrs. Osborne was invited by Rosenwald to join a team of scholars called social explorers, to the rural South to do a behavioristic study in health and welfare, thus giving her experience in research.

During the years of World War II, Mrs. Osborne opened many doors of opportunity for black nurses while serving officially as consultant on the staff of the National Nursing Council for War Service—the organization responsible for laying the groundwork for the Cadet Nurse Corps. After the war, she ran for election for the board of directors of the American Nurses Association, won and served four years, 1948–1952. In this capacity, she was one of ANA's delegates to the International Congress of Nurses in Stockholm, Sweden in 1949. While on the ANA Board, she served on the board of the American Journal of Nursing Company. Mrs. Osborne also served as a member of the Federal Citizens Committee to the United States on Education and as a member of the Advisory Committee to the Surgeon General, United States Public Health Service.

With such a rich background in education, nursing service, community health, research, and organizational affairs, it was logical that Mrs. Osborne would be invited shortly after the establishment of the National League for Nursing to join the staff (1954) in an administrative capacity. She retired 12 years later (1966) as associate general director and director of services to state leagues.

Mrs. Osborne was a prolific writer with articles to her credit in the *American Journal of Nursing, Public Health Nursing, Journal of Negro Education, Harpers, Opportunity Magazine, Crisis,* and the *Trained Nurse and Hospital Review.* Her life story has been included in many books and periodicals. She did not confine her voluntary activities to the nursing community. She extended herself to the broader community serving such organizations as the National Council of Negro Women (first vice-president); the National Urban League; the Legal Defense Fund of the National Association for the Advancement of Colored People (board); Alpha Kappa Alpha Sorority; Women's Africa Committee; the United Mutual Life Insurance Company (board); and other civic associations.

In recognition of her contributions, Mrs. Osborne received numerous honors and awards; the Mary Mahoney Award (1946) for opening opportunities for the black nurse to move into the mainstream of professional nursing; the establishment of the Estelle Massey Scholarship at Fisk University, Nashville, in recognition of her contributions to community life; nurse of the year by the New York University Division of Nurse Education (1959); Honorary Life Membership Award, Nursing Education Alumni Association, Teachers College, Columbia University (1976); and Honorary Member, Omicron Chapter, Chi Eta Phi Sorority. These are in addition to the many testimonials in her lifetime, tapes, and documentary films.

Mrs. Osborne was a great lady and a pioneer in nursing who exemplified the ideal for all nurses regardless of race . . . a lady who carried out her personal and professional responsibilities with dignity, majesty, sincerity, and warmth. In appreciation of her many contributions, Academy Fellows enter this tribute in the records of the American Academy of Nursing. (Written and presented by Mary Elizabeth Carnegie at the Annual Meeting of the American Academy of Nursing, Portland, Oregon, 1982.)

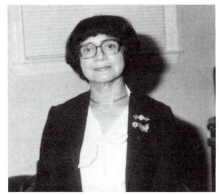

Figure 4–56   Dr. Marie Bourgeois, Honorary Fellow, AAN, 1982.

Marie Bourgeois (Diploma, Freedmen's Hospital School of Nursing, Washington, DC; Ph.D., The Catholic University of America, Washington, DC) (Fig. 4–56), was admitted to the American Academy of Nursing as an Honorary Fellow in 1982. At that time, she was assistant professor in the nursing administration major at Georgetown University in Washington, DC. She performs consultant work in nursing education nationally and internationally for directors and administrators concerned with doctoral programs in nursing and for nurses at the baccalaureate and master's level who are preparing for a career in nursing research. She has been instrumental in assisting 276 graduate nurses complete their doctoral training, providing encouragement and consultation about career patterns, goals, and the scientific merit of the doctoral degree. Currently, Bourgeois is adjunct associate professor, Graduate Program, Howard University College of Nursing, Washington, DC.

Bourgeois is one of the most recognized nurse researchers in the United States in predoctoral and postdoctoral training. As a former chief of the Research Training Section of the Nursing Research Branch, Division of Nursing, Department of Health, Education, and Welfare, she founded and administered the National Research Service Awards Fellowship Program, which provided funding for nurses in predoctoral and postdoctoral studies throughout the nation. She was the organizer of the National Conference on Doctoral Education for Nurses in 1971, which resulted in a publication entitled *Future Directions of Doctoral Education for Nurses.* The conference focused the attention of the nursing community nationally on the goals and objectives of doctoral education for nurses.

In the field of doctoral education for nurses, Bourgeois has presented numerous papers before various assemblies and has published a number of reports and articles, including "The Special Nurse Research Fellow: Characteristics and Recent Trends," published in *Nursing Research* in 1975; "Research Training Beyond the Doctoral Degree," co-authored with Phillips and Wood, in *Glowing Lamp,* 1987; and *The Fifty Year Graduates of Freedmen's Hospital Tell Their Stories, 1913–1935,* published in 1987.

Bourgeois has maintained her interest in anthropology, the field in which she did her doctoral studies. She has written several articles and has presented papers on the relationships between nursing and anthropology. She was on the board of directors of the Anthropological Society of Washington, DC, from 1973 to 1976 and became president in 1979. She is also a Fellow of the American Anthropological Association.

Bourgeois organized a workshop presented at the National Boulé of Chi Eta Phi Sorority in Washington, DC, in 1982, on "The Role of the Black Nurse in Health Care Delivery." She also organized a workshop on "The Effect of Budgetary Constraints on Black Schools of Nursing," given at the National Meeting of the Freedmen's Hospital School of Nursing Alumni in June, 1982.

For outstanding leadership in the Health Resources Administration National Research Award Programs for Nurses and for expediting the training of nurse scientists nationwide, Bourgeois received the administration's Distinguished Administrative Award. She has also received the Certificate of Merit for Distinguished Service for her work as a member of the American Nurses' Foundation Board of Trustees and she was made an Honorary Fellow, Academy of Science, Washington, DC. In 1985, she received the Black Women's Outstanding Special Service Award from the Institute for Urban Affairs and Research, Howard University, Washington, DC.

SOUTHERN COUNCIL ON COLLEGIATE EDUCATION FOR NURSING

Formal provision for interstate cooperation was built into the Constitution of the United States in 1787 (Article I, Section 10) by the Founding Fathers. This compact clause permitted the states, with the consent of Congress, to enter into agreements with each other on many matters which, at first, were mostly political in nature—settlement of boundary disputes, apportionment of water, and so forth. It was not until 1948, when the southern states entered into an interstate compact and created the Southern Regional Education Board (SREB) for the purpose of improving higher education in the South, that nursing began to benefit from this constitutional provision (Carnegie, 1968).

Nursing has been represented on the SREB at the outset with the appointment by the respective state governors of two nurses: Mary Elizabeth Carnegie, dean, Florida A&M University School of Nursing, Tallahassee; and Frances Helen Ziegler, dean, Vanderbilt University School of Nursing, Nashville, Tennessee. Through the efforts of these two, along with Alma Gault, dean, Meharry Medical College School of Nursing, Nashville, nursing became a vital part of SREB in 1950, beginning with a Committee on Graduate Education and Research in Nursing. In 1962, the collegiate nursing programs in the region, which had been focusing mostly on graduate education, began to consider a broad range of issues in nursing education and research. The need for a formal communication network among the institutions and between SREB and the institutions prompted the formation of the SREB Council on Collegiate Education for Nursing (Spector, 1987). By 1975, the council had become an independent, self-support organization within the structure of SREB. In affiliation with SREB, the council engages in "cooperative regional planning and activities to strengthen nursing education in colleges and universities in the South" (Reitt, 1987, p. 11).

In 1972, Eula Aiken (Fig. 4–57), joined the professional staff of SREB as project director. In 1990, she succeeded Audrey Spector, who had retired in 1989 as executive director, Southern Council on Collegiate Education for

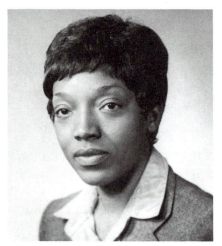

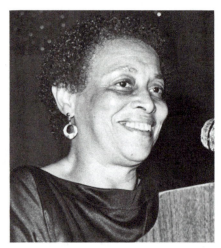

Figure 4–57   Dr. Eula Aiken, Chief Executive Officer, Southern Council on
Collegiate Education for Nursing.

Figure 4–58   Goldie Brangman, President,
American Association of Nurse Anesthetists, 1973–1974.

Nursing. For five years before then, Aiken had directed SREB's Continu-
ing Nursing Education in Computer Technology project, a Nursing Spiral
Project Grant No. DIONU24198, awarded by the Division of Nursing,
U.S. Department of Health and Human Services.

THE AMERICAN ASSOCIATION OF NURSE ANESTHETISTS

The American Association of Nurse Anesthetists (AANA), founded in
1931, is the professional organization of the nation's certified registered
nurse anesthetists (CRNAs)—anesthesia specialists who administer more
than half the 26 million anesthetics given to patients in the United States
yearly. Headquartered in Park Ridge, Illinois, the association maintains a
Washington, DC office.

From 1973 to 1974, Goldie Brangman (Fig. 4–58), director emerita,
School of Anesthesia, Harlem Hospital, New York, NY, served as president.

ASSOCIATION OF OPERATING ROOM NURSES

The Association of Operating Room Nurses (AORN) is a voluntary
organization of professional operating room nurses with both national and

international members. AORN encourages cooperative action by registered nurses to improve the quality of perioperative nursing care delivered by nurses directly working in the operating room. AORN was founded in 1949 in New York City. Today, it is home to more than 48,000 members in 50 states and 55 foreign countries and has almost 400 chapters. The Association currently employs a staff of approximately 100 people at the Headquarters building in Denver, Colorado.

In its 45-year old history, AORN has had an elected black president—Barba Edwards, who served from 1976 to 1977. At that time, Edwards was director of surgery, Archbishop Berger Mercy Hospital, Omaha, Nebraska. She now serves on the board of AORN Foundation.

PLANNED PARENTHOOD FEDERATION OF AMERICA

The Planned Parenthood Federation of America had a black president, Faye Wattleton (B.S., Ohio State University School of Nursing, Columbus; M.S., Columbia University, New York, NY) (Fig. 4–59), for 14 years—1978 to 1992. Wattleton, also a certified nurse-midwife, frequently appeared on television and spoke before large groups. She constantly traveled to keep up to date on the organization's 26,000 staff members at 860 clinics in 49 states (Great Catches, 1990).

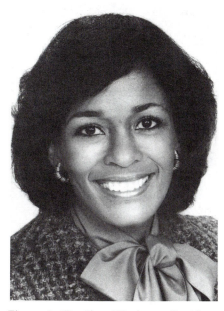

Figure 4–59 Faye Wattleton, President, Planned Parenthood Federation of America, 1978–1992.

Planned Parenthood, a nonprofit health care organization with a combined annual budget of nearly $300 million was started in 1916 by a nurse, Margaret Sanger. Sanger fought in the early part of the century for revision of archaic legislation that prohibited discussion and distributing contraceptives, and she opened the first birth control clinic in America. The federation is based on the principle that every individual has the fundamental right to choose when or whether to have a child.

Wattleton is credited with developing the organization's extensive national grassroots advocacy network that became a powerful lobbying force to block efforts to restrict and overturn women's rights to make reproductive choices. Additionally, her powerful and articulate leadership gave the organization visibility that furthered its mission and extended its reach. During Wattleton's administration, she directed the expansion of reproductive health care services for women and families from 1.1 million to about 5 million in 1990. Her strong leadership made a powerful difference in the lives of many American women and their families. In 1993, she was inducted into the National Women's Hall of Fame in Seneca Falls, New York.

THE AMERICAN ACADEMY OF AMBULATORY CARE NURSING

The American Academy of Ambulatory Care Nursing (AAACN), founded in 1978 as the American Academy of Ambulatory Nursing Administration, is an association of professional nurses who identify ambulatory care nursing as essential to the continuum of high quality, cost-effective patient care. A voluntary, nonprofit organization, it provides a forum for nurses with responsibility in ambulatory care.

The goals of the Academy are to shape professional practice and the environment, build collaborative relationships, and provide innovative thinking and vision in ambulatory care. The development and publication of *Ambulatory Care Nursing Administration and Practice Standards,* first published in 1987

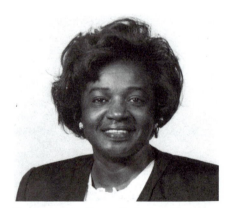

Figure 4–60   Betty Redwine, President, American Associate of Ambulatory Nursing, 1987–1988.

and revised in 1993, is evidence of AAACN's commitment to meeting these goals.

AAACN has had a black president, Betty Redwine (AD, Front Range Community College, Denver, Colorado; B.S., Regis College of Denver) (Fig. 4–60), a charter member who served from 1987 to 1988.

AAACN Viewpoint, a bimonthly newsletter, is the official publication of the organization.

CARIBBEAN AMERICAN NURSES ASSOCIATION

Conceptualized in the early 1970s by a group of nurses in New York from Jamaica, the Caribbean American Nurses Association (CANA) was formally organized in New York in 1979 with Marilyn Parker as the first elected president (Fig. 4–61). According to the constitution and bylaws adopted in 1980, CANA is composed of organizations of nurses from the Caribbean and individual members of Caribbean origin: Barbados, Belize, Grenada, Carriacou & Petit Martinique, Guyana, Panama, Jamaica, and Trinidad & Tobago.

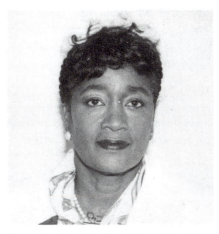

Figure 4–61 Marilyn Parker, First President, Caribbean American Nurses Association.

CANA's objectives are to: (1) become actively involved in community affairs primarily in the area of health and education; (2) become a resource group for nurses from the Caribbean; (3) become actively involved in legislation as it relates to nursing and health care; and (4) become a medium of communication among nurses from the Caribbean.

Catherine Bovell (Diploma, St. Anns School of Nursing, Trinidad & Tobago; M.A., Teachers College, Columbia University, New York), Case Manager, Montefiore Hospital Home Care Agency, Bronx, NY, is the current president of CANA.

COALITION OF AFRICAN NURSES

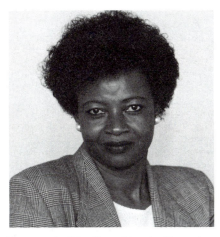

Figure 4–62 Dr. Ngozi Knongho, Founder Coalition of African Nurses.

The Coalition of African Nurses (CAN) was founded in New York in 1994 by Ngozi O. Nkongho,

R.N., Ph.D. (Fig. 4–62) to promote communication among African nurses throughout the world. At the founding meeting were nurses from Egypt, Zimbabwe, Botswana, South Africa, Mali, Morocco, Nigeria, and Ghana. Goals identified were to: (1) provide information and support on nursing and health care to African nurses in the United States; (2) develop a network among African nurses in the United States; and (3) stimulate and maintain appreciation of African cultures while integrating modern technology in health care.

CAN's objectives are to provide information to its members, develop networks among African nurses, and encourage cultural appreciation.

SUMMARY

Black nurses have always taken pride in helping to promote the professionalization of nursing. This chapter has addressed the trials and tribulations of black nurses fighting against the odds for recognition in the major national nursing organizations, particularly the American Nurses Association. Black organizations have also been included, along with a regional body that has a black chief executive, and several specialty organizations that have or have had black nurses in top leadership positions—elected or appointed. Attention is also paid to the International Council of Nurses which, in addition to board and committee representation, had a black president from Kenya from 1981 to 1985.

REFERENCES

ANA presidency is rigorous, exhilarating. (1982). *American Nurse, 14,* 15.

American Nurses' Association convention proceedings. New York: American Nurses' Association.

American Academy of Nursing Mission Statement. (1990). *Nursing outlook.* S.B. Louis: Mosley-Yearbook.

Bourne, S. T. (1989). Mabel K. Staupers Spingarn Medalist dies at 99. *Crisis, 96*(1)37, 39.

Breay, M. E., & Fenwick, E. B. (1931). *History of the International Council of Nurses, 1899–1925.* Geneva: International Council of Nurses.

Bridges, D. C. (1967). *A history of the International Council of Nurses: 1899–1964,* the first sixty-five years. Philadelphia: Lippincott.

Carnegie, M. E. (1952). Using the nursing abilities study in curriculum planning. *American Journal of Nursing, 52,* 1482–1486.

Carnegie, M. E. (1968). Interstate cooperation in nursing. *Nursing Outlook, 16,* 48–49.

Christ, E. A. (1957). *Missouri's nurses.* Jefferson City: Missouri Nurses' Association.

Dock, L. A. (1912). *A history of nursing,* (Vol. III). New York: G. P. Putnam, Sons.

First annual report of the American Society of Superintendents of Training Schools for Nurses. (1897). New York: National League for Nursing Press.

Fitzpatrick, M. L. (1975). *The National Organization for Public Health Nursing, 1912–1952, development of a practice field.* New York: National League for Nursing Press.

Flanagan, L. (1976). *One strong voice, the story of the American Nurses' Association.* Kansas City: American Nurses Association.

Fondiller, S. H. (1989). *The vision, the reality: A history of AACN's first 20 years: 1969–1989.* Washington, DC: American Association of Colleges of Nursing.

Fondiller, S. H. (1990). Nursing's journal 1900–1990. *American Journal of Nursing, 90*(10), 18, 22, 33, 40, 42, 46, 50, 56, 60, 68, 74, 80, 84, 94, 96, 98.

Gist, N. P. (1940). *Secret societies: A cultural study of fraternalism in the United States.* University of Missouri: Columbia.

Hughes, L. (1962). *Fight for freedom.* New York: Norton.

International Council of Nurses. (1966). *Basic Documents: Constitution and regulations, rules, procedures at meetings.* Geneva: International Council of Nurses.

ICN Constitution. (1993). Geneva, Switzerland.

ICNF receives funding for International Classification Standards. (1994). *Nursing Outlook, 42,* 46.

Jamieson, E. M., & Sewall, M. (1944). *Trends in nursing history.* Philadelphia: Saunders.

Kim, M. I. (1993). Overview: the International Council of Nurses: The Past, Present & Future. *Imprint, 40,* 57–60.

Marshall-Burnett, S. (1985). Fifteen years of the ICN/3M fellowship program. *International Nursing Review, 32,* 48–49.

Massey (Osborne), E. (1934). The negro nurse student. *American Journal of Nursing, 34,* 806–810.

Minor, I., & Shaw, E. (1973). ANA and affirmative action. *American Journal of Nursing, 73,* 1738–1739.

Mullen, F. (1989). *Plagues and politics: The story of the U.S. Public Health Service.* New York: Basic Books.

National Sample Survey of R.N.'s (1992). Bureau of Health Professions, Division of Nursing, Department of Health & Human Services.

National Student Nurses Association bylaws. (1972). New York: National Student Nurses' Association.

Nursing research report. (1976). Kansas City: American Nurses' Foundation.

Reitt, B. B. (1987). *The first 25 years of the Southern Council on Collegiate Education for Nursing (SCCEN).* Atlanta: Southern Council on Collegiate Education for Nursing.

Report of NOPHN council on Negro nursing. (1942). NOPHN Archive Microfilm, No. 17.

Roberts, M. M. (1954). *American nursing: History and Interpretation.* New York: Macmillan.

Seymer, L. B. (1933). *A general history of nursing.* New York: Macmillan.

Spector, A. F. (1987). Preface. *In the first 25 years of Southern Council on Collegiate Education for Nursing (SCCEN).* Atlanta: Southern Council on Collegiate Education for Nursing.

Staupers, M. K. (1951). Story of the National Association of Colored Graduate Nurses. *American Journal of Nursing, 51,* 222–223.

Staupers, M. K. (1961). *No time for prejudice.* New York: Macmillan.

Summary of proceedings, ANA convention. (1982). Kansas City: American Nurses' Association.

Smith, G. R. (1975). From invisibility to blackness: the story of the National Black Nurses' Association. *American Journal of Nursing, 23,* 225–229.

The evolution of nursing professional organizations: Alternatives for the future. (1987). Kansas City: American Academy of Nursing.

The thalamus. (1993). Newsletter of the ICN Centennial History Project. *2,* 1–2.

This is ANA. (1975). Kansas City: American Nurses Association.

Chapter
5

Stony the Road

Brown (1948) in her report, *Nursing for the Future,* pointed out that specialists in clinical nursing would be needed "if the profession is to look forward to a sound, healthy development" (p. 95). It was not until 10 years later that the American Nurses' Association (ANA) set the goal "to establish ways within ANA to provide formal recognition of personal achievement and superior performance." This was the origin of ANA's certification program, which is a part of its credentialing system (Dunkley, 1974).

Credentialing mechanisms serve to provide assurance of quality to the various publics that individuals, programs, or institutions serve. Licensing of individual nurses and state approval of schools of nursing began with the first registration laws in 1903 in North Carolina, New York, New Jersey, and Virginia. The stated purpose of the bill in North Carolina, for example, was "to secure for future nurses better education in theory and such skill in practice that the public will have confidence in the registered nurse" (Wyche, 1938, p. 95). National accreditation of educational programs came later, and the first list of schools accredited by the National League of Nursing Education was published in 1941. Today, diploma, associate degree, baccalaureate, and master's degree programs are accredited by the National League for Nursing (NLN). Certification of nurses who have specialized in a specific area of clinical practice, however, is a recent development, beginning with the certification program of the ANA. This credentialing mechanism has evolved into the American Nurses Credentialing Center

151

(ANCC). The first chair of the ANCC Commission on Certification was Dr. Beverly Clair Harris Robinson (Fig. 5–1). She has also been involved in credentialing policy issues and policy making, certification, test development, and committee appointments.

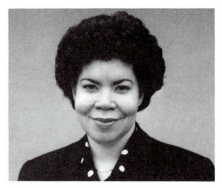

Figure 5–1   Dr. Beverly Clair Robinson, first chairperson, ANCC Commission on Accreditation.

In May 1973, ANA formally announced the initiation of its nationwide certification program to recognize excellence in the clinical practice of nursing. Unlike certification programs that merely acknowledge educational attainments, ANA certification is based on three factors: assessment of knowledge, demonstration of competence in clinical practice, and endorsement by colleagues. With the administration of certification examinations in geriatric nursing and pediatric nursing in ambulatory health care in May 1974, and a psychiatric and mental health nursing examination in September of that year, ANA launched its recognition program. In January 1975, the first nurse-practitioners certified for excellence in clinical practice were honored with a formal ceremony (Flanagan, 1976).

The American Nurses Credentialing Center was established in 1990 and currently offers certification in 21 clinical areas. Over 90,000 nurses, including a number of blacks, are currently certified by ANCC (Wharton, 1992). Certification is valid for five years at which time it can be renewed through evidence of practice and continuing education or reexamination. Most of the certification examinations require a degree for eligibility. It is anticipated that in the near future, the bachelor's degree will be required for generalist certification and the master's degree for all specialist certification.'

In the United States, as of December 1992, there were an estimated 37,963 nurses who held national certification or state recognition as nurse practitioners (NPs) or certified clinical nurse specialists (CNSs). Of the total population of certified nurses, an estimated 29,965 were certified as NPs through national certifying organizations (The American Nurses Credentialing Center, The National Certification Boards of Pediatric Nurse Practitioners and Nurses, and the National Certification Corporation for the Obstetric, Gynecologic, and Neonatal Nursing Specialist) or through State recognition processes. An estimated 10,217 of the total were nationally certified or state recognized as CNSs (Washington Consulting Group, 1994).

The first trained black nurses practiced before the profession had a credentialing system, and many were practicing before all of the states had passed licensing laws for nursing practice. In this chapter, the experiences of four such black nurses—Jessie Sleet Scales, the first black public health nurse, Elizabeth Tyler Barringer, the first black nurse employed at the Henry Street Visiting Nurse Service, Edith Carter and Emma Wilson, later at Henry Street—are reported.

In 1936, the National Association of Colored Graduate Nurses (NACGN) established the Mary Mahoney Award to be given to "a nurse who had made outstanding contributions to the nursing profession and to the community, and who also had worked to improve the professional status of the Negro nurse, thereby helping to improve intergroup and interpersonal relations within the nursing profession" (Staupers, 1961, p. 35). In 1942, an exception was made, and the award was presented to a nonnurse, Ruth Logan Roberts, who had chaired NACGN's National Advisory Council and who had given freely of her time for the improvement of the professional status of the black nurse.

After NACGN dissolved in 1951 and the function of awarding the Mary Mahoney Award was assumed by the ANA, the criteria were changed to "a person, or group of persons, who, in addition to making a significant contribution to nursing generally, has been outstandingly instrumental in achieving the opening and advancement of opportunities in nursing on the same basis to members of all races, creeds, colors, and national origins." These criteria do not limit the award to a black nurse(s) and in 1954, 1956, 1962, 1964, 1966, and 1986, the Mary Mahoney Award went to white nurses. In 1992, an American Indian nurse was the recipient (see Appendix C).

It seems fitting, also, in this chapter to elaborate on the contributions of the early black nurses who were recipients of the Mary Mahoney Award when it was presented by the NACGN, for it was these pioneers who paved the way for the black nurse of today. References to 5 of the 13 nurse recipients appear in other chapters—Adah B. Thoms, the first recipient in 1936, Mabel Northcross, Susan Freeman, Estelle Osborne, and Mabel Staupers—so they will not be included in this chapter. The 8 presented here are Nancy Lois Kemp, Carrie E. Bullock, Petra A. Pinn, Lula G. Warlick, Ellen Woods Carter, Ludie A. Andrews, Mary E. Merritt, and Eliza F. Pillars.

The origin of organized visiting nursing dates to 1859 in England. William Rathbone, a wealthy man, had employed Mary Robinson to nurse his wife during the last stages of her terminal illness. In his grief, Mr. Rathbone pondered the predicament of poor families, bereft of money and comfortable surroundings, who might be faced with long-term illness. He asked Miss Robinson to try an experiment for three months, giving nursing care to families in the poorer quarters of Liverpool. In the United States, Lillian Wald is credited with founding visiting nursing in New York in 1893 with her establishment of the first nurses' settlement house, which developed into the great organization of the Henry Street Visiting Nurse Service.

Thoms (1929), Roberts (1954), and Staupers (1961) report that **Jessie Sleet (Scales)** (Fig. 5–2) was the first black public health nurse in the United States. Miss Sleet, a native of

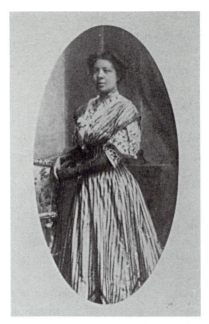

Figure 5–2 Jessie Sleet Scales, first black public health nurse.

Stratford, Ontario, Canada, and a graduate of the 1895 class of Provident Hospital School of Nursing in Chicago, had always had a strong desire to become a district nurse, a field of practice that had not been opened to black nurses. When she moved to New York, she applied to many agencies for employment in this area of practice, only to have the doors closed to her because of her race. As Morais (1967) points out in capturing the mood of the times, "That she was a graduate nurse when such nurses were a rarity meant nothing. That her skin was colored meant everything" (p. 71).

After discovering that none of the existing health organizations employed blacks, Sleet finally appealed to the Charity Organization Society. The Society's tuberculosis committee had become concerned about the high incidence of tuberculosis among the black population of the City of New York and thought that a black nurse could persuade the victims to seek treatment. With this in mind, Sleet was employed on October 3, 1900, for a two-month trial period. She performed her duties so well that after a year she was given a permanent position, which she held for nine years.

The first volume of the *American Journal of Nursing* contains a copy of Sleet's report on her work as a district nurse among black people of New York City for a two-month period in 1900. Following is an excerpt, submitted for publication by her superior:

> Visiting 41 sick families, caring for 9 cases of consumption, 4 cases of peritonitis, 2 cases of chicken pox, 2 of cancer, one diphtheria, 2 heart disease, 2 tumor, one gastric catarrh, 2 pneumonia, 4 rheumatism, 2 cases of scalp wound . . . Other cases might be spoken of, but the above is a specimen of the work . . . I cannot but feel that this house-to-house visiting, these face-to-face practical talks which I am having with the people, must bring about good results. They have welcomed me to their homes, saying, We don't know you, but we belong to the same race. They have listened to me with attention and respect, and if the advice which I gave was not always accepted, in no case was it readily rejected. (*A Successful Experiment,* 1901, p. 729)

The editor of the *American Journal of Nursing* described Miss Sleet as "a young colored woman and a trained nurse, whose genuine altruism and intelligence in social reform work has impressed with admiration her acquaintances and friends, one of whom ventures, without her knowledge, to make this record of her work."

Many black nurses performed significant roles and made valuable contributions to the development of visiting nurse service. Three who are singled out for their work are Elizabeth Tyler Barringer, Edith Carter, and Emma Wilson.

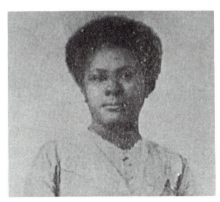

Figure 5–3 Elizabeth Tyler Barringer, first black nurse on staff of Henry Street Visiting Nurse Service.

In 1906, **Elizabeth Tyler** (Fig. 5–3), a graduate of Freedmen's Hospital School of Nursing in Washington, DC, was appointed to the staff of the Henry Street Visiting Nurse Service (renamed the Visiting Nurse Service of New York) by Lillian Wald, the founder, who also had become concerned about blacks' high morbidity and mortality rates from tuberculosis and their high maternal and infant death rates. Soon, two more black nurses were employed: **Edith Carter** and **Emma Wilson,** also from Freedmen's. A news item in the September, 1906, issue of the *American Journal of Nursing* reports:

> From Miss Dock, we learn that the Nurses' Settlement in New York is happy in several important additions to its work. A most gratifying and needed extension in the Visiting Nurse Service had been made in an upper west side region where the colored people live. Salaries have been given for two nurses who are also colored and who have settled in their district in a flat. The work is fortunate indeed in the rare ability and devotion of these two women. Besides being excellent nurses, they are both especially alive to social movements and organized preventive work. (*Nurses' Settlement News*, 1906, p. 832)

Not only did Tyler pioneer in public health nursing in New York City, but also in Philadelphia at the Henry Phipps Institute for Tuberculosis, the State and Welfare Commission of Delaware and the Essex County Tuberculosis Association in New Jersey, working to solve the health and social problems of blacks and bringing their plight to the attention of health officials.

In 1911, the first county public health agency in the United States was established in Greensboro, North Carolina, at the Guilford County Health Department, which employed a staff of nurses. To serve the black community, black nurses were employed. In 1915, a bill was passed in the legislature requiring public and private hospitals, sanatariums, and such institutions in North Carolina where colored patients were admitted for treatment and where nurses were employed to hire "colored nurses" for the care of such "colored patients" (Consolidated Statutes of North Carolina, 1915). Such bills were typical all over the country but especially in the South (black nurses were employed to care for the black patients) (Fig. 5–4).

Following are biographical sketches of eight recipients of the Mary Mahoney Award when it was being awarded by the NACGN.

In 1937, **Nancy Lois Kemp** (Fig. 5–5) became the second recipient of the prestigious Mary Mahoney Award. A charter member of the NACGN, Kemp worked with the organization until her retirement to achieve equal opportunity for black nurses. In recognition of her service to NACGN as member, treasurer, and vice-president, the organization gave Kemp an honorary life membership.

Kemp was born in Virginia and lived in Washington, DC, where she attended Howard University for two years before entering Freedmen's Hospital School of Nursing. Immediately after her graduation, she went to

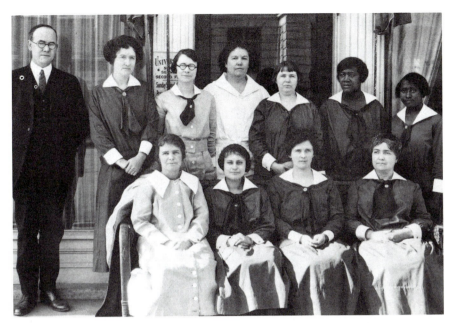

Figure 5–4 Black nurses on the staff of Guilford County Health Department, Greensboro, NC, 1924. The two black nurses in the second row are (left to right) Marian Forney Smith and Louie Booker Benton.

Philadelphia, where she practiced private duty nursing, specializing in massage treatment. When World War I began, she joined an active unit of the American Red Cross and became an instructor. She organized first aid classes and supply units.

With the influx of blacks from the South at this time, public health nurses were in great demand in northern cities. Kemp became interested in the field of public health nursing and prepared for this work by studying public health at the University of Pennsylvania. In 1922, she was appointed to the position of staff nurse at the Henry Phipps Institute, which specialized in the study, treatment, and prevention of tuberculosis. The Henry Phipps Institute, the Philadelphia Health Council, and the Whittier

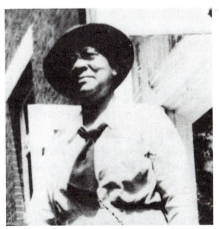

Figure 5–5 Nancy Lois Kemp, second recipient of Mary Mahoney Award, 1937.

Center jointly opened a health clinic in the northwest section of Philadelphia in 1923. Kemp served as supervisor of this dispensary for eight years, and was then transferred back to the Phipps Institute where she remained until retirement in 1940. She died three years later.

Carrie E. Bullock (Fig. 5–6) was graduated from the Scotia Seminary, Concord, North Carolina, before entering the nursing school of Provident Hospital in Chicago in 1909. A few weeks prior to her graduation from Provident, she was asked by its superin-

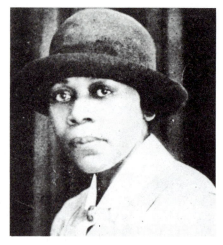

Figure 5–6   Carrie E. Bullock, third recipient of Mary Mahoney Award, 1938.

tendent to join the staff of the Chicago Visiting Nurses Association where she worked for 40 years. Beginning as a staff nurse, Bullock became assistant supervisor, and then supervisor of the Chicago Visiting Nurses' Association services to the black people of Chicago, the first black nurse to serve in such a capacity. She was thoroughly interested in her profession, reading and studying everything that might serve as a stepping stone toward a higher plane of nursing efficiency. She also took many courses at centers that sponsored extension work for nurses and social workers.

Bullock continued to serve nursing until her death in 1961. During World War II, she served on a NACGN committee created to struggle for the inclusion of the black nurse in the Army Nurse Corps. She was the first black nurse to speak on national leadership at a professional nursing meeting after the "merger" of ANA and NACGN, and she worked for unity within the integrated association.

Among the dedicated northern women who pioneered in nursing in the southern part of the United States was **Petra A. Pinn** (Fig. 5–7). "Pet," as she was known to all her friends, was a graduate of the class of 1906 from John Andrew Memorial Hospital School of Nursing at Tuskegee University in Alabama. After graduation, Pinn served as head nurse at Hale Infirmary in Montgomery, Alabama, and later became superintendent of nurses at the Red Cross Sanitarium and Training School in Louisville, Kentucky. She also worked as a metropolitan nurse in the same city.

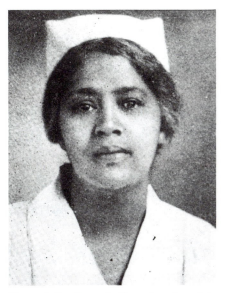

Figure 5–7   Petra A. Pinn, fourth recipient of Mary Mahoney Award, 1939.

Because of her preference for institutional work, Pinn accepted an appointment as superintendent of nurses, the Pine Ridge Hospital in West Palm Beach, Florida. After 10 years of dedicated work, making friends for the hospital, raising money, and serving without an assistant, she was obliged to retire for a much-needed rest. A year later, she accepted a position as manager of a small hospital in Miami and then worked in a number of small southern communities. She worked at Seaview Hospital in New York City before retiring to live with her family in Wilberforce, Ohio, where she remained until her death in 1958.

Pinn was a charter member of NACGN and served as its president from 1923 to 1926 and as treasurer from 1929 to 1946. While president, she tried to establish a national headquarters for NACGN, and, until this could be accomplished, she supported the registry program to help black nurses find jobs.

In 1939, Pinn accepted the Mary Mahoney Award for her contributions and dedicated service in nursing for blacks in the South. At a time when working as a nurse in the South brought problems and dangers as well as challenges, she helped maintain hospitals for blacks in Alabama, Florida, Kentucky, South Carolina, and Virginia. She was never afraid of difficult or unknown situations. She was the answer to those critics who at the time said that nurses reared in the North would not work in the South because of the indignities that black nurses suffered there and the unequal salaries that they were forced to accept. By working in spite of these obstacles, Pinn set an example for other young black nurses who subsequently made contributions to the health and well-being of blacks in the South.

Lula G. Warlick (Fig. 5–8) served the nursing profession in urban areas in the Midwest and East. After graduating from North Carolina's Scotia Seminary in 1907, she entered Lincoln School for Nurses in New York. Upon graduating in 1910, she accepted the position as head nurse in the Gynecology Department and Operating Room at Lincoln Hospital.

Welcoming the opportunity to work in another part of the country, she accepted the position of assistant superintendent of nurses at Provident Hospital in Chicago in 1911, holding this position for two years and often acting as superintendent of nurses. From Chicago, she went to Kansas City, Missouri, where she became superintendent of nurses at General Hospital No. 2, which had a bed capacity of 300. According to Christ (1957), this was the "first municipal hospital managed completely by blacks" (p. 203).

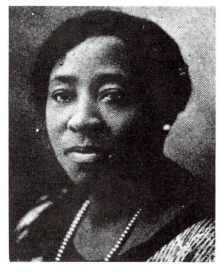

Figure 5–8   Lula G. Warlick, fifth recipient of Mary Mahoney Award, 1940.

In 1920, Warlick returned East as superintendent of nurses at Mercy Hospital in Philadelphia. When she arrived, the School of Nursing at Mercy Hospital had only 16 students and was not approved by the State Board of Nursing in Pennsylvania. As a result of her efforts, the school became a Class A school, completely approved by the State Board of Examiners. By 1929, the student enrollment had grown to 40 and the number of faculty had increased from three to nine. Lula Warlick took courses at the University of Iowa and at Columbia University in New York in order to keep her students informed of the latest developments in the nursing profession.

Warlick often spoke of her pride in the development of blacks in the nursing profession, noting that black nurses kept apace of the many changes in nursing education and that they held positions similar to those held by members of other groups. Warlick was awarded the Mary Mahoney Medal in 1940.

Ellen Woods Carter (Fig. 5–9) dedicated her professional life to improving health conditions for blacks in the South. In Virginia, North Carolina, South Carolina, and Louisiana, Carter met head-on the double standards that made her work so difficult. In addition to prejudice and the fact that her salary was less than that paid to a white nurse, she faced the indifference of blacks to their health problems. She knew that this indifference was born of frustration and neglect, a direct result of the segregation and discrimination that blacks experienced continually. Even their health care facilities were poorer than those for whites. These conditions were a

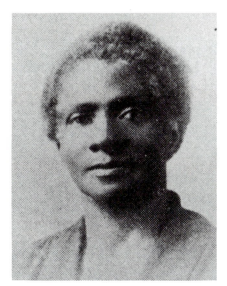

Figure 5–9 Ellen Woods Carter, 1941 recipient of Mary Mahoney Award.

challenge to Carter, and she worked to this end, doing all in her power to improve the health care of the black families with whom she worked.

Carter was graduated from Dixie Hospital School of Nursing in Hampton, Virginia, 1895. After graduation, she became head nurse at Good Physicians' Hospital in Columbia, South Carolina. This small institution was the only one in the city where black people could receive medical care. It was operated by white physicians and financed by northern white Episcopalians. She devoted herself to this position for six years and then resigned to undertake even more challenging work.

At this time, the Bureau of Child Welfare of the South Carolina State Board of Health was extending its role in a number of counties by forming classes for the instruction of midwives. Special attention was called to the instruction of black midwives, who numbered several thousand in the state. Carter was placed in Beaufort County to do midwife supervision and public health work among her own race. Beaufort County, composed of a series of small islands, had a population of 5,000 of which 4,500 were black. The blacks who inhabited the sea islands were isolated from other people and from medical services. Because communications between them and the mainland were difficult, they had to depend on the midwives for medical treatment as well as obstetric care.

When Carter started her first class in Beaufort County, only three women attended; the others were afraid or did not understand. She reported this to the local registrar, who sent an officer to round them up. After this she had no further trouble. The women came from miles around to spend the entire day learning from her, to listen to her instruction, and to see her demonstrations. Most of the midwives were unable to read or write, but they learned quickly through Carter's classes.

Another project of this remarkable nurse was her work in persuading families, especially prospective mothers, to accept care by trained physicians. While promoting care by a physician, she knew that a large number of black babies would be delivered by midwives, and she continued to work hard to improve the services they provided, making house-to-house visits to arouse the interest of each family and spreading the gospel of health through the churches and schools. Both white and black physicians helped her in her efforts to teach health and hygiene to the inhabitants of Beaufort County, where she spent 16 challenging and productive years.

After her service in Beaufort, Carter was given a trip abroad by the Bureau of Hygiene and Public Health Nursing. While in Rome, she spoke through an interpreter to a mothers' meeting, telling them about dietary measures and the proper care of infants and demonstrating her important points.

Carter knew that for any health program to be effective trained personnel would be needed. One of her favorite projects was to encourage bright young women to become nurses, conducting her own recruitment program. In 1941, when she received the Mary Mahoney Award, she could attest to 55 young women who had entered schools of nursing because of her interest and encouragement.

When nursing practice laws became a reality, not all states gave black nurses the opportunity to take the examinations to become licensed to practice nursing. Georgia was one such state. Recognition is given to **Ludie A. Andrews** (Fig. 5–10), a black nurse, who for 10 years fought the battle to gain the right for black nurses to practice nursing within the laws of the State of Georgia.

After completing the nursing course at Spelman College in Atlanta in 1906, Andrews was employed as superintendent of a hospital, connected with the Atlanta School of Medicine, built "to accommodate [sic] 12 Negro patients for the observation and training of medical students (white)" (*Spelman Messenger,* 1913, p. 8). She held this position for a number of years, even though she was denied the privilege of holding a license. In 1909, at her own expense, she instituted legal action against the Georgia State Board of Nurse Examiners. She argued that because black nurses did not have the same certification as white nurses, they

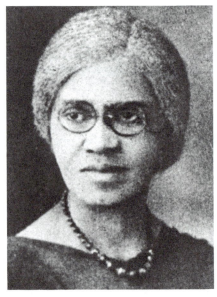

Figure 5–10   Ludie A. Andrews, 1943 recipient of Mary Mahoney Award.

would have difficulty being employed in other states. The State of Georgia offered her a license to appease her, but she refused it because other qualified black nurses were not so acknowledged. The time, effort, energy, and monies she contributed to this struggle for the rightful recognition due black nurses in Georgia were rewarded. By 1920, all black nurses who were graduated from Georgia State-approved schools of nursing were permitted to take the same examination as whites for licensure. In 1974, a black nurse, Verdelle Bellamy, a graduate of Grady Hospital School of Nursing, was appointed by Governor Jimmy Carter to the Georgia Board of Nursing Education; and a black nurse, Mary Long, served as the elected president of the Georgia Nurses' Association from 1981 to 1985. In 1985, she was elected to the board of directors of the American Nurses' Association.

It is noteworthy that in 1914, the City of Atlanta appointed Andrews to organize a school of nursing for black students at Grady Hospital. The school became State approved in 1917. Her administrative and professional capabilities in the development of the Municipal Training School for Colored Nurses were praised by officials of the City of Atlanta. In recognition of her pioneering efforts to secure registration for black nurses in Georgia, Andrews was the recipient of the NACGN Mary Mahoney Award in 1943, and the Grady Nurses Conclave presents a "Ludie Andrews Distinguished Service Award." Nurses in Georgia affectionately refer to her as the "dean of black nurses." On August 21, 1987, the Grady Alumnae Associates Conclave in Washington, DC unveiled a portrait of Andrews and presented it to Spelman College.

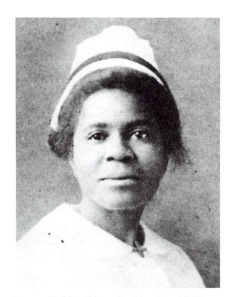

Figure 5–11   Mary E. Merritt, 1949 recipient of Mary Mahoney Award.

Mary E. Merritt (Fig. 5–11) was born in Berea, Kentucky, and received her education at Berea College. After graduation, she taught for four years in the rural schools of Kentucky. Merritt had always had an interest in caring for the sick, so when Berea College opened a small hospital for students, she decided to enter the nurses' training program there. The nursing curriculum was composed of one year of theoretical studies and one year of practical work. She and two other black women, Sarah Belle Jerman and Margaret Jones, who completed the program in 1902, were the first and only black graduates of the nursing department, since in 1904 the Kentucky law prohibited inter-racial education (Peck & Pride, 1982). Blacks would not attend Berea again until after the 1954 Supreme Court Decision. The baccalaureate program that is in operation today replaced the diploma program and the dean is a black nurse, Dr. Cora Newell-Withrow.

Because she desired additional training in a larger hospital, Merritt enrolled at Freedmen's Hospital School of Nursing in Washington, DC, in 1904. After her graduation in 1906, she returned to Kentucky as a private duty nurse for one year, then moved to Leavenworth, Kansas, where she supervised the Protective Home and Mitchell Hospital. While she was in charge, the only class of nurses ever to be graduated from Mitchell Hospital received their diplomas.

In 1911, Merritt became director of the Red Cross Hospital in Louisville, Kentucky. The hospital was founded because of the devoted work of a number of public-spirited black citizens in Louisville. They were not discouraged by a lack of funds, and under Merritt's direction, the Red Cross Hospital grew from a small, frame, rented building to a magnificent brick edifice with a well-equipped training school. In 1949, Merritt received the Mary Mahoney Award from NACGN in recognition of her outstanding 34 years of service as superintendent of nurses at the Louisville Red Cross Hospital.

Eliza Farish Pillars (Fig. 5–12) was born in Jackson, Mississippi, in 1891. She attended public schools in Jackson, then studied at Utica Junior College in Utica, Mississippi. From there she entered the School of Nursing at Meharry Medical College in Nashville, Tennessee. After graduation in 1914, she worked as an office nurse for several doctors and then worked in a number of hospitals.

In 1926, Pillars began a career in public health nursing at the Mississippi State Board of Health. During

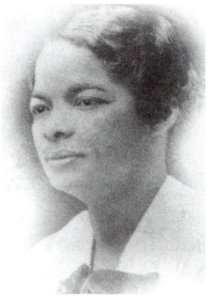

Figure 5–12   Eliza Farish Pillars, 1951 recipient of Mary Mahoney Award.

the 1920s, she was the only "accredited" public health nurse in that state. Pillars traveled into every corner and small town in Mississippi, teaching and training midwives to properly and efficiently deliver babies and take care of mothers. She gave vaccinations and inoculations against communicable diseases in schools, churches, and private homes. Wherever the people had health needs, she developed programs to meet them. In cooperation with the Mississippi State Board of Education, Pillars also taught courses in hygiene to girls in Mississippi's black high schools. Through these courses, many young women were inspired to enter the nursing profession.

Pillars, played a prominent role after Mississippi's historic 1927 flood, working diligently with the Red Cross in setting up first aid stations in Vicksburg and Natchez to take care of the flood refugees as they were brought in by boats down the Mississippi River from the Delta section of the state.

As the years passed, Pillars' eyesight weakened, and although she never became totally blind, she had to give up her work. In 1951, she became the fourteenth and last recipient of the Mary Mahoney Award given by NACGN. The organization of black Registered Nurses in Jackson, Mississippi is named the "Eliza Farish Pillars Club" in her honor. She died June 15, 1970.

SUMMARY

By definition, a pioneer is one who opens new avenues or prepares the way for others to follow. Because of the social and economic climate in the United States, many black nurses have been and still are pioneers in the health care field. In the practice areas referred to in this chapter are those black nurses who pioneered to pave the way for other black nurses. An excellent example is the story of Ludie Andrews' fight in Georgia to ensure the black nurse the right to practice her profession legally. Another example is that of Jessie Sleet Scales, who paved the way for blacks in public health nursing. More detailed accounts of many more black pioneers appear in *Pathfinders* by Thoms, and references to others are in Staupers' book, *No Time for Prejudice*. They are not repeated here. As Thoms (1929) pointed out:

> It is in the sacrifices of these early pathfinders that we see how real our life work is. Through studying the uphill struggles of the group against prejudices and misgivings the student of today learns to estimate the problems she will meet tomorrow. It is only from such a

perspective that we can guide our course in crucial times and show to the world that we are a part of the great army of consecrated women who are working toward the highest standards of nursing efficiency. (p.2)

Black nurses who forged ahead in the early 1900s exemplified courage, commitment, dedication, assertiveness, accountability, and an unwavering belief in the integrity of humankind. Today, because of these pioneers, black nurses are practicing with dignity in all areas of nursing.

REFERENCES

A successful experiment. (1901). *American Journal of Nursing, 1:* 729–731.

Brown, E. L. (1948). *Nursing for the future.* New York: Russell Sage Foundation.

Christ, E. A. *Missouri's nurses.* (1957). Jefferson City, Missouri Nurses' Association.

Consolidated Statutes of North Carolina. (1915). Raleigh.

Dunkley, P. (1974). The ANA certification program. *Nursing Clinics of North America, 9,* 485–495.

Flanagan, L. (1976). *One strong voice, the story of the American Nurses' Association.* Kansas City: The Association.

Morais, H. (1967). *The history of the negro in medicine.* New York: Publishers Co.

Nurses' settlement news. (1906). *American Journal of Nursing, 6,* 832–833.

Peck, E. S., & Pride, N. W. (1982). *Nurses in Time: Developments in Nursing Education. 1898–1981,* Berea College, Berea, Kentucky, Appalachian Fund.

Roberts, M. M. (1954). *American nursing: History and interpretation.* New York: Macmillan.

Spelman Messenger. (1913). 29, 6. Atlanta: Spelman College.

Staupers, M. K. (1961). *No time for prejudice.* New York: Macmillan.

Thoms, A. B. (1929). *Pathfinders, the progress of colored graduate nurses.* New York: Kay Printing House.

Washington Consulting Group. (1994). *Survey of certified nurse practitioners and clinical nurse specialists: December, 1992.* Washington, DC: Division of Nursing.

Wharton, C. (Ed.). (1992, Spring-Summer). *Credentialing news,* (p. 1). Washington, DC: American Nurses Credentialing Center.

Wyche, M. L. (1938). *The history of nursing in North Carolina.* Chapel Hill: University of North Carolina Press.

Chapter
6

So Proudly We Hail

T he federal government is the world's largest employer of professional registered nurses. It also provides consultant services that are helpful in improving the quality and distribution of nursing services throughout the nation. Its principal service agencies are the three military services—the Army Nurse Corps, the Navy Nurse Corps, and the Air Force Nurse Corps, the United States Public Health Service, and the Department of Veterans Affairs. In this chapter, black nurses in these agencies are discussed.

THE MILITARY

The Army Nurse Corps

Along with their sisters who nursed the soldiers in the Revolutionary and Civil Wars, the contract nurses of the Spanish-American War, under the leadership of Anita Newcomb McGee, a medical doctor, are acknowledged as the forbears of the modern Army Nurse Corps. Formally established on February 2, 1901 as a permanent corps of the Medical Department by the Army Reorganization Act of 1901, the Army Nurse Corps is the oldest of the federal nursing services. Although their initial associations with the Corps were limited to periods of international conflict when necessity forced the laying aside of racial prejudices, black nurses have served proudly and with distinction since the early days of the Corps.

Despite their honorable service in the Spanish-American War, when the Army Nurse Corps was formally established in 1901, there were no black nurses among its members. They would not serve again until 1918 when the influenza epidemic, which lasted from September 1918 to August 1919, necessitated tapping all sources of graduate nurses.

The intervening years were not, however, without activity by the black nurses desirous of serving their country. Although not specifically prohibited by regulation from joining the Army Nurse Corps, on inquiry black nurses discovered administrative hurdles. The first was the prerequisite membership in the American Red Cross, which had been designated as the primary source of reserve nurses for the military establishment by President Taft in 1911.

Adah B. Thoms, a black nurse employed in an executive capacity at Lincoln School for nurses in New York and actively involved in professional and community affairs, set about on her own not only to alert black nurses to enroll in the Red Cross, but also, through her lengthy correspondence in 1917 with Jane Delano, chairman of the American Red Cross Nursing Service, to agitate the Red Cross to remove the limitations that prevented black nurses from enrolling. These efforts led to the eventual removal of the bars. The second hurdle involved Army Nurse Corps policy, which dictated that black nurses not be accepted in the Corps because there were no separate quarters for them.

During Thoms' fight to get the color bars removed so that black nurses could serve their country, a massive influenza epidemic erupted throughout the world, causing more deaths than did the fighting (Kalisch & Kalisch, 1978). "As their doctors and nurses dropped out with the infection, army and civilian hospitals struggled with a dwindling staff until the plight of both the servicemen and their families at home was pitiful" (Dolan et al., 1983 pp. 289–290).

In a memorandum dated February 28, 1918 to Dean F. P. Keppel, Confidential Adviser, Office of the Secretary of War, Emmett J. Scott, a black man who was a special assistant in the War Department, quoted from Surgeon General William C. Gorgas' letter to him of February 14, 1918:

> Referring to your memorandum of February 12th relative to the appointment and training of colored nurses for colored soldiers, *at the present time colored nurses are not being accepted for service in the Army*

Nurse Corps as there are no separate quarters available for them, and it is not deemed advisable to assign white and colored nurses to the same posts.

After quoting the surgeon general, Mr. Scott continued in his memorandum to Mr. Keppel:

From the above, it will be seen that the whole matter of utilizing colored nurses is still very much "up in the air."

The upshot of the whole matter is that—while there are thousands of colored men who have been called to the colors as soldiers,—NO COLORED NURSES HAVE BEEN ADMITTED TO THE SERVICE, although quite a number have enrolled with the Red Cross organization as suggested, and they, together with many more well-trained, competent, and registered nurses, are ready and willing to look after sick and wounded soldiers who are now and soon will be facing shot and shell upon battlefields abroad.

I would most urgently recommend that some satisfactory way be found that will offer to colored nurses . . . the same opportunity for serving the sick and wounded soldiers, as has been so wisely and timely provided white nurses.

Waiving all discussion as to the matter of assigning white and colored nurses to the same post or quarters, it is difficult for me to understand why some colored nurses have not been given an opportunity to serve.

This vexing question is being put to me almost daily by colored newspaper editors, colored physicians, surgeons, etc., who are constantly bombarding my sector of the War Department, inquiring what has been done, and urging that something should be done in the direction of utilizing professionally trained and efficient colored nurses.

I recognize the 'problems,' but can't they be solved?

[signed] Emmett J. Scott
Special Assistant

Thus, it is noted that pressure had been put on the War Department to use the services of black nurses (Scott, 1918). The pressure of this organized campaign, coupled with the increasing need for nurses both overseas and at home, worked. In June 1918, it was officially announced that the Secretary of War had authorized the calling of black nurses in the national service. By July 1918, tentative plans were made to send black nurses in groups of 20 to several posts that had large numbers of black troops. Delays in the provision of separate quarters and dining facilities resulted in their not being officially assigned to duty until after the armistice.

The black nurses were notified by letter. Aileen Cole's letter from the American Red Cross, dated November 13, 1918, read:

> Miss Arleen [sic] Bertha Cole,
> 918 T. Street, N.W.
> Washington, D.C.
>
> Dear Miss Cole:
>
> The Surgeon General has called for a limited number of colored nurses, enrolled in the Red Cross, to be available for service about December 1.
> Your name has been selected as one who might be willing to consider an assignment, and if so, would you be good enough to notify us promptly, and also give us a permanent address where transportation may be issued.
> Miss Clara A. Rollins has been selected as the one who will be responsible for the group until they reach their posts of assignment.
> Anticipating an early reply, I am,
>
> > Yours sincerely,
> > [signed] Clara D. Noyes, Director
> > Bureau Field Nursing Service

It was followed by a form letter full of admonitions:

> It remains with you to justify our selection and to prove that the Red Cross stands for efficient service.
> You are likely to find the methods of procedure in a military hospital somewhat more formal than in a civil hospital and authority more absolute. May I urge, however, that you accept conditions without comment or criticism and make every effort to adapt yourself cheerfully and without friction to the environment . . . .

Miss Cole accepted the challenge and with 17 others formed the first contingent of black nurses: Marion Brown Seymour, Anna Oliver Ramos, Lillian Ball, Pearl Billings, Susie Boulding, Eva Clay, Aileen Cole, Edna DePriest, Magnolia Diggs, Sophia Hill, Jeanette Minnis, Clara Rollins, Lillian Spears, Virginia Steele, Frances Stewart, Nettie Vick, Jeannette West, and Mabel Williams (Maxwell, 1976).

Nine of the nurses were assigned to Camp Grant, Rockford, Illinois and nine to Camp Sherman, Chillicothe, Ohio. Their living quarters and recreational facilities were separate, but they were assigned to duties in integrated hospitals.

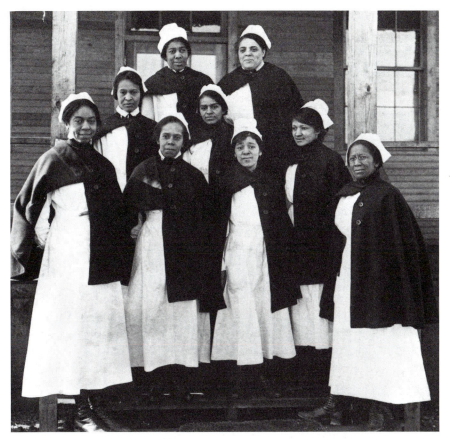

Figure 6–1   World War I black nurses at Camp Sherman, IL. Left to right: Ailene Cole, Susan Boulding, Lillian Spears, Jeanette Minnis, Sophia Hill. Center, left to right: Marion Brown Seymour, Jeanette West. Top left to right: Clara Rollins, Lillian Bell. (Courtesy U.S. Army Center of Military History)

The written testimonies of the chief nurses at Camps Sherman and Grant attest to the value of the black nurses' contributions (Fig. 6–1). Mary M. Roberts, chief nurse at Camp Sherman, wrote:

> I do not mind saying that I was quite sure, when orders came for the colored group, that I was about to meet my Waterloo. My feeling now is that it was a valuable experience for them and for me. They really were a credit to their race, for they did valuable service for our patients and it was a service that patients appreciated. I now find myself deeply interested in the problems of all colored nurses and

believe in giving them such opportunities as they can grasp for advancement . . . (Thoms, 1929, p. 164)

Of the Camp Grant group, the chief nurse said:

> Since the white and colored patients were not assigned to separate wards, these nurses were assigned to the general wards under the direction of the head nurse. They were serious-minded, quiet, business-like young women . . . . (p. 165)

Anna Oliver Ramos, a former assistant executive secretary of the National Association of Colored Graduate Nurses (NACGN) who served at Camp Grant, put it this way: "We came from good schools of nursing and we knew too well that whatever the test, we could measure up to whatever was expected of us" (Staupers, 1961, p. 99).

As they had in previous wars, civilian black nurses aided the military effort as well. The influenza epidemic so strained the ability of the Army to provide nurses that hospital commanders in the United States were granted authority to employ nurses for $75/month, one ration a day, lodging, laundry, and transportation (*Report of the Surgeon General,* 1918). Sayres L. Milliken, chief nurse at Camp Sevier, South Carolina, wrote of her black civilian nurses:

> At the peak of the influenza epidemic at Camp Sevier . . . , about fifty percent of the nurses were off duty, sick, and the hospital contained about 3,000 patients. It became necessary to employ locally [although not members of the Army Nurse Corps] every nurse who could be secured. A medical officer on duty . . . who was from the section of the country said that there were several good colored nurses who could be secured in the vicinity of Spartanburg . . . . The idea of securing the services of colored nurses did not immediately meet with enthusiasm, as fully 75 percent of the nurses were women of southern birth and had very positive objections to working with colored nurses. The need was so imperative that it was decided to employ them, furnishing them with quarters and a mess separate from the white nurses.
>
> About 12 reported for duty. They were assigned to the wards in the hospital in subordinate positions and with the exception of one or two who were not young enough to adapt themselves to the trying conditions under which everyone was working, these young women were found to be well-trained, quiet and dignified, and there was never at any time evidence of friction between the white and colored nurses. They served for a period of possibly three weeks . . . I should say that, although these nurses had no opportunity to

display executive ability, they did and can fill a valuable place in the nursing profession. (Thoms, 1929, pp. 166–167)

Other base hospitals where black nurses were assigned were Camp Funston, Kansas; Camp Dodge, Des Moines, Iowa; Camp Taylor, Louisville, Kentucky; and Camp Dix, Wrightstown, New Jersey. At these camps, a total of 38,000 black troops were located (Dunbar-Nelson, 1919).

With the armistice signed and the influenza epidemic waning, hospitals began to close in 1919, and the Army Nurse Corps, having reached 21,480 members in November, 1918, was correspondingly reduced in size. The peak of demobilization was reached in August, 1919, when 2,329 nurses left (*Report of the Surgeon General,* 1919, p. 294). Among them were the 18 black nurses. "Rumor, more or less authentic, states that over 300 colored nurses were on the battlefields, though their complexion disguised their racial identity" (Dunbar-Nelson, 1919, p. 379).

By July 1, 1920, only 1,551 nurses remained on active duty with the Army Nurse Corps. During the next 20 years the strength of the Corps remained under 1,000 members, and the issue of integration of black nurses in the Armed Forces again appeared dormant. It was during this period, however, that black nurses began the fight for integration in the professional organization—the American Nurses' Association, and into the mainstream of professional nursing (see Chapter 4).

The international anarchy that characterized the period before the outbreak of World War I reasserted itself shortly after the "War to End Wars" was over. As early as 1922, Mussolini had come to power in Italy, and by 1935 he was seeking to resurrect the Roman Empire by overrunning Ethiopia. These developments gave encouragement and comfort to Adolf Hitler, who was waiting for a chance to use his newly won authority in Germany to extend his control to neighboring nations (Franklin, 1967).

As war clouds gathered, government authorities informed the major nursing organizations—the American Nurses' Association (ANA), the National League of Nursing Education, and the National Organization for Public Health Nursing—of the need for nurses. At the 1938 biennial convention of these three organizations, it was announced that the "authorized strength of the Army Nurse Corps was increased to 675 on July 1, 1937, and on June 30, 1938, there were 674 on duty" (*Report of the Surgeon General,* 1938, p. 236).

When Europe was plunged into war in September, 1939, the policy of isolationism became more and more untenable (Franklin, 1967). Because of the war being waged in Europe, on September 8, 1939, a state of limited emergency was declared. At that time, there were 672 nurses on active duty (*Report of the Surgeon General,* 1939, p. 244). The authorized strength of the Corps was immediately increased and by June 30, 1940, there were 942 nurses in the Corps (*Report of the Surgeon General,* 1940, p. 257). An additional 15,779 nurses were enrolled in the First Reserve of the American Red Cross Nursing Service, presumably available for service if needed. On May 27, 1941, a state of national emergency was declared because of the threat of global war. Once again, it became necessary to appoint reserve nurses (Shields, 1981). When the attack on Pearl Harbor occurred, Army strength stood at some million and a half men with a Medical Department of over 130,000, including over 6,800 Army Nurse Corps members (Kriedberg & Henry, 1955).

With the Army Nurse Corps expanding its resources and services, black nurses assumed that they would be needed and began writing to the Corps for information. The NACGN alerted its members and urged that all eligible nurses enroll in the American Red Cross, the procurement agency for the military. One of the qualifications for enrollment in the American Red Cross was membership in the ANA, which was denied black nurses in the South (see Chapter 4). The Red Cross, however, established a special membership category for these nurses, permitting them to enroll if they were members of the NACGN. But in answer to their inquiries, they were informed: "Your application for appointment to the Army Nurse Corps cannot be given favorable consideration as there are not provisions in the army regulations for the appointment of colored nurses in the Corps" (Staupers, 1961, p. 100).

Waging the battle for the inclusion of black nurses in the Army Nurse Corps were the NACGN and other concerned organizations and individuals and by January, 1941, a quota of 56 black nurses to serve in the Army had been established, with the stipulation, according to Surgeon General James C. Magee, the "Negro nurse . . . would only be called to serve in hospitals or wards devoted exclusively to the treatment of Negro soldiers" (Staupers, 1961, p. 102).

With the announcement of the quota for black nurses, NACGN launched an intensive campaign, using the press and other media, for removal of the quota and against the practice of segregation and discrimination, which these young women encountered in their assignments. While the quota was still in effect, in April, 1941, a few black nurses were assigned to camps. "To date [30 June, 1941] 22 colored nurses have been assigned to Fort Bragg, N.C. and Camp Livingston, La." (*Report of the Surgeon General,* 1941, p. 245). Later that year, a small group of nurses was assigned to the Army Flying School for Negro Pilots at Tuskegee, Alabama (Staupers, 1961). Commonly referred to as the Tuskegee Airmen, the 450-man, all black unit included the first blacks allowed to serve as pilots in the Air Corps.

In 1943, the Army raised its quota of black nurses to 160, and by the end of September, 1944, there were close to 250 black nurse officers, including three captains and 30 first lieutenants (First Indorsement, 1945). But it was not until January 20, 1945, because of pressure by NACGN and others, that nurses were accepted into the Army Nurse Corps without regard to race (Hine, 1982). In fact, "the number of Negro nurses who volunteered and were commissioned in the last year of the war almost equalled the total in the army in September, 1944. In late July, 1945, there were some 500 black nurses in the Corps, including nine captains and 115 first lieutenants. They were serving in four general, three regional, and 11 station hospitals in the United States as well as in overseas areas (Groppe, 1945). It is estimated that there were a total of 8,000 black registered nurses in the country at that time.

In April, 1941, Della Raney Jackson (Fig. 6–2) of Suffolk, Virginia, the first black nurse to be commissioned in the U.S. Army (Reserve) as a lieutenant, reported for duty at Fort Bragg, North Carolina. Subsequently, in 1942, she became a chief nurse and was transferred to the station hospital at Tuskegee Air Field, Alabama. She later served as a chief nurse, Fort Huachuca, Arizona, and Camp Beale, California. In 1945, she was promoted to captain and in 1946 to major. Later she served a tour of duty in Japan. Major Raney Jackson, who has since died, was a graduate of Lincoln Hospital School of Nursing in Durham, North Carolina, and did further study at Western Michigan University, Wayne State University, the University of Michigan, and Virginia State College. In 1978, Major Jackson (retired) was honored by Tuskegee Airmen for outstanding leadership, service, professionalism, and for her historic achievements that personify the "Tuskegee Spirit." In 1989, Nancy Leftenant Colon, a retired Air Force Nurse, was elected president, Tuskegee Airmen, Inc., an organization established in 1972 to motivate and inspire young Americans to become participants in our nation's

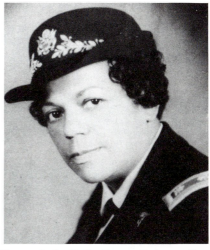

Figure 6–2   Della Raney Jackson, first black nurse commissioned in the U.S. Army Reserve, 1941.

society and its democratic process. Colon was the first black to be commissioned in the regular Army Nurse Corps. She joined reserves in February 1945, and was commissioned in the regular Army in 1948.

The first group of black nurses to be assigned to the European theater of operations arrived in England in 1944. The unit of 63 nurses, with Captain Mary L. Petty of Chicago as chief nurse, was greeted by Brigadier General Benjamin O. Davis, a black officer ("Army Nurses Tell Us," 1944). They were assigned to a hospital which treated German prisoners of war. Their commanding officer considered them to be highly efficient. A few months later, these nurses were transferred to another hospital which served as a rehabilitation center for American soldiers. For the first time, white Americans were treated by black medical personnel. This "experiment" was considered successful.

Black medical personnel were also sent to the Pacific. A hospital staffed totally by black personnel was established in North Burma to treat the soldiers building the Ledo Road. Another all-black unit was sent to the South Pacific in late 1943. Among its personnel were 15 black nurses, in addition to black physicians and black enlisted personnel who served as cooks, orderlies, drivers, and technicians. This unit saw duty in Australia (Fig. 6–3), New Guinea, and the Philippines (Department of Defense, 1982).

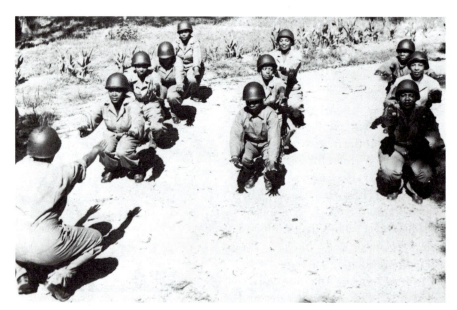

Figure 6–3 American black nurses limber up their muscles in an early-morning workout during advanced training at a camp in Australia. (Courtesy National Archives).

Another one of the 48 black nurses who joined the Army in April 1941, was Susan Elizabeth Freeman (Fig. 6–4), a 1926 graduate of Freedmen's Hospital School of Nursing in Washington, DC, with further study at Columbia University in New York and Howard University and The Catholic University of America in Washington, DC. Beginning her army career as a second lieutenant assigned to Camp Livingston, Louisiana, Sue Freeman was soon promoted to first lieutenant—the first nurse, black or white, to receive a promotion at Camp Livingston. Later, she was to become one of the first black nurses in the Army Nurse Corps to be promoted to captain.

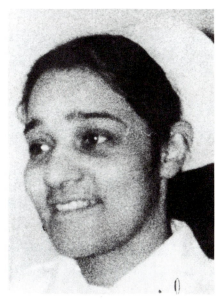

Figure 6–4   Susan Elizabeth Freeman, Chief Nurse, first overseas unit of Black nurses during World War II.

In July 1942, 60 black nurses were assigned to Fort Huachuca, Arizona, with Lieutenant Freeman as the chief nurse. She later served in Liberia in 1943 as chief nurse of the first overseas unit of 30 black nurses. While there, on November 8, 1943, she and eight other nurses received a unit commendation from the Office of the Commanding General, which stated in part, "During nearly eight months at this foreign service station, and in the face of difficult circumstances, these nurses have clearly demonstrated fidelity to duty, a sense of responsibility, and understanding of their positions as officers that is well above the average." A copy of the commendation was sent to the Surgeon General of the U.S. Army in Washington, DC. The Republic of Liberia honored Susan Freeman by making her a knight official of the Liberian Humane Order of Africa Redemption, a tribute to her success in person-to-person diplomacy with the Liberians (Staupers, 1961). By December of 1943, every nurse in the unit had contracted malaria and were returned to the United States.

Captain Freeman retired for medical reasons from the Army Nurse Corps on July 31, 1945, and received the Mary Mahoney Award that year from NACGN for service to the American Red Cross during the Ohio-Mississippi Flood of 1937 and for commanding the first unit of black

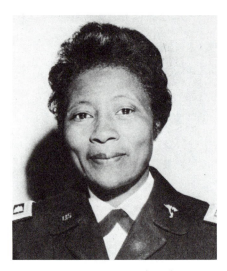

Figure 6–5   Margaret Bailey, first black nurse to attain rank of Lieutenant Colonel, 1964.

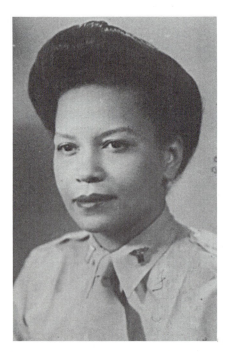

Figure 6–6   Agnes Beulah Glass Pallemon, Chief Nurse, 335th Station Hospital, Tagap, Burma 1944.

nurses overseas. Captain Freeman died in 1980 at her home in Stratford, Connecticut.

Two other black nurses who served as chief nurses in the Army Nurse Corps during World War II should be mentioned here—Margaret Bailey and Agnes Glass Pallemon.

Colonel Margaret E. Bailey (Fig. 6–5), was the first black nurse to attain the rank of lieutenant colonel (1964), having joined the army in June, 1944. Almost nine of her 27 years of service were spent outside the country—in Germany, Japan, and France. In Germany, she was head nurse on a psychiatric nursing service. In Japan, she was assistant chief nurse of the medical facility at Camp Zama and head nurse on the officers' ward. In May, 1965, Lieutenant Colonel Bailey received transfer orders for Europe to serve as chief nurse of the 130th General Hospital in Chinon, France.

In 1969, Lieutenant Colonel Bailey was assigned as health manpower training specialist to the Job Corps Health Office, Department of Labor. In January 1970, she was promoted to full colonel, again the first black nurse to hold that rank. Upon her retirement in 1971, Colonel Bailey received the Legion of Merit, the army's second highest noncombat award. In 1972, she was designated as consultant to the surgeon general of the United States Army to promote increased participation by minority group members in the Army Nurse Corps recruitment programs.

Colonel Bailey received her basic nursing education at the Fraternal Hospital School of Nursing in Montgomery, Alabama, earned a certificate in psychiatric nursing at Brooke Army Medical Center, Fort Sam Houston, Texas, and a bachelor's degree from San Francisco State College in California after having accumulated transfer credits from the University of Michigan, Kalamazoo State University in Michigan, and the University of Maryland extension in Germany.

Agnes Beulah Glass Pallemon (St. Mary's Infirmary School of Nursing, St. Louis, Missouri; Fig. 6–6) joined the Army Nurse Corps September 15, 1942 as second lieutenant and was promoted to first lieutenant a year later, 1943, at Fort Huachuca. On June 3, 1944, she was assigned principal chief nurse, Station Hospital ASF Depot, Ogden, Utah. When the 335th Station Hospital at Tagap, Burma, opened in late December, 1944, Lieutenant Glass-Pallemon was its chief nurse. In September 1946, she was promoted to captain.

As the United States entered the postwar period, blacks and whites began eradicating segregation and discrimination in the armed forces. This whole matter of blatant discrimination in the armed forces was not eliminated until Executive Order 9981 was issued by President Harry S. Truman on July 26, 1948, the first part of which stated:

> 1. It is hereby declared to be the policy of the President that there shall be equality of treatment and opportunity for all persons in the armed services without regard to race, color, religion or national origin. This policy shall be put into effect as rapidly as possible, having due regard to the time required to effectuate any necessary changes without impairing efficiency or morale.
> 2. There shall be created in the National Military Establishment an advisory committee to be known as the President's Committee on Equality of Treatment and Opportunity in the Armed Services, which shall be composed of seven members designated by the President. . . .

The order was a historic one. For the first time an American president had openly placed the force of his high office on the side of the struggle of the black for equal rights (Davis, 1966).

The protests of the sixties also served as an impetus to further improve inequities that existed. Although male nurses were first admitted to the Army Nurse Corps in 1955, it was not until September 30, 1966, with P.L. 89-609, 89th Congress, that they were commissioned in the regular army (Piemonte & Gurney, 1987, p. 51). On June 15, 1967, Lawrence C. Washington (Fig. 6–7), who happened to be black, was the first male nurse to receive a regular army commission in the Army Nurse Corps at Walter Reed Army Medical Center, Washington, DC.

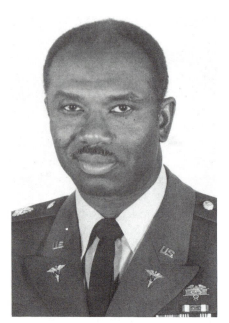

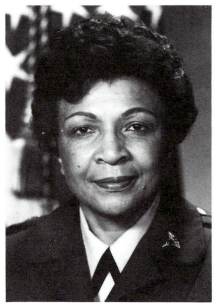

Figure 6–7 Lawrence C. Washington, first male nurse to receive a regular commission in the Army Nurse Corps, 1967.

Figure 6–8 Brigadier General Hazel Johnson-Brown, first black Chief of the Army Nurse Corps, 1979–1983. (Courtesy U.S. Army, Photograph No. p-190481)

Before Colonel Washington (Freedmen's Hospital School of Nursing, Washington, DC; M.S., The Catholic University of America, Washington, DC) entered a school of nursing, he had been an orderly and nursing assistant in civilian and military hospitals. Before retiring, he was assistant chief, Department of Nursing, William Beaumont Army Medical Center, Texas.

Ranks of the black nurses have ranged from second lieutenant to brigadier general. Tribute is paid here to Brigadier General Hazel Johnson-Brown (Fig. 6–8). In 1979, Johnson-Brown became the first black woman in the Department of Defense to achieve the grade of brigadier general and the first black to be the chief of the Army Nurse Corps. She retired from that post August 31, 1983, after 26 years of active commissioned service. Her previous major duty assignments between 1968 and 1979 had been project officer, Development Branch, Material Development Division, Surgical Directorate, U.S. Army Medical Research and Development Command, Washington, DC; dean, Walter Reed Army Institute of Nursing, Washington, DC; chief nurse, U.S. Army Medical Command, Korea; and special assistant to the chief, Army Nurse Corps.

General Johnson-Brown received her basic nursing education at Harlem Hospital School of Nursing in New York and a Ph.D. from The Catholic University of America in Washington, DC, plus honorary doctorates from Villanova University in Pennsylvania, Morgan State University in Baltimore, Maryland, and the University of Maryland, Baltimore.

Johnson-Brown, the first chief of the Army Nurse Corps to hold an earned doctorate, has been the recipient of numerous awards, among which is the Dr. Anita Newcomb McGee Medal presented by the Daughters of the American Revolution for excellence in the field of nursing for professional performance. Since retiring, Johnson-Brown has been adjunct professor, George Washington University, Washington, DC, director, Government Affairs Division, American Nurses Association, and is currently Commonwealth Professor, George Mason University School of Nursing, Fairfax, Virginia.

Clara Adams-Ender was chief, Army Nurse Corps Division, U.S. Army Recruiting Command in Fort Sheridan, Illinois from 1981 to 1984. She entered active duty in the Army in 1961 after completing her basic nursing education at North Carolina A&T State University School of Nursing in Greensboro, North Carolina. In 1969, she earned a master's degree in medical-surgical nursing from the University of Minnesota, Minneapolis, and in 1976 became the first woman in the army to earn the Master of Military Art and Science degree from the U.S. Army Command and General Staff College, Fort Leavenworth, Kansas. Her other awards include Legion of Merit, the Meritorious Service Medal with three oak clusters, and the coveted Surgeon General's "A" Professional Designation for Excellence in Nursing Administration.

From June 1984 to August 1987, Colonel Adams-Ender was chief, Department of Nursing, Walter Reed Army Medical Center, Washington, DC, the first black nurse to hold this position, bringing with her a wealth of experience in teaching, clinical practice, administration, research, and consultation. On September 1, 1987, she was promoted to Brigadier General and Chief Nurse of the Army Nurse Corps (Fig. 6–9). In 1988, she became the first Army nurse officer to be appointed Director of Personnel for the Surgeon General of the Army. During her tenure as Corps Chief, General Adams-Ender increased the strength of the Army Nurse Corps by 33 percent and initiated an upward mobility program called the Army Medical Department Enlisted Commissioning Program. In 1991, she concluded her assignment as Chief Nurse and became Commanding General of the Army post at Fort Belvoir, Virginia—the first for a woman, a nurse, and a black. She simultaneously served as Deputy Commanding General for the District of Columbia Military District. Upon retiring from this post, she established her own business in Lorton, Virginia, CAPE Associates, of which she is president and chief executive officer. CAPE (Caring About People with Enthusiasm) promotes executive and employee health and wellness.

Black nurses also served with distinction during the Korean conflict (1950–1953) where approximately 549 Army Nurse Corps officers served in support of the mission of the United States military.

Of note in the Vietnam War (1965–1975) was First Lieutenant Diane M. Lindsay (Fig. 6–10), Army Nurse Corps, who received the Soldier's Medal for Heroism in Vietnam in 1970. Lieutenant Lindsay (B.S., Hampton University School of Nursing, Hampton, Virginia), while on duty with the 95th Evacuation Hospital, happened on a berserk soldier. She and a male officer physically restrained the confused soldier and persuaded him to give up the grenade, thus preventing numerous casualties. Lieutenant Lindsay was the second nurse to be honored during the Vietnam Conflict and the first black nurse in history to receive the medal.

Brigadier General Clara Adams-Ender, then chief of the Army Nurse Corps and Director of Personnel for the Army Surgeon General and the highest ranking woman in the Army, directed the efforts of more than 20,000 Army nurses who served in the Persian Gulf area in Operation Desert Storm (1990–1991)

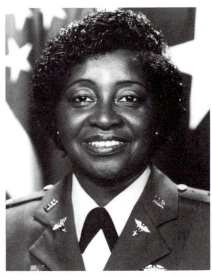

Figure 6–9 Brigadier General Clara Adams-Ender, Chief, Army Nurse Corps, 1987–1991. (Courtesy U.S. Army Visual Information Center, Pentagon, Washington, DC 20310-4800)

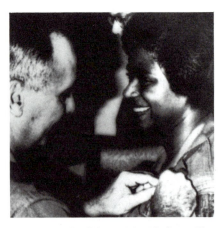

Figure 6–10 Diane M. Lindsay, First Lieutenant, Army Nurse Corps, received the Soldier's Medal for Heroism in Vietnam, 1970. (Courtesy U.S. Army Center of Military History)

and helped coordinate the efforts of more than 25,000 Army medical personnel, 2,265 of whom were nurses—from both active and reserved components. The health care personnel who went to the Desert served in 44 hospital units with 13,500 beds that were provided in these units. For her performance, Brigadier General Adams-Ender was awarded the Distinguished Service Medal. Lieutenant Colonel Barbara J. Hatcher, Ph.D. (Fig. 6–11), was one of the black nurses who served in Desert Storm. She was assistant chief nurse for clinical services, 31st Combat Support Hospital.

The Persian Gulf War, which lasted 102 days, began on August 2, 1990 when Iraq invaded and annexed neighboring Kuwait, a source of American oil, and threatened Saudi Arabia. An American military build up began in the Persian Gulf under the United Nations to protect the international interests in the region. One of the nurses who distinguished herself during the war was First Lieutenant Brenda K. Womack, who was awarded the Kuwait Medal (Fig. 6–12).

Due to the unrelenting efforts of ten years by Diana Carlson-Evans, a nurse who had served in the Vietnam War, on November 11, 1993, the Vietnam Women's Memorial was dedicated. The Memorial, honoring women in all wars, from the American Revolution to Desert Storm, is located near the Vietnam Wall at the Vietnam Veterans Memorial in Washington, DC (Fig. 6–13), entrance to Arlington National Cemetery, the nation's most hallowed resting place. Carlson-Evans felt that tributes that had existed did not acknowledge the contributions women had made.

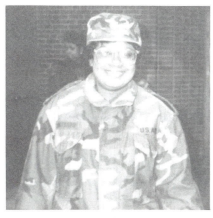

Figure 6–11 Lt. Col. Barbara Hatcher, Ph.D., R.N., reporting for duty for transfer to mobilization station enroute to the Persian Gulf.

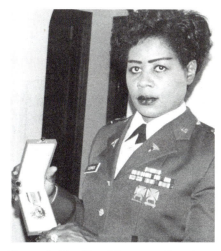

Figure 6–12 First Lieutenant Brenda K. Womack honored with the Kuwait Medal.

At the groundbreaking ceremony, General Colin L. Powell,
then chairman of the Joint Chiefs
of Staff and a Vietnam veteran who
was wounded in the war, acknowledged their suffering: ". . . for the
women who helped before the battle and for the nurses in particular,
the terror, the death, and the pain
were unrelenting . . ." The Memorial was dedicated to the 11,000
women who served in the Vietnam
War and the 265,000 women who
supported them in Japan, Guam,
the Philippines, Hawaii, and other
stateside hospitals and hospital
ships. Ninety percent of these mili-

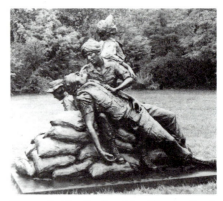

Figure 6–13   Sculpted by Glenna Goodacre of Santa Fe, New Mexico, bronze
statue depicts three American nurses and a
wounded soldier. (Courtesy Vietnam
Women's Memorial Project, Inc.)

tary women were nurses in the Army, Navy, and the Air Force Nurse
Corps.

At its 1993 biennial convention in Indianapolis, Indiana in November,
Sigma Theta Tau International honored Glenna Goodacre, the creator of
the bronze "Vietnam Women's Memorial."

Navy Nurse Corps

When President Theodore Roosevelt signed the Naval Appropriations Bill
on May 13, 1908, he signed into being the Navy Nurse Corps (Kalisch &
Kalisch, 1978). As in the case of the Army, the American Red Cross
served as the primary source of reserve nurses for the Navy. Black nurses
had the same problem of being discriminated against in terms of serving
in the Navy. The Army had a quota; the Navy's reply to black applicants
was simply, "Colored nurses are not being assigned to the Navy."

The National Association of Colored Graduate Nurses, along with concerned civic groups and individuals, while fighting to remove the quota
for black nurses in the Army, fought just as hard to get the Navy to reverse
its decision of not accepting any black nurses. Finally, in March, 1945,
after months of prodding, the Navy Surgeon General announced that the
Navy would accept a "reasonable" number of qualified black nurses and
was now recruiting for them (MacGregor, 1981). On March 8, 1945, a
few months before the cessation of hostilities, Phyllis Daley, a graduate of
Lincoln School for Nurses in New York, was sworn into the Navy Nurse
Corps as an Ensign—the first of the four black nurses who were on active

duty in the Navy during World War II. (She died in New York on October 31, 1976.)

The three other black nurses commissioned as ensigns were Helen Turner Watson (Fig. 6–14), a Lincoln School for Nurses in New York graduate; Ella Lucille Stimley of Provident in Chicago who took her oath on May 8, 1945, but was released on June 15 for reasons of physical disability; and Edith DeVoe of Freedmen's. On January 6, 1948, Edith DeVoe was augmented into the regular Navy. Approximately 11,000 nurses served in the Navy during World War II, but only four of them were black, and this presented a few problems. For example, Watson, who had been assigned to a post in Chicago, had to be housed at a YWCA branch because the Navy's policy prohibited her from sharing a room with a white nurse on its facility at Great Lakes. (Watson died September 26, 1992.)

Joan Bynum was the first black nurse to attain the rank of captain while assistant director of nursing, Naval Regional Medical Center, Yokosuka, Japan, in 1978. A native of Gary, Indiana, Captain Bynum joined the Navy shortly after receiving her bachelor of science degree in nursing, serving first at San Diego, then at Great Lakes. While in the Navy, she obtained her graduate education in pediatric nursing at Indiana University.

Marcus L. Walker (Alexian Brothers' Hospital School of Nursing, Chicago, Illinois; Sc.D., Johns Hopkins University, Baltimore, Maryland; Fig. 6–15) served four years in the U.S. Navy, 1952–1956. Walker, the first black man to graduate from a school of professional nursing in the

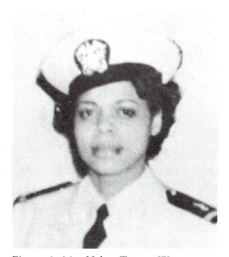

Figure 6–14   Helen Turner Watson, one of four black nurses commissioned as ensigns in U.S. Navy, 1945.

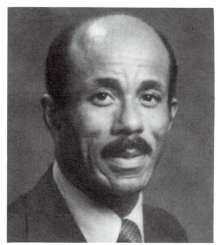

Figure 6–15   Dr. Marcus L. Walker, who served in the Navy before men nurses were commissioned.

State of Illinois, enlisted in the Navy in 1952, but because of gender, not as a commissioned officer. However, the Navy gave him assignments that were beyond the scope of enlisted hospital corpsmen—teaching nursing in the Hospital Corps School and functioning as clinical supervisor on the psychiatric units and in the operating rooms at Naval Hospital, Great Lakes, Illinois, during the Korean War.

In 1953, the Korean War ended, and Walker was assigned to the First and Third Marine Divisions, with the responsibility for establishing and evaluating two infirmaries on the marine bases, as well as supervising the nursing care provided by the hospital corpsmen.

In October 1955, Congress passed legislation to allow commissions for male nurses in the armed forces. The Army and Air Force Nurse Corps began commissioning men nurses, but the Navy decided not to do so. Walker was given the option of transferring into another branch of the service in order to be commissioned, but, having less than 6 months left of his four-year enlistment term, he chose to remain as a noncommissioned petty officer until discharge from the Navy in 1956. Ten years later, in 1965, the Navy began commissioning men in its Nurse Corps. With an extensive background in teaching, administration, clinical practice, consultation, and research, Walker, until his death in 1990, had been for 16 years on the graduate faculty of the University of Maryland School of Nursing in Baltimore as associate professor and had been Nurse Consultant, Veterans Administration Medical Center, Loch Raven, for four years.

Today, 27 percent of the Navy Nurse Corps is comprised of men, 3.5 percent of whom are black. Approximately 5.5 percent of the entire Navy Nurse Corps is comprised of black women. Black nurses have continued to attain senior rank and hold high-level positions. Six such nurses are: Captain Jacqueline Sharpe, NC, USN who serves as head, Command Education and Training at Naval Medical Center, Portsmouth, in Virginia; Captain Shirley Lewis-Brown, NC, USN who is director for nursing

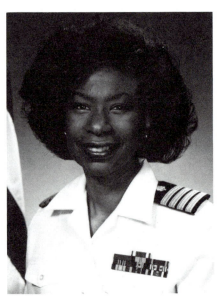

Figure 6–16 Captain Marsha Hughes-Rease, commanding officer, Naval Medical Center, Pearl Harbor, Hawaii.

service at Naval Hospital, Beaufort, in South Carolina; Captain Marilyn Day, NC, USN, an educator who serves at the Naval School of Health Sciences in San Diego, California; Captain Marsha Hughes-Rease who serves as a special assistant for the Navy Inspector General in Washington, DC; Captain Cecelia Dawegillis, NC, USN who is a nurse administrator at Naval Medical Center Oakland, in California; and Captain Julia Washington, NC, USN, who is a nurse administrator at Naval Medical Center San Diego in California.

During Desert Storm, Captain Hughes-Rease (B.S., University of Kentucky College of Nursing, Lexington; M.S., George Mason University, Fairfax, VA) (Fig. 6–16) was the most senior black woman to be mobilized. She deployed on board the USNS Comfort (T-AH 20), August 1990–April 1991, serving as department head for Medical-Surgical Nursing. Her decorations and awards received as a result of Desert Storm include: Navy Commendation Medal, National Defense Medal, Navy Unit Commendation, Southeast Asia Medal, Kuwait Defense Medal, and Sea Service Medal.

Air Force Nurse Corps

In 1942, the Army Air Forces (AAF) constituted, along with the Army Ground Forces and the Army Service Forces, one of three major commands within the War Department. With the establishment of AAF in June, 1941, the official name changed from the Air Corps to the Army Air Forces. Until 1948, officials of the War Department and the AAF reflected society's traditional racist attitude toward the participation of blacks (Osur, 1977).

The U.S. Air Force was created by the National Security Act of 1947. As the newest branch of the service, the Air Force had an open field in which to develop its own sense of purpose and identity (Willenz, 1983). Until then, as a part of the Army, the story of the black air force nurse had been incorporated in the story of the army nurse. For example, a few black army nurses, in 1941 and during the war years, were assigned to the station hospital at Tuskegee Air Field (Johnson, 1974). They also served as Army Nurse Corps nurses overseas at AAF stations.

In 1948, by Executive Order 9981, President Truman's Human Rights Proclamation directed the integration of the armed forces—the government would not discriminate. The Air Force decided to integrate immediately and by the time the Air Force Medical Service was established in July 1949, with the Air Force Nurse Corps becoming an integral part of it, integration was policy. At that time, Army nurses were permitted to transfer to the Air

Force, and 1,199 transfers were made, of which 307 were from components of the Regular Army and 892 from the Reserve. This group formed the nucleus of the Air Force Nurse Corps (Shields, 1981).

One of the black nurses who transferred from the Army to the Air Force in 1949 was Captain Abbie Sweetwine, who was promoted to her present rank in 1953 after having served at posts in this country, the United Kingdom, and Korea. Captain Sweetwine was born in Cocoa, Florida, received her basic nursing education at Brewster Hospital School of Nursing in Jacksonville, and worked as a nurse to migrants from the Bahamas and at a Veterans Administration hospital before joining the army.

Another black nurse, Lieutenant Colonel Ann Lawrence from Chadbourn, North Carolina, was the second highest ranking black woman in the Air Force in 1976. A graduate of Kate B. Reynolds Hospital School of Nursing in Winston-Salem, North Carolina, Ann Lawrence joined the U.S. Air Force in 1956. Her first assignment was to Wright Patterson Air Force Base in Dayton, Ohio. From there, she was sent to Japan for two years. After earning her master's degree in public administration from the University of Nebraska in Omaha, she spent tours of duty in Libya, North Africa, the Philippines, and Vietnam before returning to the United States.

Six black nurses have attained the rank of full Colonel or higher: Col. Mary R. Boyd (retired), Col. Clara B. Wallace (retired), Col. Margaret P. C. Nelson (retired), Col. Nora Kendall (retired), Col. Christine Spivey, and Brigadier General Irene Trowell-Harris.

Colonel Mary Rozina Boyd (St. Philip Hospital School of Nursing, Richmond, VA; M.S.N., University of California, San Francisco, Fig. 6–17) a native of Anderson, South Carolina, before retiring in 1987 as chairperson, Department of Nursing, Malcolm Grow Medical Center, Andrews Air Force Base, Washington, DC, she had held various positions— from staff nurse to chief nurse—at many bases in the United States and several foreign countries. She served as Medical Inspector, HQ USAF Inspection and Safety Cen-

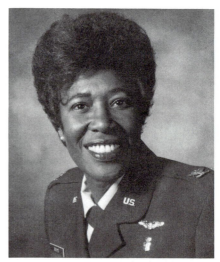

Figure 6–17   Colonel (ret.) Mary Rozina Boyd, former Chairperson, Department of Nursing, Malcolm Grow USAF Medical Center, Andrews Air Force Base, Washington, DC.

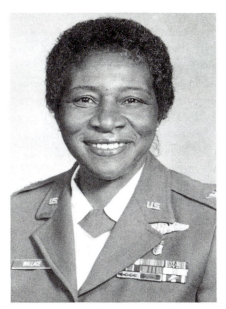

Figure 6–18 Colonel Clara B. Wallace, former Chief, Nursing Education, Randolph Air Force Base, Texas.

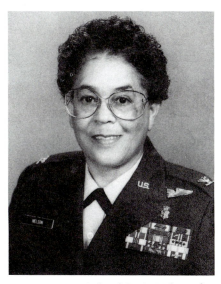

Figure 6–19 Colonel P. C. Nelson, former Nurse Staff Development Officer, Kessler Air Force Base, Mississippi.

ter. In this role, she evaluated nursing service activities in Air Force hospitals/medical centers worldwide. During this tour, Colonel Boyd served as interim team chief for a period of four months, the first time a nurse had served as chief of a medical inspection team.

Colonel Clara B. Wallace (B.S., Prairie View A&M University School of Nursing, Prairie View, TX; M.N., University of Washington, Seattle, WA, Fig. 6–18) was chief, Nurse Education, Medical Service Education Division, Directorate of Medical Service Officer Programs and Utilization Headquarters, Air Force Military Personnel Center, Randolph Air Force Base, Texas.

Colonel Wallace's military career began in February 1962, when she received a direct commission as a first lieutenant in the U.S. Air Force. Her experiences have not only been in the United States, but also in Japan, Germany, Thailand, Vietnam, and the Philippines. Her decorations include the Meritorious Service Medal, Air Force Commendation Medal, Vietnam Service Medal, Vietnam Gallantry Cross, and Vietnam Campaign Medal.

Colonel Margaret P.C. Nelson (St. Philip Hospital School of Nursing, Richmond, Virginia; M.A., Teachers College, Columbia University, NY, Fig. 6–19) was Nurse Staff Development Officer, Keesler Technical Training Center, Medical Center, Keesler Air Force Base, Mississippi. She developed, coordinated, monitored, evaluated, and implemented staff development programs which included orientation, skill training, inservice and continuing education for 306 nurses and 348 medical technicians. She also served as consultant to Headquarters Air Force Military Personnel Center and Staff Development Officers Air Force wide.

Colonel Nelson's military experience began in 1963 as charge nurse, Medical Unit, Tinker AFB, Oklahoma. Her civilian experiences before the military included nursing education, service, and administration. Among Colonel Nelson's awards are the Bronze Star Medal, the Meritorious Service Medal, and Air Force Commendation Medal.

Colonel Nora Kendall Noble (Lincoln Hospital School of Nursing, Durham, NC; B.S.N., The Catholic University of America, Washington, DC) before retiring was commander, 2803 Air Force Base Group, Newark Air Force Station, Ohio. In this capacity, she was responsible for managing base support facilities for the 2,600 military and civilians assigned to the Aerospace Guidance and Metrology Center. Colonel Kendall began her military career in 1960 at Gunter Air Force Base, Alabama. Her experiences have been in this country including Alaska, and Germany. In 1970, she served as clinic chief nurse at McGuire Air Force Base and in 1971 was selected to become the flight nurse reserve advisor at Headquarters 21st Air Force McGuire AFB, New Jersey. She assumed command of the 2803 Air Base Group July 16, 1984.

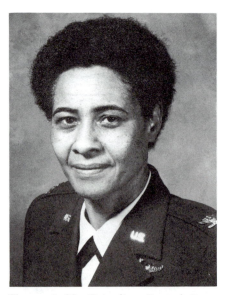

Colonel Kendall's military awards and decorations include the Meritorious Service Medal with two Oak Leaf Clusters, Air Force Outstanding Unit, Air Force Organizational Excellence Award, Air Force Longevity, Vietnam Service Medal, and the National Defense Service Medal.

Colonel Christine Spivey is stationed at Scott Air Force Base, Illinois serving as chief nurse, Scott Medical Center.

Brigadier General Irene Trowell-Harris (Columbia Hospital School of Nursing, Columbia, SC; Ed.D., Teachers College, Columbia University, NY, Fig. 6–20), in 1993 was promoted to Brigadier General at Andrews Air Force base

Figure 6–20 Brigadier General Irene Trowell Harris, Air National Guard Advisor to Chief Air Force Nurse Corps, Bolling Air Force Base, Washington, DC.

in Maryland, thus becoming the first woman general in the 357-year history of the National Guard (Army and Air Force). She began her military career in 1963 with the 102nd Airomedical Evacuation Flight unit in Brooklyn, was appointed commander of the 105th U.S. Air Force Clinic in Newburgh, New York, in 1986, and became the first nurse in Air National Guard history to command a medical unit.

THE UNITED STATES PUBLIC HEALTH SERVICE

The Public Health Service (PHS) came into being July 16, 1798, by an act of Congress. The act, signed by President John Adams, originally identified the PHS as the U.S. Marine Hospital Service, and for over 70 years the primary focus was on the care and relief of sick and injured seamen. In 1870, the Marine Hospital Service was reorganized as a national hospital system with centralized administration under a supervising surgeon given the title of surgeon general. In 1912, the Marine Hospital Service was renamed the U.S. Public Health Service. In later years, its responsibilities increased until, at the time of its transfer from the Treasury Department to the Federal Security Agency in 1939, it was charged with numerous and important responsibilities relating to the improvement and protection of the public health (Williams, 1951).

The statutory establishment of the Commissioned Corps of the PHS occurred in 1889, set up along military lines. Although PHS officers may be called by Navy rank (just as Army and Air Force officers are called by the same rank), the PHS has its own rank. The PHS and Navy uniforms are similar, but PHS has its own insignia. The uniformed corps is a mobile force of professionals subject to duty anywhere, upon assignment, to combat disease and hazards to human health.

In 1918, Congress enacted legislation for a reserve corps, making it possible to recruit professional personnel other than physicians. By 1944, the Commissioned Corps was expanded to include research scientists, nurses, and other health specialists (Abdellah, 1977). Although nurses were not appointed to the Commissioned Corps of the PHS until 1944, trained nurses were employed in the hospital nursing services of USPHS as early as 1919 and during the influenza epidemic that year, a black nurse, Charity Collins Miles, a 1906 graduate of Spelman College School of Nursing, Atlanta, Georgia, served in the PHS and received a certificate signed by U.S. Surgeon General Rupert Blue (Thoms, 1929).

Today, a black nurse, CDR. Russell L. Green (B.S.N., Tuskegee University, Tuskegee, AL; M.S.A., Central Michigan University, Mt. Pleasant, Fig. 6–21) is Commissioned Personnel Program Coordinator,

Division of Commissioned Personnel, Personnel Service Branch. He is
responsible for planning, coordinating, implementing and evaluating
PHS's promotion and assimilation
programs. Serving with Commander Green is Senior Personnel Policy
Specialist CAPT. Denise Canton
(B.S.N., Illinois Wesleyan University, Bloomington; D.N.Sc., The
Catholic University of America,
Washington, DC; J.D. Georgetown
University Law Center, Washington, DC).

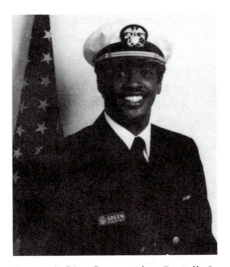

According to the January 13,
1945, issue of the *People's Voice,*
Alma N. Jackson of Richmond,
Virginia, was the first black woman
to be commissioned by the PHS. At that time (1944), she was serving as
assistant sanitarian in the all-black Public Health Service Mission to
Liberia.

Figure 6–21   Commander Russell L.
Green, Commissioned Personnel Program
Coordinator.

In 1949, the position of chief nurse officer, with the rank of assistant
surgeon general, was established (Notter & Spalding, 1965). In response
to increasing responsibilities, PHS has grown from a small nucleus of
health professionals to more than 6,500 officers of the Commissioned
Corps plus 50,000 civil service employees working in a wide variety of
health programs. As one of the seven uniformed services (Army, Navy,
Air Force, Marine Corps, Coast Guard, Public Health Service, National
Oceanic, and Atmospheric Administration) of the United States, the
commissioned corps is a specialized career system designed to attract, retain, and develop health professionals who may be assigned to Federal,
State, or local agencies or international organizations (*Commissioned Officer's Handbook,* 1994).

Today, the mission of the PHS is:

> to promote the protection and advancement of the Nation's physical
> and mental health by: conducting medical and biomedical research;
> sponsoring and administering comprehensive programs for the de-
> velopment of health resources; preventing and controlling disease
> and alcohol and drug abuse; providing resources and expertise to the
> States and other public and private institutions, and to Tribes,
> Councils and organizations concerned with the health of American

Indians and Alaska Natives, in the planning, direction and delivery of physical and mental health care services; enforcing laws to assure the safety and efficacy of drugs and protection against impure and unsafe foods, cosmetics, medical devices and radiation-producing projects; and coordinating with States, local and other Federal agencies to protect the public from exposure to toxic substances; coordinating with the States to set and implement national health policy and pursue effective intergovernmental relations; generating and upholding cooperative international health-related agreements, policies and programs and cooperating with Commissions and organizations to promote international health activities. (*Organization Manual,* Chap. H, 1990, p. 1)

Initially a part of the Treasury Department, the PHS became a part of the Federal Security Agency in 1939 and remained there until April 11, 1953, when it became the health component of the Department of Health, Education, and Welfare (DHEW), established by an act of Congress. Since the 1960s, PHS has undergone several organizational changes, including a name change from DHEW to the Department of Health and Human Services.

The Public Health Service is under the leadership and direction of the Assistant Secretary for Health who is directly responsible to the Secretary of Health and Human Services. The major activities located in the Office of the Assistant Secretary for Health (OASH) are: National AIDS Program Office, Office of Population Affairs, Office of Disease Prevention and Health Promotion, Office of Research Integrity, President's Council on Physical Fitness and Sports, Office of International and Refugee Health, Office of Minority Health, National Vaccine Program Office, Office of Women's Health, Office of Emergency Preparedness, Equal Employment Opportunity, Office of the Surgeon General, the Office of the Regional Health Administrators, and several offices providing administration and management, including the Office of Management, the Office of Health Planning and Evaluation, and the Office of Intergovernmental Affairs (*Commissioned Officer's Handbook,* 1994).

The Public Health Service consists of eight line agencies: (1) Agency for Toxic Substances and Disease Registry; (2) Substance Abuse and Mental Health Services Administration; (3) Centers for Disease Control and Prevention; (4) Food and Drug Administration; (5) Health Resources and Services Administration; (6) Indian Health Service; (7) National Institutes of Health; and (8) Agency for Health Care Policy and Research (*Organization Manual,* Chap. H, 1994).

In addition to these eight line agencies, the Public Health Service has 10 regional offices. Black nurses hold or have held key positions in most of the agencies where nurses are employed and in most of the regional offices. Because of the Privacy Act of 1974 (P.L. 93-579), it was not possible to obtain information on individual black nurses from the official files of the Public Health Service. Information presented here was obtained from the literature—books, periodicals, and newspapers—correspondence, personal interviews, and telephone interviews. Because of how the information was obtained there is the possibility that some black nurses in leadership positions have been inadvertently omitted.

The Agency for Toxic Substances and Disease Registry

Established in 1983, the mission of the Agency for Toxic Substances and Disease Registry (ATSDR) is to prevent or mitigate the adverse human health effects and diminished quality of life that result from exposure to hazardous substances in the environment. The agency works closely with state, local, and other federal agencies to reduce or eliminate illness, disability, and death that result from exposure of the public and workers to toxic substances at spill and waste disposal sites (*Organization Manual,* Chap. HT, 1989, p. 1). There are no nurses on staff.

Substance Abuse and
Mental Health Services Administration

The Reorganization Act of 1992 changed the title of Alcohol, Drug Abuse, and Mental Health Administration (ADAMHA), which had been established in 1974, to Substance Abuse and Mental Health Services Administration (SAMHSA). The mission of SAMHSA is to provide national leadership to insure that knowledge, based on science and state-of-the-art practice, is effectively used for the prevention and treatment of addictive and mental disorders (*Organization Manual,* Chap. HM, 1992).

Although there are no black nurses on the staff of SAMHSA, black nurses have been the recipients of research funding by the Agency's Center for Substance Abuse Prevention. One such nurse is C. Alicia Georges, MA, RN, lecturer, Department of Nursing, Lehman College, Bronx, NY. Georges and a fellow faculty member, Barbara Backer, collaborated on the research, "Perceptions of Eleven International Nursing Leaders of Alcohol, Tobacco, and other Drug Use and Abuse among Professional Nurses and Nursing Students in Their Countries." Georges presented a paper based on their research at the Sixth International Congress on Women's Health Issues in Gabarone, Botswana, Southern Africa, June, 1994.

The Centers for Disease Control and Prevention

The CDCP serves as the national focus for developing and applying disease prevention and control, environmental health, and health promotion and health education activities to improve the health of the people of the United States.

To accomplish its mission, CDCP:

> identifies and defines preventable health problems and maintains active surveillance of diseases through epidemiologic and laboratory investigations and data collection, analysis, and distribution; serves as the PHS lead agency in developing and implementing operational programs relating to environmental health problems, and conducts operational research aimed at developing and testing effective disease prevention, control and health promotion programs; administers a national program to develop recommended occupational safety and health standards and to conduct research, training, and technical assistance to assure safe and healthful working conditions for every working person; develops and implements a program to sustain a strong national workforce in disease prevention and control; and conducts a national program for improving the performance of clinical laboratories.
>
> CDCP is responsible for controlling the introduction and spread of infectious diseases, and provides consultation and assistance to other nations and international agencies to assist in improving their disease prevention and control, environmental health, and health promotion activities. CDCP administers the Preventive Health and Health Services Block Grant and specific preventive health categorical grant programs while providing program expertise and assistance in responding to Federal, State, local, and private organizations on matters related to disease prevention and control activities. (*Organization Manual,* Chapter HC, 1982, p. 1)

Six black nurses are on the staff of CDCP: Cheryl Blackmore, Yvonne Green, Joyce Goff, Sandra Jones, Gloria Bryan, and Pattie Tucker.

CAPT. Cheryl Blackmore (B.S., State University of New York at Buffalo; Ph.D., University of North Carolina at Chapel Hill, Fig. 6–22) is epidemiologist, Division of Reproductive Health. As a special assignment, she serves on the USPHS Black Commissioned Officers Advisory Group.

CDR. Yvonne T. Green (B.S.N., Dillard University, New Orleans, LA; M.S.N., Yale University, New Haven, CN) is assistant chief, Women's Health and Fertility Branch, Division of Reproductive Health.

CDR. Joyce Goff (B.S.N., Texas Christian University, Fort Worth; M.Ed. Georgia State University, Atlanta, Fig. 6–23) is adult immunization coordinator, National Immunization Programs.

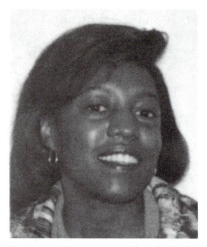

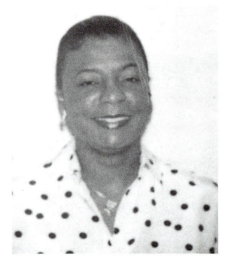

Figure 6–22   Captain Cheryl Blackmore, epidemiologist, CDCP.

Figure 6–23   CDR Joyce Goff, CDCP.

Sandra Jones (B.S.N., Prairie View A&M University, Houston, TX; Ph.D., University of Colorado, Boulder) is program analyst, Clinic Management Unit, Division of Reproductive Health. In this position she does operations research and provides technical assistance to publicly funded clinics. Since 1989, she has been assistant professor, Kuwait University.

The Food and Drug Administration

The Pure Food and Drug Act of 1906 was administered for a number of years by the Bureau of Chemistry of the Department of Agriculture. Later, FDA was established, and administration of the law was transferred to that organization (Williams, 1951).

The mission of the Food and Drug Administration is to:

> protect the public health of the nation as it may be impaired by foods, drugs, biological products, cosmetics, medical devices, ionizing and nonionizing radiation-emitting products and substances, poisons, pesticides, and food additives. FDA's regulatory functions are geared to insure that: Foods are safe, pure, and wholesome; drugs, medical devices, and biological products are safe and effective; cosmetics are harmless; all of the above are honestly and informatively packaged; and that exposure to potentially injurious radiation is minimized. (*Organization Manual,* Chap. HK-A, 1991, p. 1)

Two black nurses have been identified as holding leadership positions on the staff of FDA: CDR. Robyn Brown-Douglas and LCDR. Sharon

Murrain-Ellerbe. Robyn Brown-Douglas (B.S.N., College of New Rochelle, NY; M.A., Barry University, Miami Shores, FL) is Senior Regulatory Review Officer, Center for Food Safety and Applied Nutrition.

LCDR. Sharon Murrain-Ellerbe (B.S.N., Winston-Salem State University, Winston-Salem, NC) is consumer safety officer investigator–full performance level, Baltimore District Office, Baltimore, MD. Her assignments cover a full range of industries under FDA jurisdiction to insure conformance with good manufacturing and good laboratory practices. Areas covered include medical devices, drugs, and biologics.

The Health Resources and Services Administration

HRSA provides leadership and direction to programs and activities designed to improve the health services for all people of the United States and to assist in the development of health care systems that are adequately financed, comprehensive, interrelated and responsive to the needs of individuals and families in all levels of society. Specifically, HRSA:

> (1) provides leadership and support efforts designed to integrate health services delivery programs with public and private health financing programs; (2) administers the health services categorical grants, and formula grant-supported programs; (3) provides technical assistance for modernizing or replacing health care facilities; (4) provides leadership to improve the education, training, distribution, supply, use, and quality of the Nation's health personnel; and (5) provides advice and support to the Assistant Secretary for Health in the formulation of health policies. (*Organization Manual,* Chap. HB-OO, 1994, p. 1)

Of the major components of the Health Resources and Services Administration, black nurses hold or have held key positions in the Bureau of Health Professions and the Bureau of Primary Care.

Bureau of Health Professions.   In this Bureau are the Division of Nursing and Division of Medicine. The Bureau provides national leadership in the development of the personnel required to staff the nation's health care delivery system, targeting resources to areas of high national priority, such as increasing the supply of primary care practitioners; improving the distribution of health professionals both geographically and by specialty; ensuring the availability of adequately prepared health professionals; and ensuring access to health careers for the disadvantaged.

The **Division of Nursing** supports programs related to the development, financing, and use of educational resources for the improvement of nurse training. It supports and conducts programs with respect to the development, use, quality, and distribution of nursing personnel, to advance the health status of individuals, families, and communities. It fosters and supports projects to expand the scientific base of nursing practice and role reformulation and develops and incorporates new knowledge into practice and education. The Division provides consultation and technical assistance on all aspects of nursing to public and private organizations, agencies, and institutions, including international agencies and ministries of health.

Black nurses have held key positions in the Division of Nursing. One such nurse was Dr. Marie Bourgeois who, until her retirement in 1982, was chief, Research Training Section, Nursing Research Branch. The responsibilities of this position included administering the National Research Service Awards Program; developing policies and programs for research training; interpreting federal policies, developing contract proposals, and providing technical assistance to individuals and to public and private agencies on research projects for nursing and related fields; maintaining source material on research training; and assessing posttraining performance, educational trends and developments.

Other black nurses who have been on the staff of the Division of Nursing as consultants are Camille Alexander, Dr. Martha Lewis Smith, Dr. Alice Hilfiker, Mabel Morris, Dr. Verna Cook, Mary Whitehurst, and Dr. Doris Mosley. In 1990, Diane Thompkins served as program analyst. In 1994, Melva Owens (A.D., Community College of Baltimore, Baltimore, MD; Ph.D., George Mason University, Fairfax, VA) joined the staff as nursing consultant. Serving on the advisory committee are Alicia Georges, Dr. Rhetaugh Dumas, and Ophelia Long.

The **Division of Medicine** serves as the federal focus for the education, practice, and credentialing of medical personnel, including physician assistants. Doris Mosley (B.S., Dillard University Division of Nursing, New Orleans, LA; Ed.D., Teachers College, Columbia University, NY, Fig. 6–24) has been with the Public Health Service in various capacities since 1980. Since 1989, she has been a Public Health Analyst/Project Officer in the AIDS Education and Training Centers (AETC) Program. The AETC Program provides grant funds to eligible health professions educational programs to educate/train primary health care providers who are willing and able to care for persons with HIV/AIDS. Current trainee focus is on a multidisciplinary group of primary caregivers, including physicians, nurses, physician assistants, nurse practitioners, dentists, and dental hygienists. In addition to providing guidance and technical assistance to several of the 15 existing ETC Programs, she also serves as a key nursing education resource to the program working collaboratively with the Division of Nursing and other federal agencies and units on issues and activities of mutual interest. Mosley also serves as lead staff for minority initiatives as carried out by the ETC program in collaboration with such organizations as the National Black Nurses Association and the National Association of Hispanic Nurses. Included, also, is work with the historically black colleges and universities.

Bureau of Primary Health Care. Within the Bureau of Primary Health Care are the Division of National Hansen's Disease Programs, the Division of the National Health Service Corps, the Division of Programs for Special Populations, the Division of Scholarship and Loan Repayment, and the Division of Community and Migrant Health. LTJG. Kelly Morton, is as-

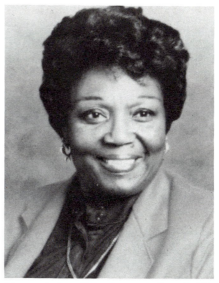

Figure 6–24 Dr. Doris Mosley, Public Health Analyst/Project Officer, AIDS Education and Learning Centers Program, Division of Medicine.

signed to the Office of Bureau Director to deal with matters pertaining to health care reform.

In 1953, the PHS Division of Hospitals operated 19 hospitals and approximately 21 outpatient clinics. During the succeeding years, declining demand for hospitalization, created mainly by the reduction in numbers of American seamen, and budgetary necessity led to the closing of some hospitals and the conversion of others to outpatient clinics.

Freedmen's Hospital in Washington, DC, a black institution that had been operating a school of nursing since 1894, had been under several federal agencies until it was placed under the direction of the PHS in 1940 and its functions transferred to the Federal Security Agency by the Reorganization Act of 1939. In 1953, all functions of the abolished Federal Security Agency were transferred to the Department of Health, Education, and Welfare (DHEW). Public Law 87-622, approved September 21, 1961, directed the transfer of Freedmen's Hospital from DHEW to Howard University, although the transfer was not completed until July 1, 1967 (*Federal Health Programs,* 1971). The name of the hospital was changed to Howard University Hospital.

As of June 30, 1971, the Federal Health Programs Service operated eight general hospitals located in Baltimore, Boston, Galveston, New

Orleans, Norfolk, San Francisco, Seattle, and on Staten Island, New York, and one hospital for the care and treatment of persons with Hansen's Disease at Carville, Louisiana (*Federal Health Programs,* 1971). In 1981 the eight general hospitals were closed, leaving only the one at Carville, the facility of the **Division of National Hansen's Disease Programs.**

The hospital at Carville which has been renamed the Gillis Long Center for Hansen's Disease, is located in Louisiana on the Mississippi River 25 miles south of Baton Rouge and 75 miles north of New Orleans. Through an act of Congress, the Louisiana Leper Home was purchased by the USPHS on January 3, 1921, from the State of Louisiana, which had operated it since 1894 as a home for persons with leprosy within the State. Today, its primary purpose is to afford leprosy patients a facility for complete evaluation and treatment. The hospital also serves as a research and training center for the disease.

Donna G. Kibble (Glendale Adventist Hospital School of Nursing, Glendale, California) is one of two black professional nurses at Gillis Long (Fig. 6–25). Since 1975, she has been a supervisor, providing management, guidance, and direction to the professional and ancillary staff.

The **Division of National Health Service Corps** (NHSC) was authorized under Public Law 91-623, the Emergency Health Personnel Act of 1970, and continued as amended under Public Law 92-585, in order "to improve the delivery of health services to persons living in medically underserved communities and areas of the United States."

The mission of the National Health Service Corps is to improve the delivery of health services in health manpower shortage areas and reduce the number of such areas by the appropriate placement of health professionals and health resources. Corps physicians, dentists, nurses, and allied medical personnel assigned to field stations are primarily commissioned personnel of the Public Health Service. Other Corps personnel may be part of the Civil Service System.

In 1990, CAPT. Joyce Elmore (Freedmen's Hospital School of

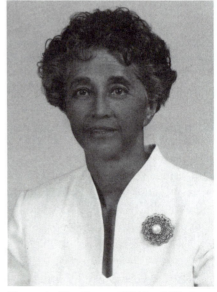

Figure 6–25   Donna Kibble, Gillis Long Center, Carville, LA.

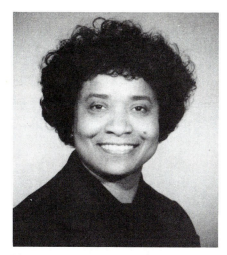

Figure 6–26   Dr. Joyce Elmore, Area/ Regional Nursing Consultant, Division of National Health Service Corps.

Nursing, Washington, DC, Ph.D., The Catholic University of America, Washington, DC, Fig. 6–26) was transferred from the office of the Assistant Secretary for Health to the National Health Service Corps as Area/Regional Nursing Consultant. In this position, she assists health professions schools in assigning students for clinical experience or placements in community health centers.

In addition to her 16 years with the PHS, Elmore's experience includes private duty, office nursing, instructor and professor in schools of nursing, dean, Chicago State University School of Nursing, director of ANA Department of Nursing Education, and consultant to the vice-president for health affairs at Howard University, Washington, DC.

The **Division of Programs for Special Populations** has two black nurses in key positions: Deborah Lynnette Parham, and Beverly Wright. CAPT. Deborah Lynnette Parham (B.S.N., University of Cincinnati School of Nursing and Health, Cincinnati, Ohio; Ph.D., University of North Carolina, Chapel Hill) is interim chief, HIV and Substance Abuse Services Branch. She is responsible for managing Title III(b) of the Ryan White CARE Act which authorizes a program to support outpatient early intervention services and clinical treatment for persons with HIV or at risk for contracting HIV.

CAPT. Beverly R. Wright (Long Island College Hospital School of Nursing, Brooklyn, NY; M.P.H., Johns Hopkins University, Baltimore, MD) is deputy branch chief, Prenatal and Child Health Branch.

In the **Division of Scholarship and Loan Repayment** is Deputy Chief Gladys Perkins (A.A., Bronx Community College, New York; MS, Hunter College, NY, Fig. 6–27).

On the staff of the **Division of Community and Migrant Health** is CDR. Regan Crump (B.S.N., Medical College of Virginia, Richmond, VA; D.P.H., Johns Hopkins University, Baltimore, MD, Fig. 6–28) who holds the title, deputy director, Policy Assistance and Development Branch. In this position he coordinates strategic planning efforts for the Branch and the Division.

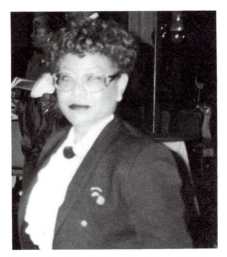

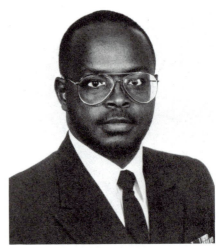

Figure 6–27   Gladys Perkins, Division
of Scholarship and Loan Repayment.

Figure 6–28   CDR Regan Crump, Division of Community & Migrant Health.

Indian Health Service

More than 800,000 American Indians and Alaska Natives depend on the Indian Health Service (IHS) for their total health needs. IHS is the only federal program that provides direct health services to the American Indians, deriving its basic authorities from the Snyder Act of 1921. Before 1955, IHS was under the Bureau of Indian Affairs. In 1955, Congress placed it under the PHS. Having been a component of the Health Resource and Services Administration, in 1988 IHS was made a line agency.

One of the largest federal agencies, IHS:

> provides a comprehensive health services delivery system for American Indians and Alaska Natives with opportunity for maximum tribal involvement in developing and managing programs to meet their health needs. The goal of IHS is to raise the health level of the Indian and Alaska Native people to the highest possible level. (*Organization Manual,* Chap. HG-OO, 1988, p. 1)

IHS operates 51 hospitals, 99 health centers, and 108 health stations. Three thousand nurses provide the major portion of health care in 24 states for American Indians and Alaska Natives. "The nurses who serve in the Indian Health Service comprise 64% of all those RNs in the Public Health Service" (Subcommittee hearings, *American Nurse,* September, 1990, p. 2).

Two black nurses hold key positions in IHS.

CDR. Arden Green (A.S.S., New York City College Department of Nursing; Ed.M., Boston University, Boston, MA) is director of nursing, PHS Chemical Dependency Treatment Center, Sacaton, AZ.

CDR. Glenda O. Jarrett (A.S.N., Norfolk State University, Norfolk, VA; B.S.N., Hampton University, Hampton, VA) is inpatient head nurse, Cherokee Indian Hospital, Cherokee, North Carolina, and serves as an assistant to the director of nursing.

National Institutes of Health

The National Laboratory of Hygiene, established in 1891, was the forerunner of NIH. The National Institutes of Health (NIH) is the steward of biomedical and behavioral research for the Nation. Its mission is science in pursuit of fundamental knowledge about the nature and behavior of living systems and the application of that knowledge to extend health life and reduce the burdens of illness and disability. The goals of the agency are to:

> (1) foster fundamental creative discoveries, innovative research strategies, and their applications as a basis to advance significantly the Nation's capacity to protect and improve health; (2) develop, maintain, and renew scientific human and physical resources that will assure the Nation's capability to prevent disease, improve health, and enhance the quality of life; (3) expand the knowledge base in biomedical and associated sciences in order to enhance the Nation's economic well-being and ensure a continued high return on the public investment in research; and (4) exemplify and promote the highest level of integrity, public accountability, and social responsibility in the conduct of science. In realizing these goals, the NIH provides leadership and direction to programs designed to improve the health of the Nation by conducting and supporting research: in the causes, diagnosis, prevention, and cure of human diseases, in the processes of human growth and development, in the biological effects of environmental contaminants, in the understanding of mental, addictive and physical disorders; in directing programs for the collection, dissemination, and exchange of information in medicine and health, including the development and support of medical libraries and the training of medical librarians and other health information specialists. (*Organization Manual,* Chap. HN-A, 1992, p. 1)

Six components of the National Institutes of Health in which black nurses are or involved are: (1) the Clinical Center; (2) the National Library of Medicine; (3) the National Institute of Nursing Research; (4) the

National Heart, Blood, and Lung Institute; (5) the National Institute of Mental Health; and (6) the Extramural Associates Program.

The Clinical Center. In 1952, the USPHS established on the grounds of the NIH in Bethesda, Maryland, a research hospital center of 500 beds called the National Clinical Center (Dolan et al., 1983). At the center, research and the clinical care of patients are closely integrated, and the nurse is not only a member of the patient care team, but also of the research team. Nurses at the Clinical Center collaborate with other health professionals to make science consistent with the highest quality of care. Apart from their roles in research initiated by scientists at the center, nurses are encouraged to use research methods to conduct studies in their own areas of interest.

Four black nurses hold key positions at the Clinical Center: Diane Thompkins, LCDR Arnette Wright, Jean Harris, and Barbara Bowens.

Diane Thompkins (B.S.N., State University of New York at Buffalo; M.S., University of Maryland School of Nursing, Baltimore) is nurse consultant, after having served briefly as program analyst with the Division of Nursing.

LCDR. Arnette M. Wright (B.S.N., Howard University College of Nursing, Washington, DC; M.A., Central Michigan University, Mt. Pleasant, MI) is chief, Basic Nursing Unit. She has 24-hour responsibility and accountability for patient care and staff activities on the pediatric endocrine/genetic unit in a research setting.

Jean M. Harris (A.A., Washington Technical Institute, Washington, DC; M.S.N., The Catholic University of America, Washington, DC) is nurse specialist for quality care.

Barbara Bowens (B.S.N., Marymount University, Arlington, VA; M.A., Trinity College, Washington, DC) is supervisory clinical nurse, Neuroscience Nursing.

The 1994 Department of Nursing Research Award at the Clinical Center went to a team of nurses who had identified the need to examine psychosocial changes in patients with Gaucher's disease receiving enzyme replacement therapy. The principal investigator was a black nurse, Olive Graham. Others on the team were Nancy Harnett, Elaine Considine, and Elaine Harrison.

National Library of Medicine. The National Library of Medicine (NLM) was established in 1836 as the Library of the Army Surgeon General's Office and remained in the military until 1956, when it was transferred to the NIH and upgraded to the National Library of Medicine.

NLM is the world's largest research library in a single scientific and professional field. Its holdings include 3.5 million books, journals, technical reports, theses, microfilms, and pictorial and audiovisual materials. Housed in the library is one of the nation's largest medical history collections, with contents dating from the 11th to the mid-19th century. NLM also houses historical documents in nursing, including those of the National League for Nursing. The nursing collection includes approximately 174 journals or serial letters and more than 2,000 book titles (Sparks, 1986).

Dorothy L. Moore (Lincoln School for Nurses, New York; M.S., School of Library Services, Columbia University, New York) is not classified as a nurse by the PHS, but as a technical information specialist. Moore also holds certificates from the National Library of Medicine Post-Graduate Associate Program in Biomedical Communications and the Health and Human Services Women's Initiate Training Program.

National Institute of Nursing Research.   On November 20, 1985, the Senate overrode President Reagan's veto of the NIH bill and established the National Center for Nursing Research at NIH. The House had voted to override the veto the week before. Steady lobbying efforts by nurses and nursing groups helped to sway the vote. It was they who convinced Congress on how vital research is to the nursing profession and to the improvement of patient care.

The National Center for Nursing Research was authorized under the Health Research Extension Act of 1985, P.L. 99-158. On April 18, 1986, Secretary Bowen of the Department of Health and Human Services announced the establishment of the National Center at NIH for the purpose of conducting a program of grants and awards supporting nursing research and research training related to patient care, the promotion of health, the prevention of disease and the mitigation of the effects of acute and chronic illnesses and disabilities (Merritt, 1986).

As part of the National Institutes of Health Reauthorization legislation, on June 10, 1993, the National Center for Nursing Research was upgraded to the National Institute of Nursing Research (NINR), making it the 17th Institute in the National Institutes of Health. According to Dr. Ada Sue Hinshaw, who had directed the Center from 1978–1994, "the establishment of the new institute reflects a recognition that nursing research is an integral aspect of nursing practice and education in and across all countries."

The Institute's purpose is to provide a strong scientific base for nursing practice, develop the knowledge and empirical basis of nursing science, and help to answer questions about how disease affects people's lives.

Serving on the Advisory Council of NINR are two black nurses; Loretta Sweet Jemmott, Ph.D., R.N., Associate Professor and Director, Center for AIDS Research, Columbia University School of Nursing, New York, and Geraldene Felton, Ed.D., R.N., Dean, University of Iowa College of Nursing, Iowa City. The Council reviews reports of research training, intramural research, and data on national needs for biomedical and behavioral research personnel. At its Fall 1993 meeting, the Council received a report from the Task Force on Minority Research and Recruitment of Minority Investigators. The Council also makes recommendations to the Secretary of Health and Human Services and directors of NIH and NINR re: the research and research training programs of the Institute. In 1994, Barbara Holder, Ph.D., R.N., was appointed a member of the Nursing Research Study Section.

On the staff of NINR is Joyce Taylor Harden (B.S.N., University of Maryland, Baltimore; Ph.D., University of Texas, Austin) who holds the position, nurse scientist administrator.

In 1993, Friends of the National Institute of Nursing Research (FNINR) was organized as a support group and by 1994 it had grown to over 350 members, representing professionals in the nursing, legal, business, academic, and association communities. On the 28-member organizing committee were four black nurses: Dr. Rhetaugh Dumas, University of Michigan, Dr. Geraldene Felton, University of Iowa; Dr. Dorothy Powell, Howard University; and Dr. Ora Strickland, Emory University. At its second annual gathering in Washington, DC in September, 1994, Dr. Rhetaugh Dumas received a special President's Award from the National Women's Hall of Fame as one leading the way into the 21st century.

National Heart, Blood, and Lung Institute. At the National Heart, Blood, and Lung Institute is a black nurse, CDR. Leslie Cook Cooper (Diploma, Henry Ford Hospital School of Nursing, Detroit, Michigan; Ph.D., University of Maryland, Baltimore), who holds the title, Nurse Epidemiologist/Health Scientist Administrator, Division of Lung Disease, Airways Disease Branch. In this position, she has the responsibility for planning, developing, and recommending awards for programs of targeted research related to the cause, treatment, and prevention of respiratory diseases.

National Institute of Mental Health. Mary S. Harper (Diploma, Tuskegee University School of Nursing, Tuskegee, AL; Ph.D., St. Louis University, St. Louis, MO, Fig. 6–29), a long-time government employee, is coordinator for long-term care, NIMH Mental Disorders of Aging Research Branch. From 1979 to 1981, Harper served as director, Office of Policy Development and Research, White House Conference on Aging. Before

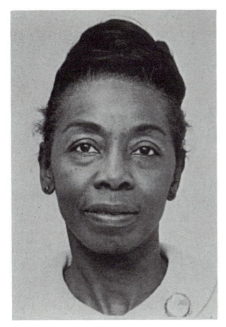

Figure 6–29 Dr. Mary Harper, National Institute of Mental Health.

then she had been with the NIMH Center for Minority Group Mental Health Programs.

Extramural Associates Program. Established in 1978, the Extramural Associates (EA) Program, administered by the Office of Extramural Research at NIH, is designed to promote the entry and participation of underrepresented minorities and women in biomedical and behavioral research. The EA Program is viewed as an investment that will yield multiple benefits to participating individuals and institutions, the NIH, and ultimately, to the vitality of health-related research in the nation. The objectives of the EA Program also coincide with NIH's goals of increasing the pool of minority and women research scientists and supporting research to address disorders which disproportionately affect these special populations.

The NIH selects, on a competitive basis, scientific faculty and academic administrators from institutions which contribute significantly to the pool of minorities and women in science. Those selected become Extramural Associates and spend five months in residence at the NIH in Bethesda, MD. The desired outcome of the EA Program is that, upon return to the home institution, each NIH-trained Associate will assume an active role to promote and expand opportunities for faculty and students to participate in biomedical and behavioral research. Among the immediate benefits the program offers is the opportunity for NIH staff and Associates to work together (NIH Extramural Associates Program, 1990). Since the program's inception, three black nurses have participated. Dr. Johnea Kelley, North Carolina Central University, Durham; Dr. Mamie Montague, Howard University, Washington, DC, and Dr. Joyce Taylor Harden, University of Texas, San Antonio.

In her final report on her EA experience, Dr. Montague wrote, "Subsequent to the EA experience, three new opportunities have become available to me: (1) the challenge of being placed in a new role as coordinator of faculty research and development within the college of nursing at my own institution; (2) the opportunity to be sponsored as a post-doctoral fellow at the University of Pennsylvania Center for Nursing Research by the Minority Fellowship Programs of the American Nurses' Association; and (3) the challenge of redefining my own research status while attempting to orchestrate a beginning research career" (Montague, 1990).

Agency for Health Care Policy and Research

The Agency for Health Care Policy and Research (AHCPR):

> provides national leadership and administration of a program to enhance the quality, appropriateness, and effectiveness of health care services, and access to such services through the establishment of a broad base of scientific research and through the promotion of improvements in clinical practice and in the organization, financing, and delivery of health care services including: (1) the effectiveness, efficiency, and quality of health care services; (2) the outcomes of health care services and procedures; (3) clinical practice, including primary care and practice-oriented research; (4) health care technologies, facilities, and equipment; (5) health care costs productivity, and market forces; (6) health promotion and disease prevention; (7) health statistics and epidemiology; (8) medical liability; (9) delivery of health care services in rural areas; and (10) the health of low-income groups, minority groups, and the elderly. (*Organization Manual,* Chap. HP-OO, 1990, p. 1)

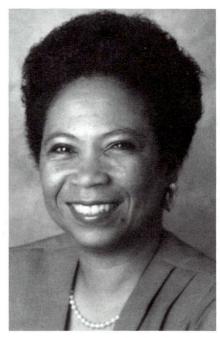

Since 1993, CDR. Ernestine W. Murray (B.S.N., Towson State University, Towson, MD; M.A.S., Johns Hopkins University, Baltimore, MD), who had been nurse consultant, Food and Drug Administration, has been Senior Health Policy Analyst, in the Office of the Forum for Quality and Effectiveness in Health Care. In this position, she integrates nonphysician

Figure 6–30   Dr. Linda Burnes-Bolton, National Advisory Council, AHCPR.

health care provider and consumer input into the development of clinical practice guidelines that will have a critical impact on the delivery of health care nationwide.

Alisan Bennett, Ed.D., R.N., Special Projects Coordinator in Nursing Education and Research at Woodhull Medical and Mental Health Center, Brooklyn, NY, serves on the panel to prepare clinical practice guidelines on the treatment of pressure sores, a followup to AHCPR's May 1992 guidelines on the prediction and prevention of pressure ulcers in adults.

Serving on the 17-member National Advisory Council of AHCPR to advise the Secretary of Health and Human Services and the Administrator of the Agency is Linda Burnes-Bolton, D.P.H., R.N., Director, Nursing Research and Development, Cedars-Sinai Medical Center, Los Angeles, CA (Fig. 6–30).

Regional Offices

The PHS Regional Offices support the PHS mission of improving the health of the nation's population by administering regional health programs and activities to ensure a coordinated regional effort in support of national health policies and state and local needs within each region. These responsibilities include the following:

> Assessing regional health requirements, assuring integration of health programs, and addressing cross-cutting program issues and initiatives to achieve program goals and meet overall regional health needs; providing a PHS focal point for responding to the needs of State and local governments, community agencies, and others involved in the planning or provision of general health and mental health services; providing a PHS focal point for emergency preparedness and emergency medical services in the regions; supporting the Department of Health and Human Services (DHHS) intergovernmental relations activities and responding to health issues emanating from State and local concerns; and administering health activities and programs to provide for prevention of health programs, improved systems and capacity for providing health care, and assuring access to and quality of general health services. (*Organization Manual,* Chap. HD, 1987, p. 1)

The ten regional offices are I–Boston; II–New York; III–Philadelphia; IV–Atlanta; V–Chicago; VI–Dallas; VII–Kansas City; VIII–Denver; IX–San Francisco; and X–Seattle. Black nurses hold key positions in nine of these regions.

Region I, Boston.   Shirley A. Smith Downie (Boston Hospital School of Nursing; M.S., Boston University School of Nursing, Boston, MA) has been regional maternal and child health nursing consultant since 1976. In this position, she has the responsibility for assessment, administration, consultation, and evaluation of federally mandated health care programs for mothers, children, and families in New England. Prior to this appointment, Downie held positions in hospitals, industry, and public health agencies in the state of Massachusetts in education, service, and administration.

Marva Nathan (St. Elizabeth Hospital School of Nursing, Youngstown, Ohio; M.S., Harvard University School of Public Health, Boston, MA) is Project Officer, Health Care Financing Administration. In this position, she monitors, directs, and evaluates Peer Review Organizations in their management of federal contracts to assure the quality of health care provided to medical beneficiaries. She also recommends approval/disapproval of the contract. One of her many past positions was instructor, Ahmadu Bello University School of Nursing, Zaria, Nigeria, West Africa.

Region II, New York.   Capt. Roberta Annette Holder-Mosley (B.A.N., Simmons College, Boston, MA; M.S.N., Columbia University, New York, NY, Fig. 6–31) is regional nurse consultant for primary care, clinical geographic representative for New York City, and regional perinatal coordinator, Division of Health Services Delivery, Resources and Clinical Services Branch. A certified nurse midwife, Holder-Mosley provides technical assistance/consultation to migrant and community health centers in relation to maternal and child health/perinatal issues in the region. A commissioned officer in the U.S. Public Health Service, she has been the recipient of five awards from the PHS since 1979.

Region III, Philadelphia.   Capt. Claudette V. Campbell (M.S.N., University of Pennsylvania School of Nursing, Philadelphia; M.P.H., Johns Hopkins University School of Hygiene, Baltimore, MD) is Associate Regional Administrator, Division of Health Care Financing Administration. She has received many commendations, the latest

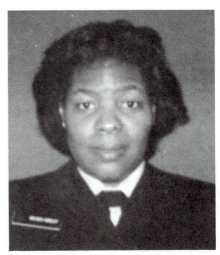

Figure 6–31   Roberta Annette Holder-Mosley, Regional Nurse Consultant for Primary Care, Region II, New York.

being the USPHS Outstanding Service Medal on December 11, 1990, in recognition of consistent outstanding performance.

Barbara Williamson (A.D., Community College of Philadelphia Department of Nursing; M.S., St. Joseph's University, Philadelphia, PA) is a nurse consultant, Survey and Certification Program Review Specialist for the Survey and Certification Review Branch, Division of Health Standards and Quality Health Care Financing Administration. In this position, she provides authoritative professional and technical expertise in the review and assessment of the quality of health care provided. She monitors and evaluates State Agency performance and effectiveness with respect to their enforcement of health and safety standards for all health care facilities/providers.

Region IV, Atlanta. CDR. Clara Henderson Cobb (B.S.N., Columbia Union College School of Nursing, Takoma Park, MD; M.S.N., Medical College of Georgia, Augusta, Fig. 6–32) is Senior Project Officer/Nurse Consultant. In this position, she serves as representative for program projects in the states of Georgia and Florida, providing technical assistance and consultation on all aspects of the projects.

Region V, Chicago. Dolores Perteet (B.S.N., Loyola University School of Nursing, Chicago; M.P.H., Yale University, New Haven, CN), has been medical review specialist with the Health Care Financing Administration, Division of Medicare, since 1987. In this position, she performs duties associated with the development and implementation of Medicare coverage policy and participates in the evaluation of fiscal intermediary medical review operations associated with claims determination. She is also assigned to work on other department initiatives associated with Medicaid funded maternal child health services aimed at decreasing maternal and infant morbidity and mortality statistics in the region.

Region VI, Dallas, Texas. Lawanda Prince Gordon (B.S.N., M.S.N., University of Cincinnati, Ohio (Fig. 6–33) is maternal and child health nursing consultant. She functions as the principal regional adviser in planning, organizing, coordinating, and evaluating MCH

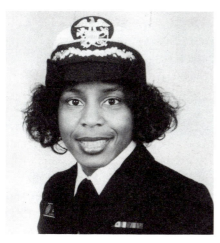

Figure 6–32 Clara L. Henderson Cobb, Nurse Consultant, Region IV, Atlanta.

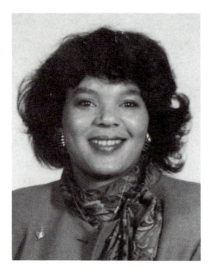

Figure 6–33 Lawanda Prince Gordon, Maternal and Child Health Consultant, Region IV, Dallas, TX.

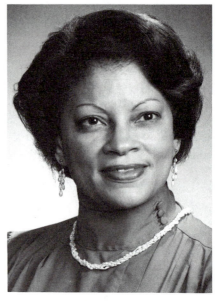

Figure 6–34 Vivian O. Lee, Regional Nursing Consultant, Region X, Seattle, WA.

nursing activities with particular emphasis on children with special health care needs.

Region VIII, Denver, Colorado. Erna S. Sanderson (St. Paul's Hospital School of Nursing, Dallas, TX; B.S., Paul Quinn College, Waco, TX) is occupational health nurse.

Region IX, San Francisco. Capt. Elizabeth J. Holcomb (B.S.N., Wagner College, Staten Island, NY) is Regional Site Manager/Occupational Health Consultant.

Region X, Seattle. Vivian O. Lee (B.S.N., University of Washington, Seattle; M.P.A., University of Puget Sound, Fig. 6–34) is the Director of the newly established Office of Women's Health. In her many years with the regional office, Lee has received 19 awards and/or promotions from the USPHS for outstanding performance in the family planning program and for special work on behalf of disabled clients and women. She has also received a national, a regional, and eight state or local awards from nongovernmental organizations for her leadership in the field of family planning.

Other Programs

In addition to assignments to regions, Public Health Service professionals are frequently detailed from the line agencies to other federal programs, such as the Bureau of Prisons, and the District of Columbia Commission on Mental Health Services.

The Federal Bureau of Prisons operates within the Department of Justice in the executive branch of the federal government. Its mission is to provide safekeeping, care, and subsistence for all inmates under the jurisdiction of the U.S. Attorney General. The Bureau of Prisons operates 47 institutions nationwide and Shirley A. Bowman (Franklin Square Hospital School of Nursing, Baltimore, Maryland; M.A., New York University, NY, Fig. 6–35) was chief nurse at the Central Office in Washington, DC from 1988 to 1992.

Since 1993, CDR. Norma Hatot (B.S.N., Hampton University, Hampton, VA; Fig. 6–36) has been serving as acting chief, Residential Placement Unit, District of Columbia Commission on Mental Health Services, Child and Youth Services Administration, St. Elizabeths Hospital.

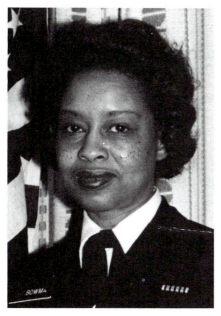

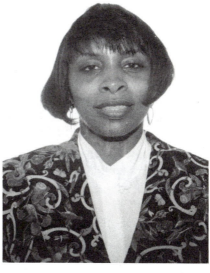

Figure 6–35 Shirley Bowman, Chief Nurse, Federal Bureau of Prisons.

Figure 6–36 Norma Hatot, Associate Chief Nurse, Forensic Inpatient Services, District of Columbia Commission on Mental Health Service.

PHS Programs Overseas

As the influence of the United States in world affairs extended beyond national boundaries, assistance from the PHS was requested for health studies in other countries (Williams, 1951).

During World War II, PHS nurses were assigned to work with the Office of Civilian Defense, the Liberian Mission, the United Nations Relief and Rehabilitation Administration (UNRRA), the Migrant Health Programs of the Department of Agriculture, and the Office of Inter-American Affairs (Williams, 1951). Black nurses of the PHS Service figured prominently in the Mission to Liberia and with UNRRA in China and South America.

Liberian Mission. With the location of the U.S. military installations in Liberia during World War II, our government became extremely interested in the public health conditions there, particularly in the problems of environmental sanitation, including malaria control (Williams, 1951).

In January, 1944, the president-elect of the Republic of Liberia requested the president of the United States to render such aid as might be available to assist the Liberian government in the solution of many of its major health problems, especially certain preventable diseases that were seriously handicapping the economic and social development of the country.

In a memorandum dated February 4, 1944, President Roosevelt wrote as follows:

> I think we should do everything possible to improve health conditions in Liberia. This should be taken up with the War department and the State department and Lend Lease. I should like to have a report on the progress. (*Cooperative Liberia-United States Public Health Program,* 1954, p. 1)

In response to the request, on March 28, 1944, the Department of State, with the endorsement of the War Department, requested the PHS to dispatch a Mission to Liberia, which was directed as follows:

> . . . to perform extra-military sanitation in cooperation with the government of Liberia for the protection of United States military personnel, including such sanitation works as may be necessary in other areas which may affect their health; to render the environs of airports free of exotic mosquito species dangerous to the United States if introduced; to advise the Liberian Government in planning for the sanitation of coastal towns, and to render such aid as may be requested by the Liberian Government in the enlargement of its public health program. . . . (Williams, 1951, p. 466)

In October, 1944, the Liberian Mission was organized under the direction of John B. West, who had been active both in appraising the health conditions in Liberia and in preparing preliminary plans and programs for the Mission. A group of four persons arrived in Monrovia in November, 1944. Shortly thereafter this group was reinforced with the arrival of Surgeon Charles West, Dental Surgeon Louis R. Middleton, Assistant Nurse Officers Theresa Colwell Jordense (Lincoln School for Nurses, New York), Virginia Ford (Kansas City General, No. 2, Kansas City, MO), and Hazel Birch (Harlem Hospital School of Nursing, New York), and Assistant Sanitarian Alma Jackson.

About this same time, the Office of Cultural Affairs of the Department of State assigned two nursing arts instructors, Vashti Hill Gilmore and Inez Butler, both graduates of Freedmen's Hospital School of Nursing in Washington, DC, to Liberia for the purpose of assisting the mission in developing a training school for Liberian nurses.

The maximum strength of the mission was reached in 1947, when 21 professional and technical persons were on active duty with the mission (Williams, 1951). Among these were Clara E. Beverly and Lillian Holly, both of Freedmen's Hospital (Beverly, 1947). Captain Beverly served as nursing arts instructor in the School of Nursing sponsored by the Liberian government. In 1949, she returned to Freedmen's, but was again assigned to the PHS Mission to Liberia in 1952, this time as director of nursing education. In 1956, she returned to Freedmen's but was again assigned to teach practical nursing at the Navajo Medical Center at Fort Defiance, Arizona.

The Mission to Liberia was taken over by the Agency for International Development (AID) in 1954. The pioneer work of the USPHS Mission to Liberia provided a valuable guide in planning health projects in other underdeveloped areas (Williams, 1951).

The United Nations Relief and Rehabilitation Administration. The United Nations Relief and Rehabilitation Administration (UNRRA) was established on November 9, 1943, in Washington, DC, upon the signing of an agreement by 44 nations, including the United States. The administration planned and administered measures for the relief of war victims through the provision of food, fuel, clothing, shelter, and other basic necessities, and medical and other services; and presented to the appropriate combined boards the overall requirements for relief (*Federal Records,* 1950). UNRRA was organized to ameliorate the tragic plight of millions of refugees and displaced persons in liberated countries (Roberts, 1954). China was one of the nations to which nurses from the USPHS were sent, and this mission included two black nurses: Florence M. Hargett and Dorothy Doyle Harrison.

Florence M. Hargett (Mercy Hospital School of Nursing, Philadelphia, PA; M.A. Teachers College, Columbia University, New York, Fig. 6–37) served as a nursing consultant from 1945 to 1947 with UNRRA Mission to China in Kwangsi, Honan, and Manchuria. During 1950 and 1951, she was director, National Tubman School of Nursing, Monrovia, Liberia. From 1952 to 1971, she served as educator/consultant for the World Health Organization in Taiwan, Egypt, Sierra Leone, and Iraq, where she was awarded the Silver Seal of the College of Nursing, University of Baghdad. She is now Professor Emerita, Seton Hall University College of Nursing, South Orange, New Jersey, where she had served on the faculty from 1973 to 1983. Included in Hargett's many publications is an article in the July–August, 1961 issue of the *International Nursing Review,* entitled "Problems of Communication for International Understanding."

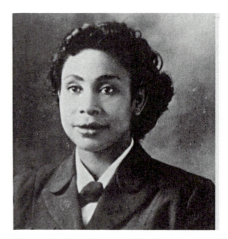

Figure 6–37   Florence M. Hargett served as a nursing consultant, UNRRA Mission to China.

Dorothy Doyle Harrison (Diploma, Mercy Hospital School of Nursing, Philadelphia, PA; Ph.D., The Catholic University of America, Washington, DC, Fig. 6–38) served two years in China, 1945–1947, as public health nurse consultant for UNRRA. Later she was appointed public health nurse consultant in the Office of Inter-American Affairs in Brazil, serving the areas of Rio de Janeiro and Belem. Her duties included the

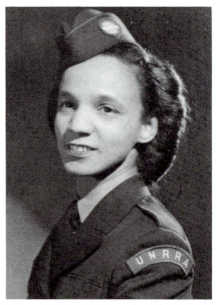

Figure 6–38   Dr. Dorothy Doyle Harrison, consultant, UNRRA in China and Brazil.

teaching of nursing and midwifery and setting up public health centers. Dr. Harrison is Professor Emerita, Howard University College of Medicine, Washington, DC, consultant to the Office of Alternative Medicine at NIH; she has a very active private practice in biofeedback.

Liquidation of UNRRA began in 1946; it was abolished September 30, 1948, but liquidation activities continued until March 31, 1949, when its remaining funds and records were turned over to the United Nations (*Federal Records,* 1950).

Point Four. Among the many midcentury international health programs that were outside the direct administrative jurisdiction of the World Health Organization was the Point Four Program, developed by governmental agencies of the United States. The Point Four Program was so named because it was based on the fourth recommendation in President Truman's inaugural address (1946) of which he said:

> This program will provide means needed to translate our words of friendship into deeds . . . By patient diligent effort, levels of education can be raised and standards of health improved to enable the people of such areas to make better use of their resources. Their lands can be made to yield better crops. (*Aspects of Point Four,* 1952)

By 1952, the program was in action in 35 countries, one of which was Liberia, and the USPHS supplied technical support and much of the personnel (Roberts, 1954). Several black nurses participated in this program, particularly in Africa.

Agency for International Development. The Agency for International Development (AID) was established November 3, 1961, by the State Department Delegation of Authority 104 as an agency within the Department of State. AID carries out nonmilitary U.S. foreign assistance programs and exercises continuous supervision over all assistance programs under the Foreign Assistance Act of 1961, the 1960 act providing for Latin American development and Chilean reconstruction, and the Agricultural Trade Development and Assistance Act of 1954. It provides assistance through development grants and research, investment guarantees and surveys, contributions to international organizations, and other activities. Under the Alliance for Progress, AID promotes technical and financial cooperation among the American Republics to strengthen democratic institutions through comprehensive national programs for economic and social development. Under Public Law 480 of 1954, AID administers certain local currency and Food for Peace programs.

Certain programs of AID and its predecessor agencies had their origin in the Economic Cooperation Act of 1948, which established the Economic

Cooperation Administration (ECA) to administer the European recovery program (the Marshall Plan). The functions of ECA were transferred in 1951 to the Mutual Security Agency (MSA), established to maintain security and provide for the general welfare of the United States by furnishing military, economic, and technical assistance to friendly nations in the interest of international peace and security. Reorganization Plan No. 7 of August, 1953, established the Foreign Operations Administration (FOA) to centralize operations, control, and direction of all foreign economic and technical assistance programs and to coordinate mutual security activities. The FOA took over the functions of the MSA, the Office of the Director of Mutual Security in the Executive Office of the President, the Technical Cooperation Administration, the Institute of Inter-African Affairs, and several other foreign assistance activities. The FOA was abolished in 1955 and succeeded by the International Cooperation Administration (ICA), which coordinated foreign assistance operations and conducted all but military mutual security programs. AID replaced ICA in 1961 (*Guide to the National Archives,* 1974).

In 1978, AID employed nurses, among whom were several black nurses, who were assigned to some of the less-developed areas of the world. They worked as a team with U.S. physicians, health engineers, and host governments to help develop efficient departments of health and a high standard of health practice. The nurses were particularly concerned with nursing education, nursing service administration, and public health. Three such nurses were Jean Martin Pinder, Clemmie Jean Smith, and Mary Mills.

Jean Martin Pinder (Highland Hospital School of Nursing, Oakland, California, M.P.H., Yale University, New Haven, CN; Fig. 6–39) started her nursing career as a public health nurse with the Department of Health, Education, and Welfare; taught public health and health education at Dillard University Division of Nursing in New Orleans, LA; and participated in a pilot multiphasic screening program as health educator for DHEW before going to Africa to develop programs for training assistant health education officers and establishing health education units within ministries of health. At her retirement in 1973, Pinder was public health advisor for the Africa Bureau of AID. While working for AID, she served as advisor and consultant to ministries of health in many foreign countries— Liberia, Ghana, Sierra Leone, Tunisia, Morocco, Botswana, and the Ivory Coast—organizing and conducting training programs, developing family planning programs, and assisting ministries of health to plan and develop expanded programs for providing primary health care to rural populations. Subsequent to retirement, from 1973 to 1978, Pinder worked as a

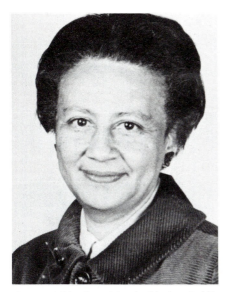

Figure 6–39 Jean Martin Pinder, Public Health Advisor, AID, served as advisor and consultant to Ministries of Health in many African countries.

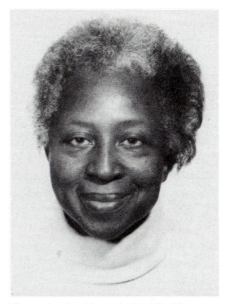

Figure 6–40 Clemmie Jean Smith, nursing advisor with AID in Pakistan and Nepal and WHO nurse educator in Africa.

consultant to the Africa Bureau and other organizations. Among her many honors was the Superior Honor Award in 1971 from AID Department of State in recognition of exceptional versatility, and persuasiveness in gaining acceptance for the implementation of new AID health and population planning programs in the face of considerable adversity.

Clemmie Jean Smith (St. Mary's Infirmary School of Nursing, St. Louis, MO; M.S., St. Louis University; Fig. 6–40), also a certified nurse-midwife, joined the International Cooperative Administration (now USAID) in 1959 as nursing advisor in medical-surgical nursing at the College of Nursing, Karachi, Pakistan, serving until 1960. From 1962 to 1964, she served as senior World Health Organization (WHO) nurse educator in His Majesty's Government School of Nursing in Kathmandu, Nepal, where she worked with one other WHO nurse, a national counterpart, and four other national nurse faculty members to raise the standards of nursing and nursing education in Nepal.

Between 1966 and 1973, Smith was WHO nurse educator in medical-surgical nursing and senior WHO nurse educator, nursing school administration at the University of Baghdad College of Nursing, a 4-year bachelor of science program in nursing. From 1973 to 1980 she was WHO nurse educator in Tanzania, East Africa. In 1983, Smith established the St. Luke's Medical Assistant school of Bulawayo, Zimbabwe, where she is currently located.

Retired in 1976, Captain Mary L. Mills (Fig. 6–41) spent more than 26 years with the USPHS beginning her career in 1946 with the Office of International Health, Public Health Service, U.S. Department of Health, Education, and Welfare; later she was detailed to the AID and its predecessor agencies. Twenty of those years were spent abroad, serving the people of Liberia, Chad, Lebanon, Cambodia, and South Vietnam. In these countries, Captain Mills helped set up maternal and child health clinics, schools of nursing, public health sanitation, and small pox and

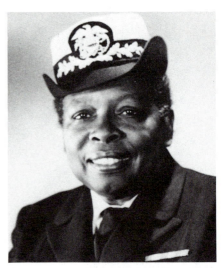

Figure 6–41 Mary L. Mills, retired Captain, U.S. Public Health Service, after having spent more than 26 years of service in the USA and other countries.

malaria eradication programs. She received several national honors for her humanitarian work in Lebanon, and other citations were awarded her by the governments of Liberia, Chad, and South Vietnam in recognition of her accomplishments in working with people in those nations. She has also represented nursing and midwifery at international nursing congresses in Mexico, Canada, Germany, Australia, Italy, and Sweden.

A native of North Carolina, Mills received her nursing diploma from Lincoln Hospital School of Nursing in Durham and a certificate in public health nursing from the Medical College of Virginia. At New York University, she earned both B.S. and M.A. degrees, and a certificate in nurse-midwifery from the Lobenstine School of the Maternity Center Association of New York. She also completed courses of study in health care administration, which led to a professional certificate from George Washington University in Washington, DC.

Since 1966, Captain Mills has been active on a number of fronts in the United States. As nursing consultant to the migrant Health Program, she was instrumental in shaping health policy to build on the strength and pride of migrant agricultural workers, frequently members of minority groups. An example of the great esteem in which she is held by her colleagues is that she was personally asked to go to Detroit after the 1967 riot to help repair communications in the burned-out areas of the city. She was able to do so with typical sensitivity and tact.

Mills has received many honors and awards, including an honorary doctor of science from Tuskegee University in Alabama, an honorary doctor of laws from Seton Hall University in South Orange, New Jersey, and the inclusion of her portrait in the Exhibit of 33 Outstanding Americans of Negro Origin in the Smithsonian Institution in Washington, DC. The portrait unveiled January 22, 1953, by Elizabeth K. Porter, President of ANA, was sponsored by the Harmon Foundation. The Foundation was established by a wealthy philanthropist to encourage blacks to achieve in the arts.

In 1971, Mary Mills received two of the nation's most coveted awards for her outstanding humanitarian service. The USPHS awarded her its Distinguished Service Award, and the Woodrow Wilson School of Public and International Affairs gave her the Rockefeller Public Service Award in the area of Human Resources Development and Protection. She was the first woman ever to be awarded the Rockefeller Award—the highest privately sustained honor for a career civil servant. This award of $10,000 was tax free. In 1972, she was the recipient of the ANA Mary Mahoney Award.

The Special Technical and Economic Mission.   In 1953, the Foreign Operations Administration (FOA), what is now the Agency for International Development (AID), Program was called the Special Technical and Economic Mission (STEM) to Southeast Asia. Laura Holloway Yergan (Harlem Hospital School of Nursing, New York; M.A., Teachers College, Columbia University, New York; Fig. 6–42) was recruited into the USPHS Reserve corps as lieutenant commander and was assigned to FOA and STEM in Indo-China (Vietnam), where she stayed until 1956 as nurse officer, nursing education advisor. Her subsequent USPHS assignments were in Beirut, Lebanon, 1956–1958; Karachi, Pakistan, 1958–1959; and Brooklyn, New York, 1959.

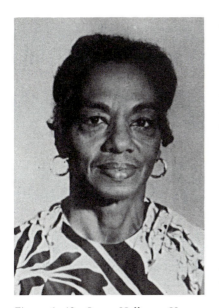

Figure 6–42   Laura Holloway Yergan, recruited into U.S. Public Health Service Reserve Corps as Lieutenant Commander, served in Indochina, Lebanon, Pakistan, Africa and Barbados.

From 1961 to 1968, Yergan was assigned by the World Health Organization to the Africa Region (Congo, Brazzaville, Nigeria, Cameroon, and Togo) and Barbados in the Caribbean Region. In 1968, she joined the faculty of the College of the U.S. Virgin

Islands where she remained until retirement as professor and director of the baccalaureate program.

Before becoming affiliated with USPHS and its foreign missions, Yergan had spent two years as director of nurses at St. Timothy's Hospital in Liberia under the aegis of the National Council of the Protestant Episcopal Church of America. For many years she served as consultant to Swaziland and Malawi.

A Proud History

At the 180th Anniversary Program of the PHS on July 26, 1978, Julius B. Richmond, M.D., assistant secretary for health and surgeon general, Department of Health, Education, and Welfare, had this to say:

> The history of the Public Health Service is a testament to our country's enduring commitment to improving the health of its people. Formed when the Nation was young, the service has grown and changed, faced new challenges, new opportunities, and new demands even as the United States evolved from an immature federation of ex-colonies to the most powerful and productive nation on Earth. Yet like the United States, the Public Health Service remains dedicated to the ideas and ideals that gave meaning and urgency to its beginnings, the belief that the vitality of the Nation depends on the health of its people and that government has a continuing responsibility to provide leadership in the effort to protect and promote health . . . .

Black nurses, too, have played and are continuing to play significant roles in the history of the PHS.

DEPARTMENT OF VETERANS AFFAIRS

Shortly after World War I, the federal government began building hospitals throughout the country for disabled veterans. With the exception of some isolated wards, little was available to meet the needs of black veterans (Morais, 1967).

Since more than 400,000 blacks had been enrolled in the armed forces during the war, the problem of providing adequate care and treatment for the disabled black veteran became acute. On August 9, 1920, the Bureau of War Risk Insurance, the Rehabilitation Division of the Federal Board for Vocational Education, and certain hospitals caring for veterans under the direction of the USPHS were transferred and combined into an independent bureau under the President of the United States, to be known as the Veterans Bureau, with a director at its head. During the same year, a committee of experts was appointed to conduct a survey of the needs of the country for hospital facilities for disabled veterans and to submit appropriate recommendations to the secretary of the treasury.

Included in the recommendations was one that stated that since approximately 300,000 of the blacks who served in the war were natives of southern states, a hospital should be provided specifically for their care and attention and should be located in that section of the country. Tuskegee, Alabama, was selected as the most suitable place for the black hospital, it being in the deep South and near the approximate center of the Southern black population. Tuskegee, already made famous by Tuskegee Institute (now University), founded by the late Booker T. Washington, was immediately acclaimed as an ideal location. In addition to the great institution endeavoring to educate black youth, there would be another institution dedicated to the rehabilitation of disabled black World War veterans (Dibble, 1943).

The officials of Tuskegee University welcomed the idea of a hospital for black veterans, but they, along with the National Association for the Advancement of Colored People (NAACP) and the National Medical Association (NMA) demanded the appointment of an all-black staff. In 1921, the Veterans Bureau and Tuskegee University agreed to the construction of a hospital on 300 acres of land owned by the University. At the cost of $2,500,000, a hospital, consisting of 600 beds in 27 permanent buildings, to treat primarily neuropsychiatric patients, was completed and dedicated on Lincoln's birthday, February 12, 1923. In the meantime, the Veterans Bureau appointed a white physician, Colonel Robert C. Stanley, as superintendent of the hospital despite a promise made to Dr. Robert R. Moton, President of Tuskegee University, that he would be consulted prior to any such appointment. Under Stanley's direction, plans were made to open the hospital "With a full staff of white doctors and white nurses with a colored nursemaid for each white nurse, in order to save them from contact with colored patients" (Morais, 1967, p. 113).

To forestall the execution of Stanley's plans, Dr. Moton wrote to President Harding on February 14, 1923, requesting him to give black physicians and nurses an opportunity to qualify for service in the hospital through special civil service examinations. After conferring with Dr. Moton, President Harding granted the request. General Frank T. Hines, director of the Veterans Bureau, was sent to Tuskegee to initiate a gradual change in the medical staff from white to black. A committee of the National Medical Association also brought this matter to the attention of the federal government. Several conferences with President Harding and General Hines resulted in agreement on the staffing of the hospital with black personnel. "It was only after a bitter fight that a Negro staff supplanted a white one at the government-supported Tuskegee Hospital for Disabled Negro Veterans" (Morais, 1967, p. 98).

Esther Juanita Bullock, a 1920 graduate of Kansas City General Hospital School of Nursing, Kansas City, Missouri, had worked at City Hospital No. 2, St. Louis, Missouri and South Side Hospital in Chicago before entering the service of the Veterans Bureau in May 1923. In June, she was assigned to the Veterans Hospital in Tuskegee, where she served as night supervisor for four months. In October, Bullock was appointed chief nurse—the first black (Thomas, 1929). Serving as assistant chief nurse was Amelia J. Gears.

Writing in the September, 1924, issue of *Crisis,* the official organ of the NAACP, W.E.B. DuBois said, "Our hats are in the air to Tuskegee and Moton . . . He and the Negro world demanded that the government hospital in Tuskegee be under Negro control. Today, at last, it is" (Fig. 6–43). In 1930, Congress enacted Public Law 536, authorizing the president to consolidate and coordinate government activities affecting war veterans into an agency to be known as the Veterans Administration (VA).

The agencies merged by executive order were the U.S. Veterans Bureau, the National Homes for Disabled Volunteer Soldiers, and the Bureau of Pensions of the Interior Department (Keough, 1981). On October 25, 1988, President Reagan signed a law which created the Department of Veterans Affairs—a cabinet level department, which became effective March 15, 1989.

Until 1941, appointments of black nurses to the VA were limited to the all-black facility at Tuskegee. It was around this time that a few black nurses were transferred from Tuskegee to other facilities. However, they were assigned to work on segregated units. For example, the group transferred to the VA Hospital in Kecoughtan, Virginia, in the early 1940s worked on wards or in buildings reserved for black veterans.

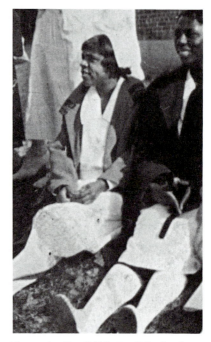

Figure 6–43 Edith English (in foreground), first black nurse to arrive at the Tuskegee VA Hospital in 1923.

During the post World War II period, the struggle for equal rights in hospital facilities was part of the wider battle to desegregate medical colleges, nursing schools, and professional bodies. The NMA was in the forefront of the fight to end discriminatory treatment in the country's hospitals. To forestall what happened at the close of the first World War, the NMA's veterans committee, together with representatives from the National Association of Colored Graduate Nurses, the Medico-Chirurgical Society of the District of Columbia, and the National Negro Publishers Association, met with General Paul R. Harvey, medical director of the VA, in October, 1945, to discuss a program for complete integration of the administration's hospital system for both patients and professional personnel. Following the meetings, Dr. Emory I. Robinson, president of the NMA stated that the VA should assist integration just as civilian hospitals were beginning to do. "We fully agree with General Hawley that there is no defense to segregation." Dr. Robinson declared. "Our Army has changed its policy and our navy has changed its policy. The Veterans Administration cannot look back. It must look forward and must change its policy" (Morais, 1967, p. 142).

To destroy the principle of segregation in the hospital system of the VA was not easy. Despite the fact that veterans were legally entitled to medical care without discrimination, 24 of the 127 veterans hospitals operating in the beginning of November 1947, had separate wards for black patients. Nineteen of them, all located in the South, refused to admit blacks except in cases of medical emergencies. Yet, in spite of such setbacks, the civil rights forces refused to abandon the battle. Finally, in October 1954, the agency ordered the end of segregation in all its hospitals. Thereafter, the order was scrupulously carried out in all veterans hospitals (Morais, 1967, p. 142).

In 1963, Beatrice L. Murray (Kansas City General Hospital School of Nursing, Kansas City, Missouri; M.S.N., Wayne State University School of Nursing, Detroit, MI), after having held various positions in governmental agencies such as the U.S. Department of Agriculture, Migratory Labor Health Association, and the VA since 1941, was enrolled as a chief nurse trainee with the VA in 1963. Upon completion of her traineeship in 1964, she was appointed chief nurse at the VA Hospital in Pittsburgh, PA—the first black chief nurse at an integrated facility. Subsequently, from 1966 to her retirement in 1981, Murray served as chief nurse at VA hospitals in Bedford, MA; Hines, Illinois; and Washington, DC.

In May, 1971, Murray represented the VA Nursing Service at the International Congress for Psychiatry and Social Change in Jerusalem, Israel, as a nurse member of the team. In 1975, she received the Honor Award from the Department of Medicine and Surgery "in recognition of outstanding performances as chief, Nursing Service in several settings, and for collaborative relationships with the academic and personnel community." (Murray died in 1991.)

In 1964, Minnie Lee Jones Hartsfield (Burwell Hospital School of Nursing, Selma, AL; M.A., Teachers College, Columbia University, New York) became the first black nurse to be appointed to the staff of Central Office of the VA in Washington, DC, having for 25 years held positions in several VA facilities, ranging from staff nurse to instructor to associate chief, nursing education.

As nursing specialist at the VA Central Office, Hartsfield's duties included assisting with gathering and analyzing significant data from VA health facilities in order to identify and justify programs, policies, and procedures needed and/or required; making visits to various health facilities to review and evaluate the standards of nursing care; assisting with recruitment and replacement of nurses in key positions; and serving as consultant as the need arose or when requested. Upon leaving Central Office in 1968, Hartsfield served as chief nurse at the VA Westside Hospital in Chicago until 1970, and chief nurse, VA Medical Center at Downey, Illinois, from 1970 to 1975.

In 1979, Liz Johnson (B.S., Texas Woman's University School of Nursing, Denton; Ph.D., University of Pennsylvania) was among five applicants selected from a pool of 254 to become a National Veterans Administration Scholar in the Chief Medical Director's Office in Washington, DC—a 2-year program. Immediately before this recognition, she had been director of nursing at the VA hospital in Baltimore, Maryland, having held other positions in the VA since 1974. Johnson (Fig. 6–44) also holds a certificate in management from the University of Baltimore.

Another black nurse, Pauline V. Skinner, was the 1988 recipient of the VA Award for Excellence in nursing. The award honors VA nursing personnel who stand out above all others in providing high quality medical care to VA patients. Skinner is a member and founder of the black nurses Association of Houston, Texas.

Today, there are no barriers, and until her retirement, December 31, 1992, the national director of nursing services was a black nurse, Vernice Ferguson (Fig. 6–45), who had been chief nurse at several VA hospitals and chief of nursing department at the Clinical Center, National Institutes of Health, Bethesda, Maryland. Ferguson, appointed director of nursing service July, 1980, brought outstanding professional knowledge and an enthusiastic spirit to lead the VA Nursing Service forward. In October 1980, Ferguson became the first nurse appointed deputy assistant chief

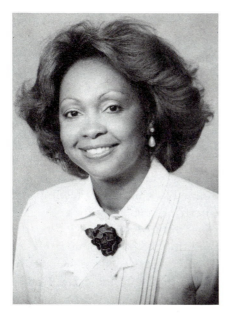

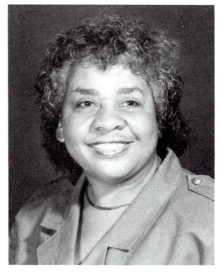

Figure 6–45 Vernice Ferguson, first nurse appointed Deputy Assistant Chief Medical Director for Nursing Programs, VA, 1980.

Figure 6–44 Dr. Liz Johnson, National VA Scholar, 1979.

medical director for nursing programs (Keough, 1981). Ferguson was succeeded by Dr. Nancy Valentine.

Today, there are 172 medical centers (formerly called hospitals), 356 outpatient clinics and community outreach clinics, 130 nursing home care units, and 35 domiciliaries. As of June 1994, the number of nursing personnel in the system totaled over 65,000 and was made up of 40,502 registered nurses, 11,221 licensed practical nurses, and 13,950 nursing assistants. The VA Nursing Service employs nurses with educational preparation reflecting every type of academic nursing education available in America today. More than 40 percent of the VA professional nurses hold baccalaureate or higher degrees. About 30,000 RN and LPN nursing students affiliate with VA medical centers for nursing experience each year.

SUMMARY

Black nurses have served in every conflict in which our nation has been involved, beginning with the Revolutionary War. As indicated in this chapter, black nurses fought for the right to participate as nurses and as citizens during World War I and World War II. Solely because of the color of their skin, they were not accepted in the Army Nurse Corps until after the armistice was signed, signaling the end of World War I. With persistence and cooperation of many white and black Americans, black nurses did gain acceptance in the Army Nurse Corps on a quota basis in 1941, and hundreds served during World War II, although assigned mostly to segregated units. Four black nurses were finally accepted in the Navy Nurse Corps during the last months of World War II. Black nurses distinguished themselves in the Korean War, the Vietnam War, and most recently in Operation Desert Shield/Desert Storm. They are now serving all branches of the armed services, being assigned without discrimination.

In the Public Health Service can be found black nurses at practically all levels of positions, holding commissioned officer ranks from the equivalent of ensign in the Navy and Second Lieutenant in the Army to Captain in the Navy and Brigadier General in the Army in this and other countries.

The Department of Veterans Affairs, the last of the federal agencies to integrate its professional staff, has done so completely and a black nurse has held the highest nursing position—deputy assistant chief medical director for nursing programs.

REFERENCES

Abdellah, F. G. (1977). U.S. Public Health Service's contribution to nursing research—Past, present, future. *Nursing Research, 26,* 244–249.

Adams-Ender, C. L. (1993). The future of minorities in military nursing. *Imprint, 40,* 51–53.

Army nurses tell us. (1944). *American Journal of Nursing, 44,* 998.

Aspects of Point Four Program. (1952). Department of State Bulletin, September 22.

Beverly, C. E. (1947). Nursing schools in Liberia. *American Journal of Nursing, 47,* 530–531.

Brief history St. Elizabeths Hospital. (1984). Washington, DC: Public Health Service, U.S. Department of Health and Human Services.

Commissioned Officer's Handbook. (1994), CCPM Pamphlet No. 62. Washington, DC: Public Health Service, U.S. Department of Health and Human Services.

Cooperative Liberia-U.S. Public Health Program under the Joint Liberian-U.S. Commission for Economic Development. (1954). Republic of Liberia, National Public Health Service.

Davis, J. P. (ed) (1966). *The American Negro reference book.* Englewood Cliffs: Prentice-Hall.

Department of Defense. (1982). *Black Americans in defense of our nation.* Washington, DC, The Department.

Dibble, E. H. (1943, Sept.). Care and treatment of Negro veterans at Tuskegee. *Journal National Medical Association.*

Dolan, J. (1968). *History of nursing,* 12th ed. Philadelphia: Saunders.

Dolan, J., Fitzpatrick, M. L., & Herrmann, E. K. (1983). *Nursing in society; A historical perspective,* 15th ed. Philadelphia: Saunders.

Dunbar-Nelson, A. (1919). Negro women in war work. In E. J. Scott (Ed.) *The American Negro in the World War*. Washington, DC: The Author.

Federal Health Programs Service Operations Manual. (1971). Transmittal Letter No. 45, September 23. Washington, DC.

Federal Records of World War II, Vol I, Civilian Agencies. (1950). U.S. Government Printing Office, National Archives, Pub. No. 51-7. Washington, DC.

First Indorsement. (1945). Memorandum from The Surgeon General to Office of Secretary of War, Attention: Mr. Truman Gibson, Jr., Civilian Aide to the Secretary of War, Jul 26, Washington, DC: National Archives.

Frank, M. E. V., & Piemonte, R. V. (1985). The Army Nurse Corps: A decade of change. *American Journal of Nursing, 85,* 985–988.

Franklin, J. H. (1967). *From slavery to freedom,* 3rd ed. New York: Alfred Knopf.

Grant, M. (1975). *Handbook of community health*. Philadelphia: Lea & Febiger.

Groppe, LTC E. (1945). Memorandum to Truman Gibson, Civilian Aide to the Secretary of War, Jul 26, Washington, DC: National Archives.

Guide to the National Archives of the United States. (1974). Washington, DC: National Archives and Records Service, General Services Administration.

Highlights in the History of the Army Nurse Corps (1975). Washington, DC: The Historical Unit, U.S. Army Medical Department.

Hine, D. C. (1982). Mabel K. Staupers and the integration of black nurses in the armed forces. In J. H. Franklin, & A. Meier, (Eds.) *Black Leaders of the Twentieth Century*. Chicago: University of Illinois Press.

Johnson, J. J. (1974). *Black women in the armed forces, 1942–1974*. Hampton: The Author.

Kalisch, P., & Kalisch, B. (1978). *The advance of American nursing*. Boston: Little, Brown & Co.

Keough, G. (1981). *History and heritage of the Veterans Administration Nursing Service, 1930–1980*. New York: National League for Nursing Press.

Kreidberg, M. A., & Henry, M. G. (1955). *History of military mobilization in the United States Army, 1775–1945*. Washington, DC: Government Printing Office.

MacGregor, M. J., Jr. (1981). *Integration in the armed forces*. Washington, DC: U.S. Army Center of Military History.

Maxwell, P. E. (1976). *History of the Army Nurse Corps, 1775–1948*. Unpublished Manuscript. Maintained by the Army Nurse Corps Historian, U.S. Army Center of Military History, Washington, DC.

Merritt, D. H. (1986). The National Center for Nursing Research, *Image: Journal of Nursing Scholarship,* Vol. 18, No. 3, Fall 84–85.

Montague, M. C. (1990). Final report of the EA experience. Bethesda: National Institutes of Health.

Morais, H. (1967). *The history of the Negro in medicine*. New York: Publishers Co.

NIH Extramural Associates Program (1990). U.S. Department of Health and Human Services. National Institutes of Health.

Notter, L., & Spalding, E. (1965). *Professional nursing: Foundations, perspectives, and relationships*. Philadelphia: J. B. Lippincott.

Organization Manual. (1990). PHS Chapter H. Washington, DC: Public Health Service.

Organization Manual. (1994). PHS Chapter H. Washington, DC: Public Health Service.

Organization Manual. (1990). PHS Chapter HP-OO. Washington, DC: Public Health Service.

Organization Manual. (1991). PHS Chapter HK-A. Washington, DC: Public Health Service.

Organization Manual. (1989). PHS Chapter HT. Washington, DC: Public Health Service.

Organization Manual. (1988). PHS Chapter HG-OO. Washington, DC: Public Health Service.

Organization Manual. (1987). PHS Chapter HD. Washington, DC: Public Health Service.

Organization Manual. (1992). PHS Chapter HM. Washington, DC: Public Health Service.

Organization Manual. (1994). PHS Chapter HB-OO. Washington, DC: Public Health Service.

Organization Manual. (1982). PHS Chapter HC. Washington, DC: Public Health Service.

Osur, A. M. (1977). *Blacks in the Army Air Force during World War II.* Washington, DC: Office of Air Force History.

Piemonte, R., & Gurney, C. (1987). *Highlights in the history of the Army Nurse Corps.* Washington, DC: U.S. Army Center of Military History.

Report of the Surgeon General. (1918). U.S. Army to the Secretary of War. Washington, DC: Government Printing Office.

Report of the Surgeon General. (1919). U.S. Army to the Secretary of War. Washington, DC: Government Printing Office.

Report of the Surgeon General. (1938). U.S. Army to the Secretary of War. Washington, DC: Government Printing Office.

Report of the Surgeon General. (1939). U.S. Army to the Secretary of War. Washington, DC: Government Printing Office.

Report of the Surgeon General. (1940). U.S. Army to the Secretary of War. Washington, DC: Government Printing Office.

Report of the Surgeon General. (1941). U.S. Army to the Secretary of War. Washington, DC: Government Printing Office.

Roberts, M. M. (1954). *American nursing: History and interpretation.* New York: Macmillan.

Scott, E. J. (1918). *Memorandum to Dean F.P. Keppel, Confidential Advisor, Office of the Secretary of War.* Record Group 407, Washington, DC: National Archives, Feb. 28.

Shields, E. A. (Ed.). (1981). *Highlights in the history of the Army Nurse Corps.* Washington, DC: Government Printing Office.

Sparks, S. M. (1986, March–April). The U.S. National Library of Medicine: A Worldwide nursing resource. *International Nursing Review, 33,* 47–49.

Staupers, M. K. (1961). *No time for prejudice.* New York: Macmillan.

Subcommittee hearing brings praise to IHS nurse. (1990, September). *American Nurse,* 2.

Thoms, A. B. (1929). *Pathfinders, The progress of colored graduate nurses.* New York: Kay Printing House.

Willenz, J. A. (1983). *Women Veterans: America's forgotten heroines.* New York: Continuum.

Williams, R. C. (1951). *The United States Public Health Service 1790–1950.* Bethesda: Commissioned Officers Administration, USPHS.

Chapter
7

Nursing in the Caribbean

Although not yet a member of the International Council of Nurses (ICN), reference is made in this chapter to Belize, a Caribbean country in Central America, because in 1994 its nurses celebrated 100 years of formal nursing education in their country. A former British colony (British Honduras), for 25 years nursing education has been effectively conducted by Belizean nationals who were prepared both in Belize and abroad. Unfettered by outside regulations, but cognizant of the diversity of existing educational patterns, Belizean nurses have developed a nursing education system which distinctively addresses the nation's health care needs (Fig. 7–1).

The nine black English–speaking countries in the Caribbean that have membership in ICN are presented in alphabetical order: Bahamas, Barbados, Bermuda, British Virgin Islands, Grenada, Guyana,

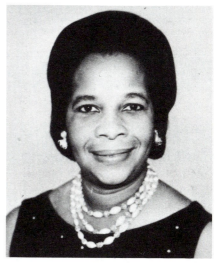

Figure 7–1   Hazel M. Wright, first native-born, nationally prepared Principal Nursing Officer of Belize, 1970. (Courtesy Eleanor Herrmann)

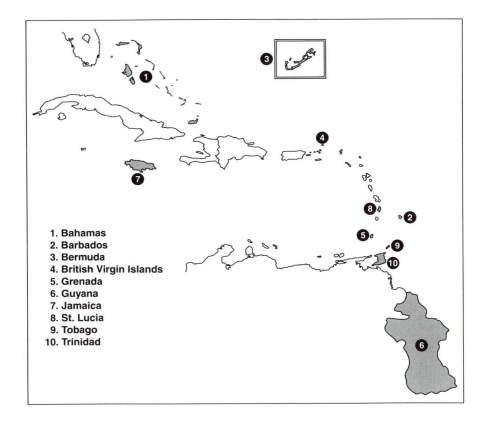

1. Bahamas
2. Barbados
3. Bermuda
4. British Virgin Islands
5. Grenada
6. Guyana
7. Jamaica
8. St. Lucia
9. Tobago
10. Trinidad

Jamaica, St. Lucia, and Trinidad & Tobago, followed by a brief overview of the Caribbean Nurses' Organization.

BAHAMAS

The Bahamas is the most northern group of islands in the West Indies, located between Florida and Haiti. Consisting of 5,380 square miles, it is slightly larger than New Jersey and Connecticut combined. Christopher Columbus discovered the Bahamas in 1492 when he first landed in the Western Hemisphere. It became a British Crown Colony in 1717 and has been an Independent Commonwealth since July 10, 1973, with executive authority vested in the British monarch. Its independence was achieved through a series of constitutional and political steps. In 1989, the population of 243,933 consisted of blacks of African descent—85 percent and

European—15 percent, with a literacy rate of 93 percent (*Background Notes*, April, 1990).

A school of nursing was established in 1902 at Bahamas General Hospital. The matrons and sisters traditionally came from the United Kingdom and the School was associated with the British system. The first Bahamian nursing sister, Hilda Brown, was appointed in 1953 and in 1960 became the first Bahamian matron.

The practice of nursing in the Bahamas had been controlled by law which dated back to 1926. It was not an act for nurses, but for midwives. At that time, however, all nurses were registered as midwives and most of them were employed by the government under the Ministry of Health. The current law was passed in 1971—a statutory instrument to regulate the education and practice of nurses and midwives in the Commonwealth of the Bahamas.

In 1947, the nurses formed an association. Having met the criteria for membership in the International Council of Nurses, the Nurses Association of the Bahamas was admitted to the ICN in 1973. The Association also has membership in the Caribbean Nurses Association (1968) and the Commonwealth Nurses Federation.

BARBADOS

Located in the Caribbean, Barbados occupies 166 square miles and is about three times the size of Washington, DC. Its population of 253,800 (1988 estimate) consists of blacks of African descent—80 percent; mixed—16 percent; and European—4 percent. British sailors landed in Barbados in 1625 and the first British settlers arrived in 1627 or 1628 and colonized and controlled the Island until 1966 when it became a Commonwealth with a Governor General representing the British monarch (*Background Notes*, May 1990).

Historically there have been two nursing schools in Barbados—the Tercentenary School of Nursing, Queen Elizabeth Hospital at which both general nursing and midwifery were taught and the Psychiatric School of Nursing, Psychiatric Hospital which had both a 3-year basic psychiatric nursing program and an 18-month post-basic psychiatric program. In April, 1985, the general and midwifery programs were transferred to the Barbados Community College, Division of Health Sciences. In 1987 psychiatric nurse training recommenced both at basic and post-basic levels at the Psychiatric School of Nursing.

Nurses in Barbados organized themselves into a national association in 1936, with Eunice Gibson serving as its first president. Incorporated in 1943, this is the second organization in the Caribbean. A year after, in 1937, the Barbados Registered Nurses Association (BRNA) was formed with 12 nurses as members, BRNA launched the District Nursing Service—a voluntary service funded since 1944 by voluntary contributions along with government assistance. Having met the requirements for membership in the International Council of Nurses, the Barbados Registered Nurses Association was admitted to the ICN in 1957 in Rome, Italy.

The Caribbean Nurses Organization, established in 1957, held its tenth biennial conference in Barbados in 1976 with nurses from 26 countries speaking four different languages, but committed to a common goal—nursing care of people. Nursing in Barbados had moved from colonial to independent status; therefore, senior positions moved from colonial to national hands. At this meeting the leadership was completely within Caribbean nursing.

At the ICN Congress in Seoul, Korea in 1989, Dame Nita Barrow (Fig. 7–2), then Ambassador to the United Nations from Barbados, a nurse from the Caribbean who was to become the Governor General of Barbados in 1990, delivered the keynote address. It was at this Conference Dame Nita became the second recipient of the Christine Reimann Prize, the Nobel Prize of Nursing. She was cited for her notable contributions to the development of health care and nursing, not only in the Caribbean, but also internationally. She is also considered one of the world's leading authorities on public health and health education.

Since 1989, membership in the Barbados Registered Nurses Association has increased over 500 percent due to registration of the organization as a nursing-controlled union. Increased funding resulted in more

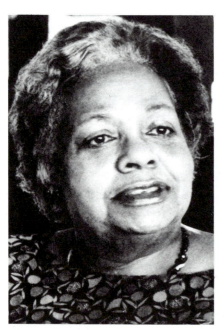

Figure 7–2   Dame Nita Barrow, Governor General of Barbados. (Courtesy ICN)

continuing education, greater image promotion, and increased compensation packages.

At the 1993 ICN Congress in Madrid, Spain, Peggy Rickinson was one of the panelists who addressed the "Importance of Local Leaders." Eleane Hunte of St. Michael, Barbados, was elected to the Board of Directors at the same conference. In 1992, Lyman A.R. Phillips was awarded the ICN/3M Fellowship for baccalaureate education.

BERMUDA

Discovered in 1503 by Spanish explorer, Juan de Bermudez, Bermuda is a group of about 360 coral islands of 20.6 square miles in the Atlantic Ocean located 650 miles east of North Carolina. Its population is 61 percent black of African descent and 39 percent white and others. Bermuda has been a British colony since 1620—the oldest self-governing colony in the Commonwealth. However, it did not have a formal constitution until 1968 (*Background Notes,* April, 1988).

Health services in Bermuda are provided at general and psychiatric hospitals. Public health nurses are employed by the oldest established health service, the Public Health Department, and District nursing is run by the Welfare Society.

In 1958, one school of nursing in Bermuda, under the aegis of King Edward VII Memorial Hospital closed. There are no schools of nursing in Bermuda today. Those interested in pursuing nursing as a career must go abroad for their education and most of the graduate nurses are from the United States, Canada, the United Kingdom, and New Zealand. In 1969, a nursing law was passed providing for a Nursing Council to regulate and control nursing practice and to maintain a register of qualified nurses.

Until 1967 there had been two nurses associations—one for whites, the other for blacks. Amalgamation of the two to include all nurses on the island was a precondition for membership in the International Council of Nurses. Upon accomplishment of this, the Bermuda Registered Nurses Association (BRNA) was admitted to the ICN in 1969 in Montreal, Canada. By 1990, Bermuda had also become a member of the Caribbean Nurses' Organization.

In 1991 Patrice Dill, a psychiatric nurse, received the "Nurse of the Year Award" from the Minister of Health and Social Services at a special ceremony launching the week's International Nurses' Day Festivities. The next day, a proclamation announcing "Mental Health Week" was read by the Bermudian Premier on the steps of City Hall.

THE BRITISH VIRGIN ISLANDS

The Virgin Islands are a group of islands at the eastern extremity of the Greater Antilles, divided between Great Britain and the United States of America. Those of the group which are British number 46, of which 11 are inhabited and have a total area of about 59 square miles. The British Virgin Islands are hilly, being an extension of the Puerto Rico and the U.S. Virgin Islands archipelago. The 1991 Census showed a total population of 16,115 (*Whitaker's Almanack,* 1993).

Until 1994, when an associate degree program was established in nursing at the Community College, there was no nursing program in the British Virgin Islands. All nurses there had received their education abroad—usually in Jamaica, the U.S. Virgin Islands, Barbados, or the United States. A few now hold university degrees.

Currently, the Chief Nursing Officer is Rita Frett-Georges (Fig. 7–3) who was graduated from the University Hospital School of Nursing in Jamaica, pursued postgraduate training in midwifery and psychiatric nursing in Scotland, and earned a Master of Arts degree in Clinical Psychology in Puerto Rico. Frett-Georges, the first psychiatric nurse and clinical psychologist in the territory not only revolutionized the concept of mental care as opposed to mental illness in the BVI, but was the founder of the BVI Mental Health Association, founding member and president for six years of the BVI Nurses Association, and is Vice-President of the Caribbean Nurses Association.

In 1989 the Nursing Council, which had been dormant since 1974, was revived with the chief nursing officer as chairperson. A registry was also instituted, which in 1993 showed "a total number of 93 nurses practicing in the Islands: 60 trained and 33 untrained. Eighty-two percent of nurses work for the Ministry of Health. They are qualified to practice in a range of specializations from General Nursing and Midwifery, through to Administration and Management and are employed in grades ranging from Registered General Nurses,

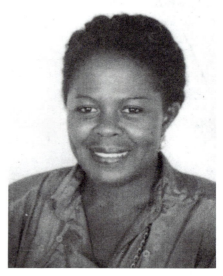

Figure 7–3   Rita Frett-Georges, Chief Nursing Officer.

Nursing Supervisors, Directors of Nursing Units and Chief Nursing Officer. The year 1996 will mark the 75th Birthday . . . of Organized Health Services and Nursing in the territory" (Frett-Georges, 1993, p. 15).

The British Virgin Islands Nursing Association (BVINA) was founded in 1971 and is considered the official representative by the government on all issues concerned with nursing and nurses. In 1983, to commemorate Nurses Week, the BVINA requested and the government approved and released four special stamps recognizing nurses.

BVINA, which had applied for ICN membership in 1990, was granted provisional membership in 1991, which was formally ratified at the ICN Congress in Madrid, Spain in 1993. It is the only organization representing nurses and is also an active member of the Caribbean Nurses' Organization.

GRENADA

Grenada, "The Isle of Spice," is the largest of the three islands (Grenada, Carriacou, and Pétit Martinique) comprising the independent State of Grenada. About twice the size of the District of Columbia, it is situated 12 degrees north of the Equator. Its population, estimated in 1989 to be 98,000, are mainly blacks of African descent along with a few East Indians and Europeans.

Christopher Columbus discovered Grenada in 1498 during his third voyage to the new world. He named the island "Concepcion." The origin of the name "Grenada" is obscure; however, legend has it that the Spanish renamed the island after the City of Grenada in Spain. Grenada remained uncolonized for more than 100 years after its discovery. Because British efforts to colonize the island were unsuccessful, a French Company purchased it from Great Britain in 1650. One hundred years later it was captured by the British. Although Grenada has been independent of Great Britain since 1974, it recognizes the British monarch and is governed under a parliamentary system inherited from the British (*Background Notes*, November, 1990).

Through the efforts of such pioneer nurses as Monica Agnes Clyne, nursing educational standards were raised, laws were enacted staturizing nursing certification, and a professional nursing association was organized. Grenada is a small country, hence membership in the Grenada Nurses Association (GNA) is small—only 250 members in 1990. The Association, however, serves its members by having educational sessions and by representing the nurses' interest to the government. It also provides a focus for nursing activities. Its leadership is strong and highly respected (Fig. 7–4).

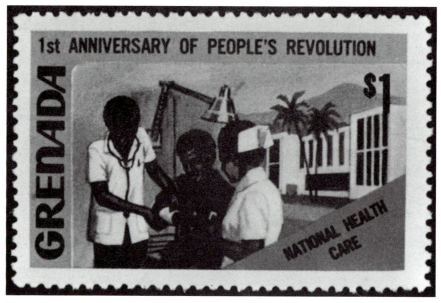

Figure 7–4   Nurses at work in Grenada. (Courtesy JFE Nursing Stamp Collection)

In spite of its size and other handicaps, the Grenada Nurses Association met the criteria for membership in the International Council of Nurses and was formally admitted in 1993 at the Congress in Madrid, Spain. The president of GNA is Luret Clarkson.

GUYANA

Formerly British Guiana, Guyana, the only English-speaking country in South America occupies 83,000 square miles—about the size of Idaho, and is bounded by the Atlantic Ocean, Brazil, Surinam, and Venezuela. Its population, estimated in 1986 to be 756,072, is composed of East Indians—49.6 percent, blacks of African descent—30.4 percent, mixed—14.1 percent and European and Chinese—0.5 percent. "Guiana" was the name given the area sighted by Columbus in 1498. The Dutch settled there in the late sixteenth century and the British became de facto rulers in 1796. When British Guiana became independent on May 26, 1966, its name was changed to "Guyana." It became a Republic on February 23, 1970 and adopted a constitution in 1980 with a modified parliamentary government (*Background Notes,* May, 1989).

In Guyana there are general hospitals, specialized hospitals, health centers, health stations, and private hospitals. The health care personnel consist of traditional physicians, dentists, general nurses, midwives, and assistant nurses. Dispensers make up another category of health care providers— men with nurse training who dispense commonly used drugs. A nursing officer is on the permanent staff of the Secretariat. In 1953 an ordinance for the registration of nurses and midwives was passed and the Nursing Council of Guyana was established. The Nursing Council, inaugurated in 1954, is responsible for authorizing the establishment of nursing schools and for examining and licensing nurses. Nursing education programs are controlled jointly by the Ministry of Health and the General Nursing Council (*Nursing in the World,* 1977). The 1977 amendment to the ordinance made the Principal Nursing Officer the Chairman of the Council.

The nursing education system today is British in structure. There are four schools of nursing. The government-owned Georgetown and New Amsterdam schools of nursing offer three programs—a basic three-year general nursing program, a one-year basic midwifery program, and a two-year program for assistant nurses. The three-year basic program at St. Joseph Mercy Hospital School of Nursing is private. The Charles Roza School of Nursing of the Bauxite Mining Town is semi-private and offers a three-year basic general nursing program and a one-year midwifery program. The University of Guyana offers a post-graduate program for tutors and administrators.

The inaugural meeting to form a nurses association was held in 1928 with the following objectives: to raise the standards of nursing in the Colony and to assure that nursing is practiced by a duly qualified person. This organization was the first professional nurses association established in the Caribbean region.

In the 1950s, the then British Guiana Nurses Association joined the Caribbean Nurses Organization and for 20 years it worked to qualify for membership in the International Council of Nurses. This was realized in 1961 at the ICN Congress in Australia.

JAMAICA

The third largest island in the Caribbean, Jamaica occupies 4,411 square miles comprising part of the Great Antilles chain in the Northern Caribbean Sea with Cuba, Puerto Rico, and the island shared by Haiti and the Dominican Republic. Its population of 2.5 million consists of: blacks of African descent, 76.3 percent; Afro-European, 15.1 percent; Chinese and Afro-Chinese, 1.2 percent; East Indian and Afro-East Indian, 3.4 percent; Europeans, 3.2 percent; other 0.9 percent. Jamaica was discovered in 1494 by Columbus on his second voyage to the New World and settled by the Spanish during the early 16th century. In 1655, British forces seized the island and in 1670, Great Britain gained formal possession through the Treaty of Madrid. On August 6, 1962, Jamaica became independent, but stayed in the Commonwealth. The 1962 constitution established a parliamentary system of government based on the British model. On the advise of the prime minister, Queen Elizabeth II appoints a governor general as her representative in Jamaica (*Background Notes,* February, 1990).

Although there had always been women who performed nursing duties (for example, Couba Cornwallis and Mary Seacole, see Chapter 1), formal training of nurses did not begin in Jamaica until 1890 with the establishment of the Deaconess Institution by Enos Nuttall, Anglican Bishop of the Island. Beginning with two recruits practical training was given in the Public Hospital under those sisters who were trained English nurses with the aid of the medical staff. By 1910 there were three established training institutions in Kingston, the capital city.

Today there are three diploma programs and one generic baccalaureate program including a program for registered nurses that prepare professional nurses. Whereas for many years Jamaican nurses had to go out of the country (England, Scotland, Canada, and the United States) to obtain advanced nursing education, such courses are now offered in Jamaica at the University of the West Indies, along with a baccalaureate program in nursing. Syringa Marshall-Burnett heads the Advanced Nursing Program at the University (Fig. 7–5). In addition, she is Deputy President of the Senate, Upper House of Parliament, Government of Jamaica.

The late forties and early fifties were historically significant for Jamaican nursing. By the end of the 1950s, Jamaican nurses had effectively demonstrated their determination to chart their own professional directions and strengthen Caribbean alliances. Such outstanding milestones as establishing a professional organization in 1946 with Nita Barrow (now Dame Nita) as its first president, a medium through which nurses could be heard, along with the institution of an official journal *The Jamaican Nurse* in 1961, with Gertrude Swaby as its first

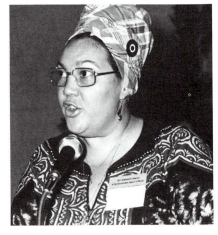

Figure 7–5 Syringa Marshall-Burnett addressing the ICN Congress in Tokyo, Japan 1977. (Courtesy ICN)

editor, successfully engineering passage of a bill for state registration; and fostering creation of a General Nursing Council to direct and monitor professional practice were indeed creditable. As a consequence of assertive action, basic education for the preparation of general, mental, and midwifery nurses was greatly improved. There is much evidence that input from external sources enhanced many of their campaigns, but professional development was due to the collective efforts and determination of Jamaican nurses themselves (Ho Sang, 1984). Having met the criteria for membership, Jamaica was admitted to the International Council of Nurses in 1953 at the Congress in Brazil, and has been actively involved ever since with representation on ICN Committees, the board of directors, and staff. In 1969, Dr. Mary Jane Seivwright, well prepared in education and research, joined the ICN staff as nurse advisor (Fig. 7–6). She also served on the board from 1973 to 1977. Syringa Marshall-Burnett has also served on the board of directors from 1977–1985. Merel Hanson, Jamaica's principal nursing officer, served on the board from 1985–1993 and was elected 3rd vice-president of ICN from 1989–1993. She also served as chairperson of ICN's Socioeconomic and Welfare Committee (Fig. 7–7). In 1991, the Council of National Representatives of the ICN held its meeting in Jamaica.

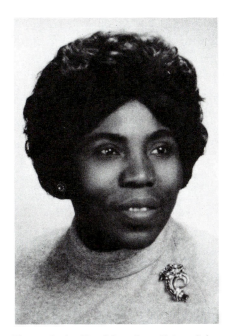

Figure 7–6   Dr. Mary Jane Seivwright, nurse advisor to ICN, 1969. (Courtesy ICN)

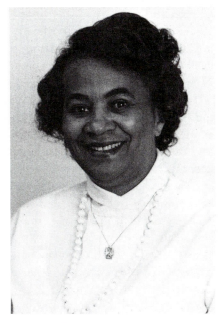

Figure 7–7   Merel Hanson served on ICN Board of Directors, 1985–1993. (Courtesy ICN)

Three Jamaican nurses have been recipients of the ICN/3M fellow-ships: Valerie Hardware in 1990 for study toward a bachelor's degree, Dotnie Smith in 1992 to complete a master's degree, and Rupertia Elizabeth Smith in 1990 for study toward a master's degree in public health.

ST. LUCIA

Occupying 238 square miles, St. Lucia in the West Indies, lies about 24 miles south of the French Island of Martinique and 21 miles northeast of St. Vincent, in the middle of the windward group. Its population consists of 140,000—African descent, 90.3 percent; East Indian, 3.2 percent; Caucasian, 0.8 percent; and mixed, 5.5 percent. The first known inhabitants of St. Lucia were the Arawaks, believed to have come from northern South America to settle in St. Lucia around 200–400 AD. The Arawaks were replaced by the Caribs. European discovery of the island is thought to be either 1492 or 1502 by Juan de la Cosa. The French established a settlement in 1651; it was controlled later by the British. As an associated state of the United Kingdom from 1967 to 1979, St. Lucia had full re-sponsibility for internal self-government, but left its external affairs and defense responsibilities to Great Britain. This ended on February 22, 1979 when St. Lucia achieved full independence. Ties to Great Britain, however, remain as the nation recognizes Queen Elizabeth II as titular head of state and is an active member of the Commonwealth (*Background Notes,* June, 1987).

For a number of years, St. Lucia had two diploma programs in nurs-ing—St. Jude and Victoria Hospital. St. Jude eventually closed and the one at Victoria Hospital was moved to the Sir Arthur Lewis Community Col-lege in 1989. This three-year course is the only one preparing students for entry into nursing.

The St. Lucia Nurses Association was organized in 1946, sought mem-bership in the International Council of Nurses and was admitted in 1975. The government recognizes the Nurses Association for all matters con-cerned with nursing and it has representation on the Nursing Council. It is also a member of the Caribbean Nurses' Organization. The Association has grown in strength over the years and has been representative of the various categories of nursing personnel on the island. It is registered as a trade union and now holds full bargaining rights for nurses.

In 1981, Eleanor Grant Collymore was the recipient of the ICN/3M fellowship to pursue a master's degree.

TRINIDAD AND TOBAGO

The second largest of the English-speaking West Indian islands, Trinidad and Tobago occupies 1,980 square miles and is about one and one-half times the size of Rhode Island, with a population of 1,279,920 (1988 estimate): African, 43 percent; East Indian, 40 percent; mixed, 14 percent; European, 1 percent; Chinese, 1 percent; others 1 percent. Trinidad and Tobago are the southernmost islands of the Lesser Antilles chain in the Caribbean. Geologically, it is an extension of the South American continent. Trinidad has an area of 1,864 square miles; Tobago lies 19 miles northeast of Trinidad and has an area of 116 square miles. Trinidad and Tobago's cosmopolitan society is mainly comprised of people of African and East Indian origin.

Trinidad was discovered by Columbus in 1498 on his third voyage to the Western Hemisphere. At that time, Trinidad was inhabited by several Arawak Indian tribes, who were destroyed later by early European settlers. The Spanish made the first successful attempt to colonize Trinidad in 1592 and it continued under Spanish rule until it was captured by the British in 1797. Trinidad was ceded formally to the United Kingdom in 1802.

Tobago has changed hands more often than any other West Indian island. Dutch, French, and English expeditions captured it from each other during its early colonial history, before it was finally ceded to the United Kingdom in 1814. Trinidad and Tobago were merged in 1888 to form a single colony, which obtained full independence on August 31, 1962 and joined the British Commonwealth of Nations (*Background Notes,* April, 1989).

During the nineteenth and early part of the twentieth centuries, the medical profession was solely responsible for the training nurses received at the Colony's hospitals. At the opening of the Port of Spain Colonial Hospital in 1858, it was reported that there were nine nurses on the staff—a "head nurse and eight other nurses" (Waterman, 1958).

At the turn of the century, nurse training at the hospitals was three years in length. In 1913, for the first time, an attempt was made to formalize the training nurses received; that is, a syllabus was prepared to instruct pupils similar to that used in English hospitals (*Rules for Colonial Hospitals,* 1938). Midwifery was considered a fundamental part of the education and training of nurses. So on completion of the three-year program in general nursing, graduates were expected to proceed to the one-year midwifery course.

A new era of nursing education began with the introduction of legislation for the establishment of a Nursing Council in 1950, which was given the responsibility for the education of nurses in the country. The period of training in general nursing became 3¼ years. Created in 1950, the Council deals with training, examination, and registration of nurses.

The British presence in the nursing service officially began in 1895 with the recruitment of an English nurse to serve as nursing superintendent of the Colonial Hospital, Port of Spain, and lasted for 64 years when independence was attained in 1962.

The first Trinidadian trained nurse to be accepted to pursue the sister-tutor's course at the University of Edinburgh, Scotland, in 1954 was Lucy Agatha Fields. On her return to Trinidad, her involvement in nursing education, and as a member of the education committee of the Nursing Council, led to significant changes in the country's nursing syllabus. The changes were designed to meet the needs of the country's health care delivery system, rather than continue the slavish copying of what obtained in English hospitals (Grayson, 1989). Today, nursing education has moved from the hospital to a College of Nursing within the framework of the National Institute of Higher Education Research Service and Technology.

The Trinidad and Tobago Registered Nurses Association was established in 1930 and was admitted to membership in ICN in 1953 at the Congress in Brazil. Two nurses from Trinidad and Tobago have been elected to the Board of Directors of ICN—Jean Grayson (Fig. 7–8) in 1989 in Korea and Yvonne Pilgrin (Fig. 7–9), executive secretary of TTRNA in 1993 in Spain.

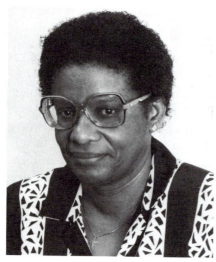

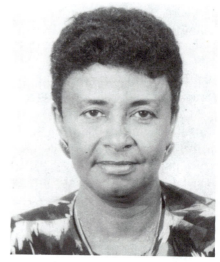

Figure 7–8   Dr. Jean Grayson, elected to ICN Board of Directors in 1989. (Courtesy ICN)

Figure 7–9   Yvonne Pilgrin elected to ICN Board of Directors, 1993.

The Association has always promoted continuing education for its members, hosting seminars and workshops, and the like. In 1988, the Trinidad and Tobago Registered Nurses Association hosted the workshop which was held in Tobago. It was sponsored by ICN/Florence Nightingale Foundation, and the W.K. Kellogg Foundation to implement "The Regulation of Nurses." There were 28 participants from 14 countries including Belize, Guyana, Lesotho, Botswana, Swaziland, and Zimbabwe.

Jean Grayson, one of the Association's active and outstanding members was the recipient of the 1977 3M Nursing Fellowship for baccalaureate and masters education study in the United States. In 1989, Grayson was awarded the doctoral degree at Teachers College, Columbia University, New York. Her dissertation was on the history of nursing in Trinidad and Tobago.

THE CARIBBEAN NURSES ORGANIZATION

In 1957 Mavis Harney, of the Certified Nurses Association of Nurses and Midwives in Antigua, invited Caribbean colleagues to a nurses conference. Thirteen nurse delegates representing nine territories met in Antigua for a stimulating professional, social, and cultural program. So satisfied and motivated were the participants that they decreed the activity worthy of regular repetition and full Caribbean participation. Harney served as a temporary president and is recognized as the founder of CNO.

Grenada hosted the 1959 conference, with the theme, "Nursing Education for the Unification of Nursing Services in the Caribbean." From its inception, CNO has reached out to all nurses in the territories and countries of the Caribbean and to Caribbean nurses residing in the United States.

The oldest regional organization in the Caribbean, CNO has concerned itself with the improvement of basic nursing education and has: tirelessly supported university education for nurses; instituted biennial awards to recognize nursing excellence; established an honor roll dedicated to those nurses recognized as change agents, visionaries, spokespersons, and advocates; published a newsletter and a journal, *The Caribbean Nursing Chronicle*; encouraged and supported the growth of national nurses associations, especially in small island states and territories; served as a catalyst to bring the region's nurses together enabling them to share and exchange ideas, address issues, and speak with a unified voice; provided Caribbean nurses outside the region with an organizational link; and provided a regular forum for continuing education on important regional/international issues.

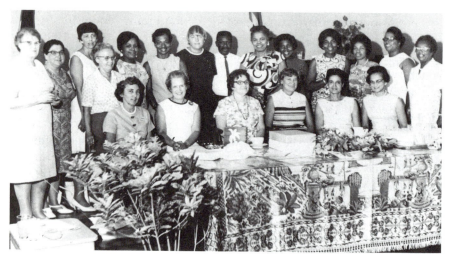

Figure 7–10   Biennial conference, Caribbean Nurses Organization, Kingston, Jamaica, July 1968. Gertrude Swaby, founding Editor of *The Jamaican Nurse* is seated far left, front row.

CNO has a membership of 27 national nurses associations and one group, divided into four regions. It has convened 19 biennial conferences (Fig. 7–10), the last of which was held in Bermuda in November, 1994.

SUMMARY

As in the United States and other countries, the education of nurses in the nine Caribbean countries presented in this chapter had its origins in hospitals. Because all of these countries had been British colonies, their nursing programs had been patterned after the British system. The trend today, as indicated in several of the countries, is toward university education for nurses.

Two of these countries—Jamaica, and Trinidad and Tobago—were the first black countries in the world to become members of the International Council of Nurses, having been admitted in 1953 at the Congress in Brazil.

Of significance, also, is the formation of the Caribbean Nurses Organization with a membership of 27 countries, enabling them to share and exchange ideas, address issues, and speak with a unified voice.

REFERENCES

Background Notes (Newsletter). (1987–1990). Washington, DC: U.S. Department of State, Bureau of Public Affairs, Office of Public Communications.

Grayson, J. H. F. (1989). *The Nurses Association of Trinidad and Tobago.* Unpublished doctoral dissertation. Teachers College, Columbia University, New York.

Ho Sang, P. E. H. (1984). *The development of nursing education in Jamaica, West Indies: 1900–1975.* Unpublished doctoral dissertation. Teachers College, Columbia University, New York.

Nursing in the world. (1977). Tokyo: International Foundation of Japan.

Rules for colonial hospitals. (1938). Port of Spain and San Fernando.

Waterman, I. D. (1958). A century of service. *Caribbean Medical Journal, 20,* 36.

Whitaker's almanack. (1993). London: J. Whitaker and Sons, Ltd.

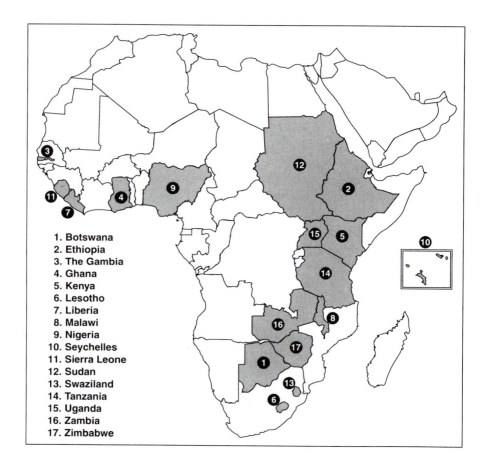

1. Botswana
2. Ethiopia
3. The Gambia
4. Ghana
5. Kenya
6. Lesotho
7. Liberia
8. Malawi
9. Nigeria
10. Seychelles
11. Sierra Leone
12. Sudan
13. Swaziland
14. Tanzania
15. Uganda
16. Zambia
17. Zimbabwe

Chapter
8

Nursing in Africa

efore presenting the English-speaking black African countries that
have membership in the International Council of Nurses, tribute
is paid to two black nurses on the continent for their pioneering
efforts: Samora Machel in Mozambique and Cecilia Makiwane in South
Africa.

Machel led the freedom fight in Mozambique against Portugal. After
independence was won in 1975, he was elected the new Republic's president (Fig. 8–1). He was killed in an airplane accident a few months later
and was replaced by Joaquim Chissano.

In 1908, Makiwane became South Africa's first black professional registered nurse and pioneer of black nurses there. In 1977 a statue of her was
sculpted and unveiled on the grounds of Victoria Hospital in Lovesdale
(Fig. 8–2).

Africa is a continent that covers nearly 12 million square miles, almost
as large as North America and Europe combined and nearly twice the size
of South America. Presented here are accounts of nursing in just 17 of the
many countries on that vast continent: Botswana, Ethiopia, The Gambia,
Ghana, Kenya, Lesotho, Liberia, Malawi, Nigeria, Seychelles, Sierra
Leone, Sudan, Swaziland, Tanzania, Uganda, Zambia, and Zimbabwe.
These are followed by a brief overview of two regional organizations:
West African College of Nursing and East, Central, and Southern African
College of Nursing, plus a description of the Kellogg Project in Southern
Africa.

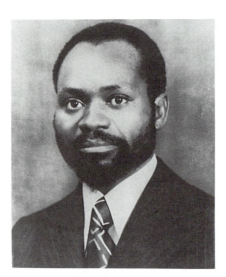

Figure 8–1 Samora Machel, freedom fighter and first President of Mozambique.

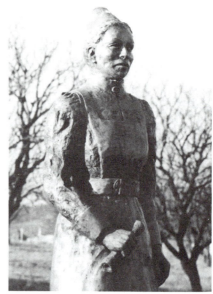

Figure 8–2 Cecilia Makiwane, South Africa's first black professional registered nurse.

BOTSWANA

The Republic of Botswana occupies 224,710 square miles and is about the size of Texas, Kenya, or France. It shares borders with Namibia in the west and north, Zambia and Zimbabwe in the northeast, and South Africa in the east and south. Its population of 1,255,700 (1989 estimate) consists of blacks—89 percent; whites—1 percent; and others—10 percent. By the 1700s, the ancestors of today's African population were established as self-sufficient herders and farmers or hunters and gatherers in the region which is now Botswana. The people's first contact with Europeans came through missionaries in the early nineteenth century when the territory was torn by intertribal warfare. Following appeals by Botswana for assistance, the British government, in 1885, proclaimed the country to be under British protection. In June, 1964 the British government accepted proposals for a form of self-government for Botswana that would lead to independence. Botswana adopted a constitution in March 1965 and on September 30, 1966, became independent. Its government is a parliamentary democracy with a president who is chief of state and head of government. Botswana has one of the best known human rights records in the world. The country's small white minority and other minorities participate freely in the political process (*Background Notes,* October, 1990).

The introduction of health facilities in Botswana and the introduction of institutionalized health care for the African population set the stage for a demand for trained African nurses to take care of their own people. The first health facility built for the African population was the Seventh-Day Adventist Hospital at Kanye in 1922. In 1925, the first three candidates were admitted to the hospital for work and training. The entry requirements for training were a Standard Six qualification (Grade eight) and certification for physical fitness. The training was to be two years long (Selelō-Kupé, 1993).

In 1978, the University of Botswana opened its doors to the nursing profession with the admission of eight nurses. The program, which led to a Bachelor of Education, was developed for registered nurses wishing to work as teachers in schools of nursing. The degree program for registered nurses was the first of its kind in all of Africa south of the equator (Selelō-Kupé, 1993).

In 1980, the Department of Nursing Education was formed under the leadership of Dr. Harriett Karuhije, a black nurse from the United States (Fig. 8–3). The Department of Nursing Education enjoys autonomy at the University and is currently headed by a native of Botswana, Dr. Sheila Dinotshe Tlou. Since 1980, the program has admitted students from Lesotho, Swaziland, Zimbabwe, and Malawi. With monetary assistance from the W. K. Kellogg Foundation, the Department of Nursing is currently developing a master's program in nursing.

In 1981, a family nurse practitioner program was established, offered through the National Health Institute of Botswana. It is the result of a collaborative effort between the Ministry of Health of the government of Botswana and the United States Agency for International Development. This one-year, post-basic nursing program evolved

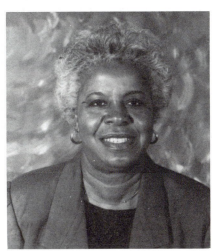

Figure 8–3   Dr. Harriett Karuhije from USA, nurse consultant to the University of Botswana.

from a national commitment to expand and upgrade primary health care services. The curriculum, based on service needs and reflecting national development priorities, has been designed to increase the relevance of nursing education to the social and health needs of the people (Ngcongco & Stark, 1986).

A Nursing Board and Nursing Council were established in 1964. These two bodies authorize the nursing schools and the training facilities for nurses and midwives, control the educational programs, hold the state examinations, and are also responsible for the registration of successful candidates of nurses and midwives.

Botswana, Swaziland, and Lesotho now have a joint examining board for nurses. With independence of the three countries, this has become a collectively agreed-upon examination board which provides for the legal establishment of nursing councils in each country. The last group of Botswana nurses from Kanye Nurse Training School took their examination under Nurses Examination Board of Botswana, Lesotho, and Swaziland in May 1988.

In 1989, Kanye SDA College of Nursing affiliated with the University of Botswana and their examinations are controlled by the Board of Affiliation for Health Institutions under the University of Botswana.

There had been no professional organizations in Botswana until 1969 when the Nurses Association of Botswana (NAB) was founded. The Association is recognized as a negotiating body for the profession. It became a member of the International Council of Nurses (ICN) in 1973. Botswana is represented on the board of directors of ICN by Dr. Selelō-Kupé, former chief nursing officer, Ministry of Health, who is serving her third term (Fig. 8–4). NAB owns its own headquarters, a hostel, and a day care center. Writing in the first edition of the Association's Newsletter, in 1970, Dr. Selelō-Kupé expressed the country's nursing philosophy, indicating that the nursing philosophy of any country must be in accordance with the cultural beliefs of the people of the country regarding illness and care of the sick.

The ICN-administered 3M fellowship has gone to two nurses from Botswana: Kgomotso Kenaope Badimela in 1986 and Kelesitse Tiala in 1988.

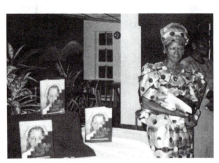

Figure 8–4   Dr. Selelō-Kupé (left) displays her book on the evolution of black nursing in Botswana.

ETHIOPIA

Occupying 472 square miles—the size of Texas, Oklahoma, and New Mexico, Ethiopia is located on the Horn of Africa and is bordered on the northeast by the Red Sea, on the east by Djibouti and Somalia, on the south by Kenya, and on the west and northwest by Sudan. It has more than 40 different ethnic groups. Ethiopia is the oldest independent country in Africa and one of the oldest in the world. Herodotus, the Greek historian in the fifth century BC, describes ancient Ethiopia in his writings. The Old Testament of the Bible also records the Queen of Sheba's visit to Jerusalem. According to legend, Menelik I, son of King Solomon and the Queen of Sheba, founded the Ethiopian empire (*Background Notes,* July, 1988).

Nursing education in Ethiopia dates back to only 1941 when Princess Tsehai, Her Imperial Majesty (HIM) third daughter of the Emperor, H.I.M. Haile Selassie I, returned to Ethiopia after having been trained as a nurse in the United Kingdom. She died in the service of her country in 1942 (*The Ethiopian Woman,* 1960).

In 1953, the first nurses were graduated from an Ethiopian nursing school—the Red Cross School of Nursing in Addis Ababa. In 1954, a Nursing Council was established. In 1960, a Nursing Division was established in the Ministry of Public Health and by 1963 the total number of nursing personnel was 319 graduate nurses, including foreign nurses. Of this number, about 85 had had post-basic training either abroad or in Ethiopia where midwifery training was available. By 1974, the number of registered nurses had increased to 1,200. The Haile Selassie I University in Addis Ababa started a Department of Nursing in 1961—courses for graduate nurses in ward administration, bedside nursing, and public health nursing were offered. With the trend toward specialization, courses to educate nurse specialists have been introduced: infectious diseases, gastrointestinal disorders, neurology, pediatrics, midwifery, education, and anesthesia. All nurses are registered upon completing their basic program and passing a national licensing examination. Registration is for life.

The Ethiopian Nurses Association was admitted to membership in ICN in 1957 in Rome and is the second oldest association member in Africa. In 1975, during the presidency of Emawayish Gerima, the Association launched its nursing journal and one of its members, Wengelarvit Beyina, received the ICN/3M fellowship.

A native of Eritrea (then part of Ethiopia), Ghebrehiwet Tesfamicael joined the staff of the International Council of Nurses in 1994. After receiving a diploma in nursing and teaching, Tesfamicael worked his way up the career ladder from staff nurse to clinical supervisor to senior instructor at the Menen School of Nursing in Asmara. He later earned a Bachelor of Science in Nursing from the University of Indiana; a master's degree from Liverpool University, U.K.; and a Ph.D. from the University of South Hampton, U.K. At ICN headquarters in Geneva, Switzerland, he serves as a nurse consultant.

In 1994, Nigisti Gebreslassie, instrument nurse at Police Force Hospital and secretary of the Ethiopian Nurses Association, presented a paper at the research congress in Sydney, Australia, sponsored by Sigma Theta Tau International and the Australia Royal College of Nursing (Fig. 8–5).

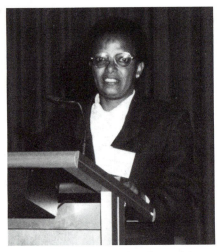

Figure 8–5　Nigisti Gebveslassie delivering a paper in July 1994 at a research congress in Australia, sponsored by Sigma Theta Tau International and the Australia Royal College of Nursing.

THE GAMBIA

Located on the west coast of Africa, The Gambia occupies 4,361 square miles—slightly more than twice the size of Delaware, with a population of 855,000 (1991 estimate). Approximately 2,500 non-Africans live in The Gambia including Europeans and many families of Lebanese origin. Once a part of the Empire of Ghana and the Kingdom of Songhais, in the fifteenth century, The Gambia was a part of the Kingdom of Mali. In 1783, the Treaty of Versailles gave Great Britain possession of The Gambia and in 1881 it became a British Crown Colony. Full internal government was granted in 1963 and in 1965 independence was achieved and it became a constitutional monarchy within the British Commonwealth. On April 24, 1970, The Gambia became a republic following a majority-approved referendum (*Background Notes,* December, 1992).

In 1954, there were only two hospitals in the country. Other health care work was done from health centers, which may have had a few beds, mostly maternity, and small dispensaries. The government was the sole employer of nurses, who were mostly men. However, Julia Williams, a locally trained nurse who subsequently had pursued post-basic education in the United Kingdom, the United States, and elsewhere was matron of the nursing service for the whole country.

Until 1969, there was no systematic nursing education program in the country. Individuals—male and female—were prepared on the job at various levels and called dressers/dispensers. They also provided primary care without supervision in rural areas. Nurses trained outside the country, usually in the United Kingdom, were designated as State Registered Nurses and held supervisory positions.

In 1969, a basic nursing program was started in Banjul for both genders, three years in length, and requiring completion of secondary school for admission. The fourth year was devoted to midwifery for the women and pharmaceutics for the men. It was not until 1972 that legislation was passed regarding education, registration, examinations, and a code of ethics. The Ministry of Health, Labour, and Social Welfare Medical and Health Department of Gambia is the authority responsible for accrediting nursing schools, as well as recognition of educational programs. In 1991, the Nurses and Midwives Council of The Gambia was established, with Thomas A.B. King as registrar.

The Gambia Nurses Association was founded in 1963, with Julia Williams as president. Williams was also matron of Royal Victoria Hospital. She not only showed great leadership, but had the support of some very fine nurses. All nurses in the country belong to the Association, which sponsors inservice education programs, workshops, and educational programs for its nurses. In 1965, The Gambia Nurses Association became a member of the International Council of Nurses when it met in Frankfurt, Germany. The Gambia has a unique program in higher education for nurses in that it is attached to a high school instead of a university—The Gambia College of Nursing and Midwifery, Banjul, with Francis Sair as the Principal/Lecturer.

GHANA

Known as the Gold Coast until 1957, Ghana occupies 92,000 square miles in West Africa—about the size of Illinois and Indiana combined—a few degrees north of the Equator. In 1989, its population was estimated as 14.8 million (it is now nearly 16 million). The first contact between Europe and the Gold Coast dates from 1470 when a party of Portuguese landed. When Ghana gained its independence on March 6, 1957, it had been under the control of Great Britain. (Just as the Supreme Court Decision—Brown

v. Board of Education—in 1954 sounded the death knell for legal segregation in the United States, the independence of Ghana marked the beginning of the end of Colonial rule in Africa.) The Peace Corps program in
Ghana is the oldest in the world. In 1990, there were some 100 volunteers
there—more than half in education; others in agriculture, rural development, and fisheries (*Background Notes,* February, 1990).

Formal nursing education was first introduced in Ghana in 1899 when
a British ward sister was sent to Accra to start a training program. Previous to this mission, colonial medical officers had enlisted the help of male
orderlies and instructed them in simple nursing procedures. Gradually,
more females were encouraged to enter the nursing field. The basic education of these candidates varied, but the highest was ten years of schooling.
In 1928, a midwifery training school was established and in 1931 legislation
for training, examination, registration, and practice of midwifery came into
being and the Midwives Board was formed to administer the ordinance. By
1944, it became necessary to plan for the establishment of a higher grade
nurse training and to standardize the various grades that already existed.
The first state-registered training program began January 1945 (Walter-
Holtz, 1969). Dr. M. Elizabeth Carnegie visited the College of Nursing
in Accra in 1960 (Fig. 8–6).

In 1945, a new system evolved. Girls with the West African School
Certificate were recruited and trained in the British pattern and awarded
the State Registered Nurse certificate. The training of public health nurses

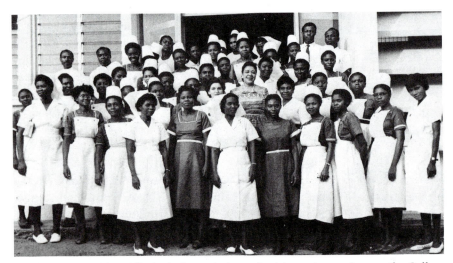

Figure 8–6   Dr. Mary Elizabeth Carnegie (center) with nursing students at the College
of Nursing in Accra, 1960.

began in 1952. In 1970, the basic nursing program was changed to emphasize promotive and preventive health care. Nursing is no longer confined to the hospital, but has moved into the community to provide comprehensive care in the form of curative, promotive, and preventive services as well as rehabilitation (Akita et al., 1979).

The first university-based nursing institution was established at the post-basic diploma level in 1963, one year before the first medical school. A basic baccalaureate program was established eventually in 1980, when the University of Ghana introduced a combined basic and post-basic nursing degree program. The University of Ghana's Department of Nursing is in the process of developing a master's degree program in nursing.

In Ghana, nursing is well integrated into the administrative structure of the government, with a chief nursing officer. The Nursing Council of Ghana regulates the profession. There are about 9,000 nurses in the country of whom 3,000 are professional nurses. With the exception of those in private practice, all nurses in Ghana are civil servants. A nursing division within the Ministry of Health has contributed to the harmonious development of specialties in Ghana.

The Ghana Registered Nurses Association (GRNA), organized in 1960 with Docia Kisseih (Fig. 8–7) as president, is the sole association recognized to deal with the welfare of nurses and speak for them. GRNA was admitted to membership in ICN in 1961 at its Congress in Australia. Docia Kisseih, who earned her doctorate at Boston University, was elected to the ICN Board of Directors in 1965 and reelected as first vice-president in 1973. Presently, GRNA is concentrating on four program areas: nursing regulation and the setting of standards, a building project, socioeconomic welfare, and continuing education for its members. In 1991, GRNA became involved in the ICN AIDS Project, which has not only strengthened ICN/GRNA relationships, but has provided increased visibility to its members.

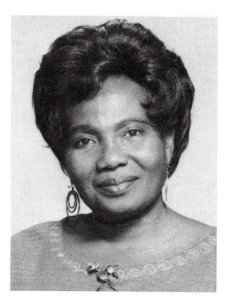

Figure 8–7   Dr. Docia Kisseih, first President, GRNA.

Three nurses from Ghana have been recipients of the ICN/3M

fellowships: Wilberforce Adade, who was awarded the bachelor's degree in Ghana in 1989; Mary A. Opare, who was awarded the bachelor's degree in 1991; and Faustina Oware-Guyekye in 1992 for baccalaureate education.

In 1991, Ghana hosted a four-day conference with 200 attendees including ministers of health, finance, and social affairs and planning, and discussed ways to integrate health programs in all economic policies and development strategies. Developed at the conference was a plan for action to make health the central objective in all development strategies.

KENYA

Kenya occupies 224,960 square miles and is slightly smaller than Texas. It is astride the equator on the East Coast of Africa and is bounded by Somalia, Ethiopia, Sudan, Uganda, Lake Victoria, Tanzania, and the Indian Ocean. Nairobi, its capital, has become a hub of communications, international conferences, and commercial and industrial activities in East and Central Africa. Fossils found in East Africa suggest that protohumans roamed the area more than 20 million years ago. In 1988, the population was estimated to be 21.6 million, with non-Africans making up only 1 percent of the population.

The colonial history of Kenya dates from the Berlin Conference of 1885, when the European powers first partitioned East Africa into spheres of influence. In 1895, the British government established the East African Protectorate and soon after opened the fertile highlands to white settlers. The settlers were allowed a voice in government even before it was officially made a British Colony in 1920, but Africans were not allowed any direct political participation until 1944. Kenya gained its independence from Great Britain in December, 1963 (*Background Notes,* January, 1988).

Having been under British rule before independence, it is understandable that nurses in high positions had been British. Today, all leadership positions in nursing in the country are filled by Kenyan nurses. The present chief nurse officer in the Ministry of Health is a Kenyan African. Kenya has two levels of nurses: first level are Registered Nurses; the second level are Enrolled Nurses. Their practice is controlled by the Nursing Council which was established in 1949 by an Act of Parliament. Registration is required only once and is good for life.

In addition to basic diploma programs in nursing, a post-basic education program and a WHO-sponsored University program was established

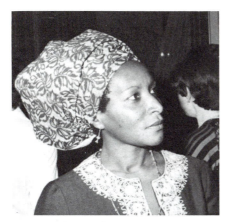

Figure 8–8   Eunice Muringo Kiereini, first black President of ICN. (Courtesy ICN)

in 1968 offering a Diploma in Advanced Nursing. In 1989, the first B.Sc. Nursing students were admitted to the private University of East Africa, a four-year program for high school graduates. Another such program opened in Nairobi in 1992. The nursing profession of Kenya plays a very fundamental role in society and the education of nurses forms a significant part of the overall educational system. Thus the nursing curriculum reflects the educational philosophy of society as a whole (Mule, 1986).

The National Nurses Association of Kenya (NNAK) is the organization representing all nurses in Kenya and has been publishing its own journal since 1972. Having met the criteria for membership in the International Council of Nurses, NNAK was admitted to ICN in 1961 at its Congress in Australia. And in 1979, the ICN Council of National Representatives held its meeting in Kenya.

In 1981, for the first time, a black nurse was elected President of the International Council of Nurses—Mrs. Muringo Kiereine, having served on the ICN Board of Directors (Fig. 8–8). In 1985, Tel Aviv University conferred an honorary degree on Kiereine.

LESOTHO

Lesotho in southern Africa occupies 11,718 square miles—about the size of Maryland. It is one of the two countries in the world completely encircled by another country—the Republic of South Africa. The other country is San Marino in Western Europe. Basutoland, now Lesotho, was sparsely populated by bushmen until the end of the sixteenth century. Between the sixteenth and nineteenth centuries, various clans from surrounding areas gradually formed the Basotho ethnic group. In 1818, Moshoeshoe I consolidated the various groupings and became their king. During his reign (1823–1870), a series of wars with South Africa (1856–1868) resulted in the loss of extensive lands. He appealed to Queen Victoria for assistance and in 1868 the country was placed under British protection. Independence was gained from Great Britain on October 4, 1966 (*Background Notes,* Nov., 1990). In 1993, according to Lesotho population sheet, the population was estimated at 1,980,814 including 1,700 Europeans and 900 Asians.

Many people live in valleys and areas inaccessible by road and are dependent on clinics, government and mission district hospitals, and flying doctors' service. The Private Health Association of Lesotho is responsible for coordinating the work of mission hospitals and clinics. It provides about half of the health services and nursing education for midwives, registered nurses, and nursing assistants.

Since independence in 1966, Lesotho nurses have been in senior posts in government health services, nursing education, and the community. Nurses are a powerful force in Lesotho and recognition of the value of their contribution to health care is apparent.

There are three three-year schools of nursing that admit high school graduates, the largest of which is the National Health Training College (NHTC) in Masaru, the capital city. Each has a program for midwives which requires an additional year. In addition, there are also the following post-basic nursing programs: nurse clinician, psychiatric nursing, public health nursing, ophthalmic nursing, and nurse anesthetist. All are based at NHTC.

Nurses had been going to the Republic of South Africa and to countries of the British Commonwealth for post-basic experience. Many now go to the University of Botswana and the United States of America for degree programs.

The Lesotho Nursing Association was founded in 1966. Having met the requirements of the International Council of Nurses, it was admitted to membership in 1981. LNA takes a positive role in special health projects.

In 1993, a W. K. Kellogg Foundation sponsored program on primary health care was held in Lesotho with some of the consultants coming from the United States (Fig. 8–9).

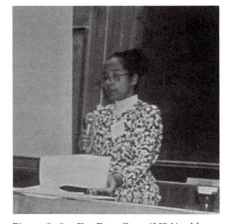

Figure 8–9   Dr. Faye Gary (USA) addressing participants at a W. K. Kellogg Foundation-sponsored program on primary health care, 1993.

LIBERIA

Occupying 43,000 square miles, Liberia lies at the southwestern extremity of the western bulge of Africa and is bordered by Sierra Leone, Guinea, and the Ivory Coast. It has a 370-mile long coastline on the Atlantic Ocean and its population of 2 million includes 16 distinct ethnic groups and descendants of emancipated slaves from the United States. Some 15,000 foreigners reside in Liberia, most of whom are members of the Lebanese and Indian trading communities. About 3,000 U.S. citizens live there, mostly U.S. government employees and dependents, missionaries, and business representatives.

The history of modern Liberia dates from 1816 when the American Colonization Society, a private U.S. organization, was given a charter by the U.S. Congress to send freed slaves to the west coast of Africa. The U.S. government, under President James Monroe, provided funds and assisted in negotiations with native chiefs for the ceding of land for this purpose. The first settlers landed at the site of Monrovia in 1822. In 1838, they united to form the Commonwealth of Liberia under a governor appointed by the American Colonization Society. In 1847, Liberia became Africa's first independent republic, with a constitution modeled after that of the United States. The United Kingdom officially recognized the Republic of Liberia in 1848, as did France in 1852, and the United States in 1862. Liberia has been a leader in pan-African affairs and played an important role in the founding of the Organization of African Unity (*Background Notes*, Sept. 1987).

The Government Hospital was established in 1927 by three Liberian nurses—Jeanette Howard, Lucille Todd, and Magdalene Cooper, two of whom had completed the diploma program at Lincoln School for Nurses in New York. They had persuaded the Liberian government to let them convert a large house into a much-needed hospital (Carnegie, 1960; Bernard, 1994). Howard had also attended Meharry Medical College in Nashville where she studied to be a nurse anesthetist.

In 1929, Jeannette Howard married Charles E. Cooper, Liberia's first Consul General to Great Britain. She accompanied him there. Returning to Liberia in 1932, she found the Government Hospital closed. She persuaded community leaders and the Liberian Government to reopen the hospital, succeeding in her efforts in 1934. She was appointed superintendent of nurses with Lucille Todd as assistant superintendent.

Serving her country and people as superintendent of nurses from 1934 to 1953, Jeannette Cooper translated her devotion and commitment to helping and caring for the sick into monumental realities: establishing the first Liberian nursing school, creating the Board of Nurse Examiners in 1947 which is responsible for registration and licensing of nurses for practice, constructing the first building in Liberia designed as a hospital, and erecting the first quarantine facility.

After the death of her first husband, Jeannette Cooper married Charles D. B. King, former President of Liberia. She then began devoting her efforts to reorganizing and achieving international recognition for the Liberian Red Cross Society, which she had organized in 1949. She rendered her people and country outstanding patriotic and unparalleled service as president of that organization for three decades until her retirement in 1979.

In 1964, King was awarded the Florence Nightingale Medal for distinguished service to the nursing profession—the first African nurse to receive that distinction. In 1974, she was decorated by the government of Sweden for constructive and conspicuous assistance rendered to the international relief effort, mobilized during that year to relieve the sufferings of millions of people affected by drought in Africa's sahil region.

In 1975, King received from a grateful and appreciative government her country's highest medal of distinction, Grand Commander, Order of the Pioneers, for untiring and dedicated service to her people and country. She was also honored by the issuance of a Liberian postage stamp—the first in her profession to be so honored by her country. She died on April 18, 1985 (Bernard, 1994).

Due to the civil war that has been raging in Liberia for 14 years, there is no accurate count of the number of health care facilities still in existence. Hospitals, health centers, clinics, and health posts, had numbered over 200 before the war. One hospital in Monrovia had been devoted to maternal-child care (Fig. 8–10).

There are six institutions that train nurses and midwives—three of these train professional nurses: Cuttingham University College of Nursing Division (baccalaureate) which was established in 1964; Tubman National Institute of Medical Arts (diploma); and Winifred J. Harvey's School of Nursing (diploma). Approximately 500 professional nurses are working in Liberia, 41 with bachelor's degrees and 15 with master's degrees in various nursing disciplines (Davis et al., 1992).

The Liberian Nurses Association (LNA) is one of the professional organizations for nurses in the country and was admitted to membership in the International Council of Nurses in 1957 when it met in Rome. Elouise Duncan, who had been the president of LNA, was elected to the ICN Board of Directors in 1973 and re-elected in 1977. In 1982, Martha Kair

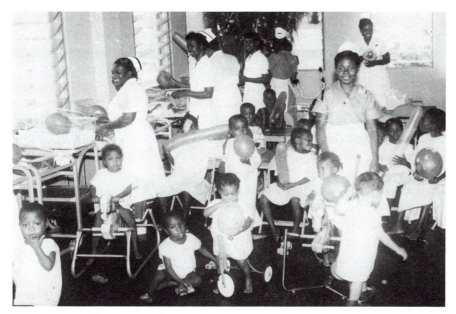

Figure 8–10 Christmas at the Carrie V. Dyer Maternal and Child Welfare Center, Monrovia, 1959.

Bellek, B.S.N., M.S., FWACN, who had been chair, Cuttingham University College of Nursing, was appointed Minister of Health and Social Welfare, Liberia.

MALAWI

Formerly Nyasaland, Malawi in Central Africa occupies 45,747 square miles and is about the size of Pennsylvania, with a population of 8.2 million (1988 estimate)—blacks, Asians, and Europeans. The country is divided into three regions (North, South, and Central) and 24 administrative districts. Although the Portuguese reached the area in the 16th century, the first significant Western contact was the arrival of explorer David Livingstone along the shore of Lake Malawi in 1859. Subsequently, Scottish churches established missions in Malawi. One of the objectives was to end the slave trade that continued there as late as the end of the nineteenth century. Malawi's independence was gained from Great Britain July 6, 1964, becoming a member of the Commonwealth. Two years later, a new constitution was adopted and it became a republic. Its capital city is Lilongwe (*Background Notes,* Feb., 1989).

All government health services in Malawi are free. Each of the 24 districts has a government hospital. Below the district hospital is a rural hospital, followed by health centers and health posts which are located in the community (Fig. 8–11). At the Ministry of Health is a Nursing Division with a Chief Nursing Officer responsible for placement of staff in government services and administration of nursing services at the national level. Nursing personnel (registered and practical) form the largest work force in all health care facilities and, in most cases, the nurses work with minimum support from physician services.

In-country nursing education is a relatively new phenomenon in Malawi. In 1955, one year after independence, the National School of Nursing was established. Five years later, the first class of Registered Nurse-Midwifery students was admitted. In 1979, the School became the fourth constituent of the University of Malawi and named Kamuzu College of Nursing in honor of the first president, His Excellency Ngwazi— Dr. H. Kamuzu Banda.

Prior to 1965, all Malawian trained nurses were products of mission schools and similar to practical nurses. Those who became registered nurses were educated outside the country, usually in Great Britain and South Africa. In 1985, the first men were admitted to the College of Nursing.

The course of study is four years and focuses on delivery of primary health care in urban and rural areas. There is a strong emphasis on

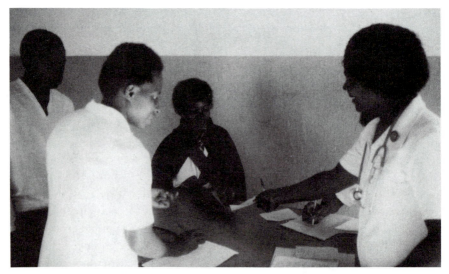

Figure 8–11   Limbe Health Center, Malawi, 1985. (Courtesy, Nan Green)

community health and management of disease. The first three years are designed to prepare a graduate who can competently practice in a variety of rural or urban settings as a nurse, manager, leader, teacher, and resource person. At completion of this program the student is awarded a diploma in nursing. The fourth year, a certificate program, builds on the knowledge acquired in the diploma program and focuses on developing skills and knowledge received to practice midwifery. The midwifery program is a mandatory year of study for all graduates so that all are prepared to provide services to pregnant women.

In 1990, ten graduates of the College of Nursing were admitted to a newly developed B.Sc. Program which is two years in length. They have been prepared to function as teachers in the Enrolled Schools (schools of practical nursing) located throughout Malawi. This program is significant because it will give access to higher education to a larger number of nurses who can be educated in their own country (Essoka & Marks, 1993). Registered nurses also participate in the program and they require three years to complete the curriculum. It is hoped that this program will eventually be converted into a basic bachelor's nursing degree (BSN) replacing the diploma.

The National Association of Nurses of Malawi was founded by Lucy Kadzamira in 1979. The Association applied for membership in the International Council of Nurses in 1980. In 1981, Malawi was admitted to the ICN at the Congress in Los Angeles. In 1985, the Association began publishing its official journal, *The Malawian Nurse.*

NIGERIA

Nigeria occupies 356,700 square miles—about the size of California, Nevada, and Arizona combined. The most populous country in Africa, Nigeria accounts for one-quarter of sub-Saharan Africa's people—250 ethnic groups, making an estimated total of 115 million people. Following World War II, in response to the growth of Nigerian nationalism and demands for independence, successive constitutions legislated by the British government moved Nigeria toward self-government on a representative, increasingly federal, basis. Nigeria was granted full independence from Great Britain on October 1, 1960 under a constitution that provided for a parliamentary form of government. In October 1963, Nigeria altered its relationship with the United Kingdom by proclaiming itself a federal republic and promulgating a new constitution (*Background Notes,* April, 1991).

Nurse training began in Nigeria with the provision of medical and health service by the army for army personnel only. These services later extended to civil servants and their relatives. The health of the rest of the nation was largely in the hands of indigenous herbalists and "traditional doctors." Government efforts at providing health services were later supplemented by the work of missionaries who began to arrive about 1860. Thus mission dispensaries, maternity centers, and later hospitals for civilians in remote areas were started. The first group of trained nurses from abroad were Roman Catholic nuns who began the earliest efforts to train Nigerian nurses (Pratt, 1968).

Nigeria had had diploma programs in nursing at hospitals, but it was not until 1964 that a program leading to a bachelor's degree was established at the University of Ibadan, Faculty of Medicine and the University of Nigeria, Enugu Campus in 1982. The University of Ife, in 1977 began a generic program leading to B.N.Sc. At the government's request, the program was assisted by WHO, UNICEF, and the Rockefeller Foundation. WHO provided teaching materials and other assistance, and the Rockefeller Foundation provided the building.

For a long time there were two recognized grades of training and registration—two categories of state-registered nurses (from the United Kingdom and the University College Hospital) and the Nigerian Registered Nurses.

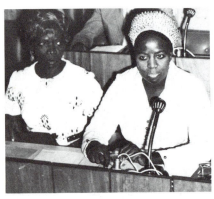

Figure 8–12   Symposium on Priorities in National Health Planning, University of Ibadan, Nigeria, 1973. Kofoworola Pratt, Chief Nurse, Ministry of Health (left); Adetoun Bailey (right), Registrar, Nursing Council. (Courtesy Anne Davis)

The Professional Association of Trained Nurses of Nigeria was established in 1938 and was referred to as the Nigerian Union of Nurses. In 1961, Nigeria was admitted to membership in the International Council of Nurses at their meeting in Australia, with Kofoworola Pratt as its president. Pratt (Fig. 8–12) was later to become the third vice-president of ICN. In 1978, the National Association of Nigeria Nurses and Midwives was founded when 13 nursing associations composed of the various specialty groups united to become the present organization to speak for the majority of nurses and midwives in the country.

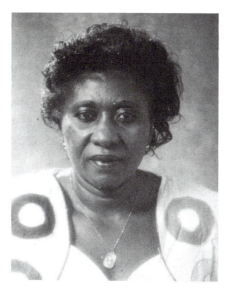

Figure 8–13 Grace Madubuko, 1980 3M Scholarship recipient.

The Nursing and Midwifery Council of Nigeria was established by decree No. 89, 1979 with A. Bailey as the first registrar; V. Udenze is the current registrar. There are 60 approved schools of midwifery in Nigeria, 56 approved schools of basic nursing and six schools of psychiatric nursing. There are about 10 public health schools. PHC [sic] is being integrated into the standardized basic nursing curriculum with family planning and population control.

The National Association of Nigerian Nurses and Midwives has sponsored numerous continuing education programs for its members, including participating in an ICN/UNICEF project on "Social Mobilization of Communities," with workshops in 20 states.

In 1979, Kola Oyedepo was the recipient of a 3M Fellowship to pursue doctoral studies in Nigeria. He earned the doctoral degree in 1988. In 1980, Grace Madubuko was the Nigerian winner of the 3M Scholarship Award (Fig. 8–13).

SEYCHELLES

Located in the Indian Ocean, the Republic of Seychelles occupies 171 square miles and comprises an archipelago of 92 tropical islands. Its population of 67,000 (1988 estimate) is classified as creole—a mixture of Asians, Africans, and Europeans. The Seychelles remained uninhabited for more than 150 years after they became known to Western explorers. The islands appeared on Portuguese charts as early as 1505, although Arabs may have visited there much earlier. A French expedition in 1756 gave the islands their present name. The Seychelles islands were captured and freed several times during the French revolution and the Napoleonic wars, then passed officially to the British under the Treaty of Paris in 1814. On August 31, 1903 Seychelles became a separate British crown colony. Negotiations with the British resulted in an agreement by which the

Seychelles became an independent sovereign republic on June 29, 1976 (*Background Notes,* Nov. 1989).

Basic health services are provided in clinics and health centers. While all health care services are free in government-owned institutions, within the private sector, health services are offered on a fee-for-service basis.

Because there is no university on the island, doctors are recruited from abroad. There is one school of nursing—a three-year program plus a year of midwifery, based on the British system. The Polytechnic Institute, which houses the school of nursing, comes under the Ministry of Education. There is no university program in the country but plans are being made to link the School of Nursing with a university in another country. There is a Nursing Council and nurses are registered for life. Registration is the major function of the Council.

The Nurses Association of the Republic of Seychelles (NARS) was formed in 1977 and admitted to membership in ICN in 1980. The Association, which is the recognized association for all nurses registered in the Republic, is involved in health education projects and works in close collaboration with other management organizations on different projects. It is also fully acknowledged and supported by the government and serves as a consultative body on health policy.

SIERRA LEONE

The Republic of Sierra Leone occupies 27,925 square miles—slightly smaller than South Carolina. It is located in the southwestern part of the great bulge of West Africa, with a 210-mile Atlantic Ocean coastline. Eighteen ethnic groups make up the population of 3.7 million (1985 estimate). About 60,000 are creoles, descendants of black settlers from Great Britain or North America. In addition about 20,000 Lebanese, 500 Indians, and 2,000 Europeans reside there. Among the first European contacts with Sierra Leone were British colonists. The Portuguese were the first to visit in 1462, followed by the English in 1562 in search of slaves. In 1808, the area was annexed as a British colony. In the early nineteenth century, Sierra Leone served as the education center of British West Africa. Fourah Bay College, established in 1827, rapidly became a magnet for English-speaking Africans on the west coast. For more than a century, it was the only European-style university in black Africa.

The 1951 constitution provided the framework for decolonization and independence came in April, 1961. Sierra Leone became a parliamentary system within the British Commonwealth (*Background Notes,* July, 1986).

Health services in Sierra Leone are under the administration of the Ministry of Health and Social Services, which employs most of the nurses. All nurses are under Civil Service.

When the country became independent in 1961, there were 12 district hospitals and two government training schools for nurses—three years in length plus 15 months post-basic training for midwifery training. Ten years later, there were three programs for the educational preparation of professional nurses and their auxiliaries—all governed by legislation and administered by the Nurses Board of Sierra Leone, which approves the establishment of schools, controls educational programs, and conducts qualifying examinations. In the 1980s, nurses were beginning to enroll in post-basic courses offered in Ghana and Nigeria, rather than in Great Britain. Sierra Leone, however, does have a one-year, university-based, post-basic program in community health. It is made up of a three-month certificate and nine-month diploma component.

The National Nurses Association of Sierra Leone (NNASL) was established in 1962, with Josephine Demby as president. It was admitted to membership in ICN in 1965 when it met in Frankfurt, Germany. The Association is officially registered as a non-profit, professional organization and has relationships with many organizations, the most important of which is the West African College of Nursing which is an agency of the West African Health Community, a body linking the five West African countries.

Nurses from Sierra Leone have been able to benefit from scholarships offered by the World Health Organization, the West African College of Nursing, and the International Council of Nurses (ICN). In 1984, the 3M Fellowship administered by ICN went to Cynthia Cecilia Ayodele Pratt for masters study in the United States; her degree was awarded in 1987. Another honor occurred when Edith Jarrett, assistant secretary of the Sierra Leone Nurses Association, was invited to participate in the Commission on Human Rights which was inaugurated in 1985. She was elected to the Board of this Commission and continues to be an active member. In 1973, the President of NNASL was Iyatunde Marie Palmer (Fig. 8–14).

In 1993, two U.S. Army Reserve civil affairs officers, Major Marie O. Mosley, a black nurse, and Major Richard J. Indrieri, a veterinarian, were deployed to Sierra Leone to support a joint U.S. and Sierra Leone military medical assistance exercise in this former British colony. Both soldiers were assigned to medical outreach teams that provided medical and dental screenings, preventive medical care, and the immunization of Sierra Leone nationals. Major Mosley (Fig. 8–15) was responsible for primary care,

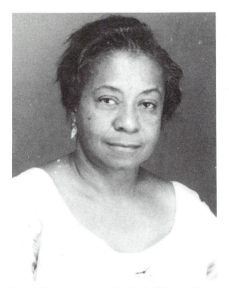

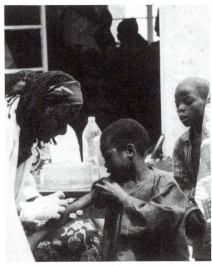

Figure 8–14   Iyatunde Marie Palmer, President, NNASL. (Courtesy ICN)

Figure 8–15   Dr. Marie Mosley, U.S. Army nurse, immunizing Sierra Leone Nationals.

immunizing children against communicable diseases, and supporting the village of Lungi and the capital city of Freetown.

SUDAN

Sudan occupies 967,500 square miles in Africa—about one-third the size of continental United States. In 1989, it was estimated that its population was 25 million, and consisted of two distinct cultures—Arab and Black African. Sudan was a collection of small, independent states from the beginning of the Christian era until 1820–1821 when Egypt conquered and unified the northern portion of the country. In 1899, Sudan was proclaimed a condominium under British-Egyptian administration. While maintaining the appearance of joint administration, the British formulated policies and supplied most of the top administrators.

In February 1953, the United Kingdom and Egypt concluded an agreement providing for Sudanese self-government and self-determination. Sudan achieved independence on January 1, 1956. The United States was among the first foreign powers to recognize the new state (*Background Notes,* March, 1991).

The Ministry of Health in Sudan is responsible for medical and public health services throughout the country. A few missionary institutions supplement the services. Rural midwifery services are also provided.

The Sudan medical services date back to 1898 when the country was reoccupied by Anglo-Egyptian troops, and the services were provided by military staff. By 1900, a few small civilian hospitals were opened and staffed by civilian doctors. Male orderlies who could read and write Arabic were enlisted to be trained in nursing because women, with a few exceptions, due to cultural and conventional patterns, were not available. As hospital services expanded, expatriate nurses were introduced; the first, a British nurse in 1907, and by 1939 there were 90 expatriate registered nurses, British and Egyptian, in the country.

In 1925, the first hospital for women was opened in Omdurman and women were required to staff the services. A training program for female nurses started in 1926 at the hospital—two years in length and the matron of the hospital, a British nurse, was responsible for the preparation of the first Sudanese women in nursing. As more hospitals were opened, they in turn became recognized as training schools for nurses.

In 1948, a Central Nursing Council was formed in order to control and coordinate training for nurses. A Nurse Registry was formed and the length of training was extended to three years. Until 1950, all teaching was done by British nurses. Then a course was introduced to prepare Sudanese nurse instructors. In 1965, the total number of schools, including those in mission hospitals, was 40 and the total number of nurses was 25,000, mostly men.

The Khartoum College of Nursing was established in 1955 by the combined efforts of the Sudanese government and the World Health Organization which contributed help until 1965. The College was placed under the Ministry of Health until 1973. From 1973 on, the College became one of 18 specialized colleges under the Ministry of Education, Department of Higher Education's General Council. At graduation, students receive a diploma from the Khartoum College of Nursing. In 1975, a post-basic course of one year was started in the Higher Institute of Midwifery. Nurses go abroad for other post-basic preparation.

Between 1958 and 1964, the government banned organizations of any type. With the new government in 1964 the professions organized themselves and nurses formed their organization in 1965, which was approved by the government. The Sudan Professional Nurses Association's constitution specifically states that the Association "will include professional nurses without regard to religious beliefs, race, or color." The Association was admitted to membership in the International Council of Nursing in 1976.

SWAZILAND

The area occupied by Swaziland, Africa's smallest nation, is 6,704 square miles, slightly smaller than New Jersey. It is bordered on three sides by the Republic of South Africa and shares a 70-mile border with Mozambique. Its population (1988 estimate) is 750,000, 47 percent of whom are under the age of sixteen. The great majority of the people are Swazi, with some Zulu and non-African inhabitants. The whites consist of English, Afrikaäns, and Portuguese. In 1903, Great Britain formally took over the administration of the country. In 1921, Swaziland's first legislative body, an advocacy council of elected white representatives, was established. Its purpose was to advise the high commission on purely non-Swazi affairs. Swaziland became independent on September 6, 1968 (*Background Notes,* May, 1990).

There are 10 main hospitals in Swaziland and numerous clinics. There is also a Nursing Council, legally established under an act by the government to establish basic regulations and standards for registering and licensing nurses.

There had been only two schools of nursing—the Swaziland Institute of Health Sciences in Mbabani and one associated with Raleigh Fitkin Memorial Hospital—a mission hospital under the auspices of the Church of the Nazarene. The latter graduated its first nurses in 1931. In 1956, a separate nursing college was established with a 4-year course. Examinations for the graduates are prepared by the Nursing Education Board of Botswana, Lesotho, and Swaziland. There is a separate midwifery course of one year for nurses or two years for non-nurses.

Swaziland Nurses Association was established in 1965 and admitted to membership in the International Council of Nurses in 1975. The Association has sponsored and participated in many educational programs for its members. One such project, sponsored by ICN in 1988

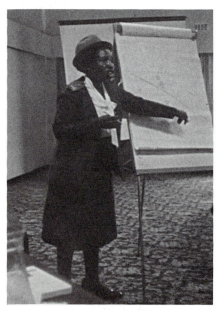

Figure 8–16 Public health nurses in Swaziland. (Courtesy W. Holzemer)

was on "Improving the Health of Mothers and Children Through Community Involvement."

In 1990, Swaziland hosted a four-week course on "Curriculum Development: Techniques of Teaching and Evaluation," offered by the College of Nursing and the Office of International Health, Howard University, Washington, DC (Fig. 8–16). Twenty-one educators participated in the course: five each from Botswana, Lesotho, Zimbabwe, and six from Swaziland. In-country consultation was provided by the Office of the Chief Nurse, Ministry of Health and the Bursar's Office, University of Swaziland. Full-time secretarial support and transportation were provided by the Ministry of Health (Adderly-Kelly et al., 1992).

TANZANIA

Tanzania is the result of the union of Tanganyika and Zanzibar in East Africa, formed in 1964 after each became independent. The mainland of Tanzania is 363,000 square miles, slightly smaller than New Mexico and Texas combined, with a population of 26 million (1988 Census). Northern Tanganyika's famed Olduvai Gorge has provided rich evidence of the area's prehistory, including fossil remains of some of humanity's earliest ancestors. The discoveries made by Dr. and Mrs. L.S.B. Leakey, and others, strongly suggest East Africa as the site of human origin. The coastal area first felt the impact of non-African influences as early as the eighth century with the arrival of Arab traders. Traders and immigrants came later from Persia (now Iran), Portugal, and India. European exploration of Tanganyika's interior began in the mid-nineteenth century. German colonial rule ended with World War I. Control of most of the territory passed to the United Kingdom under a League of Nations Mandate. After World War II, Tanganyika became a United Nations Trust territory administered by the United Kingdom. Zanzibar had been an early Arab/Persian trading center and fell under Portuguese domination in the sixteenth and early seventeenth centuries. The United Kingdom's early interest in Zanzibar was motivated by commerce and British determination to end the slave trade (*Background Notes,* May, 1992).

After independence, the late Lucy Lameck (Fig. 8–17) one of the three women members of Parliament appointed by President Julius Nyerere as parliamentary secretaries in the Ministry of Community Development was a nurse. After completing her basic nursing education in Moshi, she completed a post-basic course at Ruskin College, Oxford, and then studied political science at Western Michigan University,

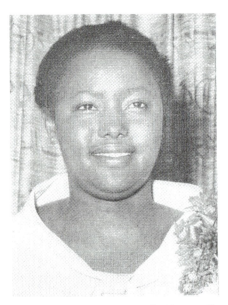

Figure 8–17 Lucy Lameck (deceased), Junior Minister for Health in Tanzania. (Courtesy Delta Sigma Theta)

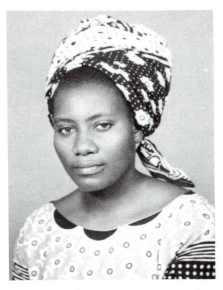

Figure 8–18 Ellen Evelyn Zablon, first President of the National Nurses Association of Tanzania. (Courtesy ICN)

U.S.A. (MacDonald, 1966). She was once a Junior Minister for Health in Tanzania.

A Nursing Council was formed in 1952 by an ordinance which empowered it with the responsibility for controlling nursing education, registration, and practice.

In 1964, there was one government school of nursing and midwifery at Muhimbili Hospital. In 1989, with assistance from the Canadian International Development Agency through Dalhousie University School of Nursing, a bachelor of science in nursing program for registered nurses was established. A baccalaureate nursing program has also been established at Muhimbili Medical University College of Health Services of the University of Dar-es-Salaam.

Founded in 1971, the National Nurses Association of Tanzania (TARENA) is recognized by the Registrar of Associations as the body which speaks for nursing in the country. The government, through the Ministry of Health, has been very supportive of TARENA which has 25 branches (mainland only), some with 80 percent membership. The Nurses Association of Tanzania was accepted for membership in the International Council of Nurses in 1973. The first president of the Association was Ellen Evelyn Zablon (Fig. 8–18).

In 1978, Pauline Mella, the current (1994) president of TARENA, won a 3M nursing fellowship to pursue a bachelor's degree in the United States. She was awarded the degree in 1981 from St. Louis University in Missouri. She also serves as a member of the ICN Professional Services Committee for 1994.

In 1992, the Tanzania Midwives Association (TAMA) was formed with Joyce Safe as president. TAMA is intended to speak for midwifery in the country.

UGANDA

Sometimes called the jewel of Africa, Uganda occupies 94,354 square miles in East Africa and is about the size of Oregon. Its population in 1989 was 17 million: Africans—99 percent, Europeans, Asians, and Arabs—1 percent. Arab traders moving inland from the Indian Ocean coastal enclaves reached the interior of Uganda in the 1830s and found several African kingdoms with well-developed political institutions dating back several centuries. For a number of years, Uganda was under a British protectorate. This began to change formally in 1955, when constitutional changes leading to Uganda's independence were adopted. In 1966, the Prime Minister suspended the constitution, assumed all government powers, and removed the President and Vice-President. In 1967, a new constitution proclaimed Uganda a republic, gave the President greater power, and abolished the traditional kingdoms (*Background Notes,* March, 1991).

Uganda owes its beginnings in nursing to missionaries. In 1896, Sir Albert Cook, a medical doctor, set out for Mombasa from England on a long safari to Uganda. His aim was to begin medical work on invitation of King Mwamga in the country. In his party was Catherine Timpson, a nurse, whom he later married. He and his wife, Lady Cook, brought healing and friendship as well as the gospel to the people of Uganda (Musoke, 1968). Lady Cook began midwifery training at Mengo in 1919. Various Roman Catholic nursing orders also began to train midwives in 1921 and nurses in 1938 at Nsambya Hospital. The first government school of nursing for the Uganda trained nurse was at Mulago Hospital, the teaching hospital attached to Makerere College.

Almost all of the nursing service in Uganda is supplied by the government. The majority of the nurses and midwives are trained by schools attached to mission hospitals and all follow a basic curriculum approved by the Uganda Nurses, Midwives, and Nursing Assistants Council. The Nursing Council by law controls the training, registration, and discipline of nurses.

With funding from the Rockefeller Foundation, Case Western Reserve University, Frances Payne Bolton School of Nursing, Cleveland,

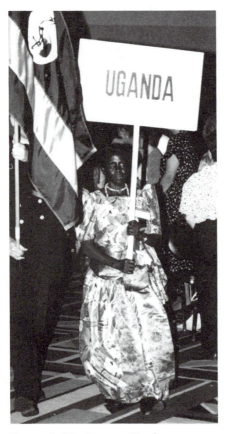

Figure 8–19 Dorcus Katali represents Uganda at a Sigma Theta Tau International Research Conference at Ohio State University, Columbus OH, 1992.

Ohio, USA, is involved in a project started in 1993, to implement a B.Sc.N. program at Makerere University in Kampala through consultancy in needed areas of instruction and administration of the program.

The Uganda National Association of Registered Nurses and Midwives was organized in 1964 and admitted to membership in ICN in 1969 at the Congress in Canada. It is the only official organization of professional nurses and midwives in the country. It is vigorously engaged in a nationally expanded immunization program to enhance the government's efforts to eradicate the major preventable diseases that annually claim many lives of children. Uganda was also the site for a national evaluation of an AIDS control program in 1988, sponsored by WHO, with ICN as a collaborator.

In 1990, Specious Mbabali won the 3M Fellowship for masters study in Great Britain. In 1992, Dorcus Katali presented a paper at the Sigma Theta Tau International Research Conference at Ohio State University. Katali, a nurse and midwife, trained in Great Britain and Australia, is executive director, Uganda National Association of Registered Nurses and Midwives (Fig. 8–19). Also in 1992, Selina Rwashana, principal nursing officer in the Ministry of Health and vice-president of UNANM, presented an abstract for the conference at Florida State University, Boca Raton.

ZAMBIA

Zambia, formerly Northern Rhodesia, occupies 290,585 square miles, slightly larger than Texas with 8 million people (1991 estimate). There are more than 70 tribal groups plus British expatriates, South Africans, and a small Asian population, most of whom are Indians. Three of its neighbors are Zimbabwe, Mozambique, and Angola. It also shares a border with Namibia. The indigenous hunter-gatherer occupants of Zambia began to be displaced or absorbed by more advanced migrating tribes about 2,000 years ago. Except for an occasional Portuguese explorer, the area lay untouched by Europeans for centuries. After the mid-nineteenth century, it was penetrated by Western explorers, missionaries, and traders. David Livingstone first saw Victoria Falls in 1855. In 1888, Northern Rhodesia was proclaimed a British sphere of influence and the administration was transferred to the British Colonial Office in 1924 as a protectorate. Controversy began around 1953 when the Africans made insistent demands for greater participation in government coupled with European fears of losing control. On October 24, 1964, Northern Rhodesia became the Republic of Zambia—the first British territory to become a republic immediately upon attaining independence (*Background Notes*, September, 1992).

Until Zambia became independent of Great Britain in 1964, there were no registered nursing schools in the country. In 1965, a basic three-year school of nursing was established in Kitwe. All but one faculty were British. The one Zambian tutor, Mary Chibungo Zyongwe, had received her post-basic education in Montreal, Canada, and the United States.

A Nursing Act passed in 1970, provided for a General Nursing Council responsible for registration of nurses. Practically all of the European nurses in Zambia had been trained and had had advanced studies in South Africa, the United Kingdom, or Southern Rhodesia. Nursing services were provided by the government, missions and mines, in hospitals and clinics by nurses and newly established community health nurses. The Flying Doctor Service, a statutory body set up and financed by the government, provides quickly a doctor and a nurse and an air ambulance for everybody in need in places inaccessible by road.

Northern Rhodesia Nurses Association, now Zambia Nurses Association (ZNA), was accepted into membership by ICN in 1953, before independence, hence there were no African members. Today, all of the executive officers are Zambian registered nurses. Under its leadership there is a university nursing program, continuing education in clinical specialties, and post-diploma programs in teaching.

ZNA has organized and participated in workshops and seminars, publishes a journal, and has the support of radio, television, and the press. In addition, while Kaunda was President of Zambia, Madame Kaunda, the First Lady, was a Patron of the Association.

In 1970, supported by WHO, the Zambian Nurses Association organized a regional conference and invited nurses from neighboring

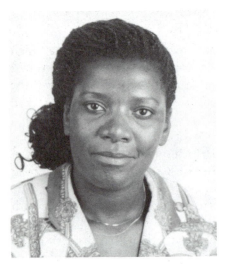

Figure 8–20   Annete Mwansa Nkowane of Zambia.

countries. The conference, with the theme, "The Role of the Nurse in the Promotion of Health and the Underlying Philosophy and Purpose of Basic and Post-Basic Nursing Preparation to Enable Her to Meet this Role," was unique because it was the first to be organized in that area by a nurses' association in membership with ICN.

Annette Mswansa Nkowane (Fig. 8–20), a native of Zambia who had earned her diploma in general nursing at Lusaka School of Nursing in 1978 and a Bachelor of Science in Nursing at the University of Zambia in 1990, received a Master of Arts from Webster University in Geneva, Switzerland, in 1993. Her master's research project was "Optimization of Community Health Nurses in Developing Countries." She is currently nurse consultant, Health Department, International Federation of Red Cross and Red Crescent Societies, Geneva, Switzerland, responsible for the development and field testing of *First Aid in the Community: A Manual for Trainers of Red Cross and Red Crescent Volunteers in Africa.*

ZIMBABWE

Formerly Southern Rhodesia, Zimbabwe occupies 151,000 square miles—slightly larger than Montana. In June 1987, the population of over 99 percent black was estimated to be 8.8 million, with less than 1 percent being white, colored (mixed race), and Asian. A landlocked country in south-central Africa, Zimbabwe is bordered by Zambia on the north, Mozambique on the north and east, South Africa on the south, and Botswana on the west. Archeologists have found stone-age implements and pebble tools in several areas of Zimbabwe, suggesting human habitation for many centuries. The ruins of stone buildings also provide evidence of early civilization.

In the sixteenth century, the Portuguese were the first Europeans to attempt colonization of south-central Africa, but the hinterland lay virtually untouched by Europeans until the arrival of explorers, missionaries, and traders some 300 years later. In 1888, Cecil Rhodes obtained a concession for mineral rights from local tribal chiefs. In that year the area that became Southern and Northern Rhodesia was proclaimed a British sphere of influence. In 1923, Southern Rhodesia was formally annexed by the United Kingdom. After years of strife, the British government formally granted independence to Zimbabwe on April 18, 1980. The United States was the first nation to open an embassy in Salisbury on that day (*Background Notes,* March, 1988).

The Ministry of Health and Child Welfare is committed to the provision of primary health care for everyone in Zimbabwe, including the most remote communities. Health care is free for those earning less than a stipulated amount of income. The system encourages community participation in every kind of health program.

Training of black African nurses started in 1958, with one of the country's diploma programs—the one for black nurses only. Today, there is a baccalaureate program for registered nurses with a well-prepared and experienced faculty. The goal is to have nursing within the system of higher education.

With a $1.5 million grant from the W. K. Kellogg Foundation, Case Western Reserve University (CWRU) Frances Payne Bolton School of Nursing in Cleveland, Ohio, is engaged in a collaborative project in the establishment of a Master of Science in Nursing Distance Learning Program with the University of Zimbabwe. Responding to the need for nurses in leadership roles in the Zimbabwean health care and education systems, the nursing education program will grant the country's first graduate nursing degree. Beginning in 1993, the three-year project is directed by Dr. Doris Modly and Joette Clark of CWRU.

The Zimbabwean Ministry of Health opened the door for collaboration in 1986 through its "Zimbabwe Health for All Action Plan," in which was cited the need for greater numbers of better skilled health care team personnel to meet the needs of Zimbabwe and the region.

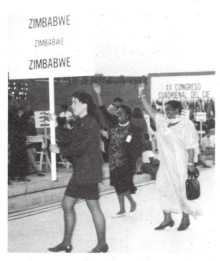

Figure 8–21 Representative from Zimbabwe at opening ceremony of the International Congress of Nurses, in Madrid, Spain, 1993.

Southern Rhodesia (now Zimbabwe) was admitted to ICN membership in 1953 (Fig. 8–21). Due to circumstances in the country beyond their control (apartheid), the nurses in the association withdrew from ICN and dissolved their organization to facilitate the admission of a new organization. The Nurses Association of Zimbabwe, established in 1980, which was absorbed into ICN in 1983, with a membership of 4,000. For the quadrennial, 1989–1993, Joyce Kadandara, deputy secretary, Health Support Services, Ministry of Health and Child Welfare, served on the ICN Professional Services Committee.

The first national congress of the Zimbabwe Nurses Association (ZINA) was held in 1982. This was the first opportunity that black nurses had to participate. Although a predominantly black organization now, white nurses have been welcomed and invited to join.

The Nurses Association is recognized and respected by the government and health authorities as the only professional association representing nurses in the country. A nurse with a doctorate is responsible for the education of all health personnel in the country and a nurse with a masters' degree is responsible for nursing services. Many Zimbabwe nurses have been educated in the United States, the United Kingdom, and South Africa and several are in the Ministry of Health.

In Zimbabwe, nurses comprise 75 to 80 percent of the health care personnel. Nurses' increased responsibilities have paralleled the country's development, particularly after independence in 1980 when the health service system was recognized as part of the country's emphasis on decentralization. Under the new system, each community has become responsible for the health care of its members and nurses are being called upon to implement, monitor, and evaluate nursing activities at all levels of the health care system (Kadandara, 1989). Zimbabwe can boast of the fact that nurses are included in the country's delegation to the World Health Assembly held yearly in Geneva, because most countries have never included a nurse.

WEST AFRICAN COLLEGE OF NURSING

The West African College of Nursing (WACN) is a specialized agency of the West African Health community and consists of fellows from five English-speaking countries in West Africa: The Gambia, Ghana, Liberia, Nigeria, and Sierra Leone. Efforts are being made to strengthen collaboration with Francophone nursing colleagues in readiness for the management of the proposed West African Health Organization.

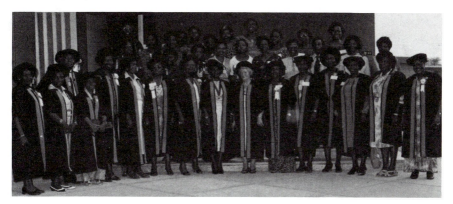

Figure 8–22   West African College of Nursing conference attendees.

The College was established in 1981 in Banjul, The Gambia, and is headquartered in Lagos, Nigeria, located within the Secretariat of the West African Health Community, the parent organization. The College was established with the belief that this would enhance the educational facilities for basic registered nurse training programs and for continuing post-basic courses across the sub-region.

Some of the objectives of the College are: (1) to promote excellence in nursing education at basic and post-basic levels and maintain the standards of practice of nursing within the community; (2) to formulate and support nursing education programs; (3) to contribute to the improvement of health care within the West African sub-region; (4) to plan and implement continuing education programs for nursing personnel; and (5) to promote and encourage research in nursing.

In 1991, WACN celebrated its tenth anniversary and held its biennial meeting in Bakau, The Gambia. Papers presented focused on the outlook of nursing education and practice, continuing education, and research. The Fellows set as their goal the development of health centers to train nursing students in primary health care (Fig. 8–22).

In 1993, Virginia Aristodemus-Davies, of Sierra Leone, was elected President of the West African College of Nursing. WACN's eleventh scientific session was held in Accra, Ghana, in March 1994.

EAST, CENTRAL, SOUTHERN AFRICAN COLLEGE OF NURSING

The East, Central, Southern African College of Nursing (ECSACON) is a professional body of nurses within the Commonwealth Regional Health

Community comprising the 12 member states of Botswana, Kenya, Lesotho, Malawi, Mauritius, Namibia, Seychelles, Swaziland, Tanzania, Uganda, Zambia, and Zimbabwe. It is not a physical structure, but a regional coordinating agency that provides a unique forum that speaks authoritatively for the nursing profession in the region on issues affecting nursing and health. It has a Council of National Representatives which is an executive arm of the College upon which the management of the College is vested. The College is headed by the president and assisted by the vice-president. The day-to-day activities are carried out by the College Secretariat headed by the executive secretary. The main objective of ECSACON is to promote and maintain excellence in nursing education, practice, administration, and research for improving health care to the community.

In 1993, ECSACON held its first 5-day workshop in Nairobi for chief nursing officers and senior nurse leaders, with 12 countries participating. The conference focused on strengthening administrative skills and capabilities in the provision of health services, including primary care.

KELLOGG FOUNDATION
SOUTHERN AFRICA PROJECT

The W. K. Kellogg Foundation of Battle Creek, Michigan, established in 1935, has been a major supporter of nursing at home and abroad. In

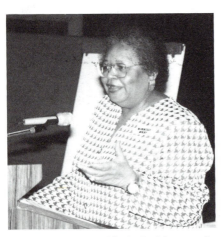

1988, its interest was broadened as a result of a meeting conducted in Tobago by the International Council of Nurses which brought together not only nurses from the Caribbean, but from four countries in southern Africa as well—Botswana, Lesotho, Swaziland, and Zimbabwe. At this meeting, in addition to reviewing the regulatory structure governing nursing education and practice, which was the purpose of the meeting, the nurses from the African countries recommended that a meeting of representatives of the four countries be convened within their region to identify areas in which

Figure 8–23   Dr. Gloria Smith, coordinator of Health Programs and Program Director, W. K. Kellogg Foundation, at the 1992 conference in Southern Africa.

they might work to strengthen nursing. Such a networking conference was held in March 1988 in Botswana with the overall goal being to improve primary health care nursing. Since then, a fifth country, South Africa has joined the project.

Plans were made to not only hold annual conferences, but to have consultants from the United States work with the nurses in each country. In addition, the Foundation has supported a number of nurses to study outside the region. To reach the goal of self-sufficiency, the need has been recognized to prepare an adequate number of nurses and nurse leaders for education and practice within the region; i.e., to prepare a critical mass of nurses at the baccalaureate level and to establish graduate programs to prepare nursing educators and leaders. To this end, the Kellogg Project in Southern Africa continues (Fig. 8–23). The 1994 conference was held in January in Zimbabwe.

SUMMARY

As can be seen from the discussion of nursing in the 17 African countries presented in this chapter, there seems to be a common thread running through all of them. For example, all but two countries—Liberia and Ethiopia—had been under British colonial rule before independence; the nursing schools had been founded in hospitals, many of which had been organized by missionaries; and the professional nursing associations were developed by the nurses themselves as a means of upgrading their status, having a catalyst for continuing education, exchanging ideas, and enjoying fellowship with like organizations in other countries, such as those with membership in the International Council of Nurses.

Nursing education in Africa is also changing gradually from being hospital-based and controlled, to being more community focused and educational institution-controlled.

REFERENCES

A decade of West African College of Nursing, past, present, and future. (June 1992). *West African College of Nursing Journal, 4,* 1.

Adderly-Kelly, B., Bradford, G., & Mitchum-Davis, A. (1992). A faculty development initiative in Africa. *Association of Black Nursing Faculty Journal, 3,* 10–15.

Akita, A., Agbleze, P., & Samaras, J. (1979). Environmental and social change: The effects on nursing practice. *International Nursing Review, 26,* 10–16.

Background Notes. (1986–1992). Washington, DC: U.S. Department of State, Bureau of Public Affairs, Office of Public Communications.

Bernard, J. S. (1994). Personal communication.

Carnegie, M. E. (1960). Flying trip to West Africa. *Nursing Outlook, 8,* 144 +.

Davis, B., Marlin, B., & Daniel, E. D. (1992). Professional nursing and Operation Smile International. *Association of Black Nursing Faculty Journal, 3,* 10–15.

Essoka, G., & Marks, L. D. (1993). Hunter-Bellevue Professor shares expertise in Central Africa. *Newsletter: Hunter-Bellevue School of Nursing, 9,* 1, 3.

Ethiopian Woman, 1960, Vol. I, 1–2.

Kadandara, J. C. (1989). Making the case for nurses as managers of nursing resources. *International Nursing Review, 36,* 109–112.

MacDonald, A. (1966). *Tanzania: Young nation in a hurry.* New York: Hawthorne Books.

Mule, G. K. (1986). Nursing education in Kenya: Trends and innovations. *International Nursing Review, 33,* 83–86.

Musoke, A. S. B. (1968, July). Uganda's nurses and the hospitals they work in. *International Nursing Review, 15,* 254 +.

Ngcongco, V. N., & Stark, R. D. (1986). The development of a family nurse practitioner program in Botswana. *International Nursing Review, 33,* 9–14.

Osei-Boateng, M. (1992). Nursing in Africa today. *International Nursing Review, 39,* 175–180.

Pratt, K. (1968). Professional association of trained nurses of Nigeria. *Nigerian Nurse, 1,* 1–2.

Selelō-Kupé, S. (1993). *An uneasy walk to quality: The evolution of Black nursing education in Botswana.* Battle Creek, Michigan: W. K. Kellogg Foundation.

Walter-Holtz, S., & Dier, K. (1969). Development in nursing education in Ghana. *Ghanian Nurse, 5,* 14–16.

Bibliography

Abedo, E. O. (1976). The survival of the nursing profession in today's Nigeria. *Nigerian Nurse, 8,* 7–9.

Adeloye, A. (1977). Nursing in Nigeria: Improvement and the future. *Nigerian Nurse, 9,* 29–31; 51.

Akinsanya, J. A. (n.d.). *An African Florence Nightingale, A Biography of Kofoworola Abeni Pratt,* Ibadan, Nigeria: Vantage Publishers.

Allen, M. E., Nunley, J. C., & Scott-Warner, M. (1988). Recruitment and retention of Black students in baccalaureate nursing programs. *Journal of Nursing Education, 27*(3), 107–116.

American Nurses' Association Hall of Fame. (1976). Kansas City: The Association.

Banks, J. (1986). Stress management for black nurses. *Journal of the National Black Nurses Association, 1*(1), 61–65.

Barrow, N. (1968). The role of the nurse in the changing Caribbean. *International Nursing Review, 16,* 167–171. (Reprinted from the *Jamaican Nurse,* 1968, March/April.)

Beck, F. S. (1971). Background of nursing south of the Sahara. *International Nursing Review, 18,* 263–270.

Bell, P. L. (1993). "Making do" with the midwife: Arkansas' Mamie O. Hale in the 1940s. *Nursing History Review, 1,* 55–69.

Bessent, H. (1987). Doctorally prepared nurses in mental health, *Journal of the National Black Nurses' Association, 1,* 36–40.

Bessent, H. (1989). Postdoctoral leadership training for women of color. *Journal of Professional Nursing, 5,* 279–82.

Best, T. (1992, February 25). Mary Seacole: Pioneer Red Cross Nurse. *Carib News,* New York, p. 23.

Beverly, C. E. (1947). Nursing schools in Liberia. *American Journal of Nursing, 47,* 530–531.

Brown, J., et al. (1971). Public health nursing: experience at Cuttingham College in Liberia. *International Nursing Review, 18,* 99–112.

Buckley, J. (1980). Faculty commitment to retention and recruitment of Black students. *Nursing Outlook, 28,* 46–50.

Callista, A. (1993). Women of "exceptional merit": Immigration of Caribbean nurses to Canada. *Canadian Journal of Women and the Law, 6,* 85–101.

Campinka-Bacote, J. (1988). The black nurses' struggle toward equality: An historical account of the National Association of Colored Graduate Nurses. *Journal of the National Black Nurses' Association, 2,* 15–25.

Capers, C. F. (1985). Nursing and the Afro-American client. *Top Clinical Nursing, 7*(3), 11–17.

Carnegie, M. E. (1962). The path we tread. *International Nursing Review, 9,* 25–33.

Carnegie, M. E. (1965). The impact of integration on the nursing profession. *Negro History Bulletin, 28,* 154–155.

Carnegie, M. E. (1984). Black nurses at the front. *American Journal of Nursing, 84,* 1250–1252.

Carnegie, M. E. (1987, March/April). Blacks in nursing. *The Black Collegian, 17,* 109–114.

Carnegie, M. E. (1974). The minority practitioner in nursing. *Current Issues in Nursing Education.* New York: National League for Nursing.

Carnegie, M. E. (1988). *Making choices, taking chances: Nurse leaders tell their stories.* Schorr, T. M. & Zimmerman, A. (Eds.). St. Louis, MO: C. V. Mosby. pp. 28–42.

Carnegie, M. E. (1990, February). Blacks in nursing: An update. *American Nurse, 22,* 6.

Carnegie, M. E. (1992). Black nurses in the United States: 1879–1992. *Journal of the Black Nurses Association, 6,* 13–18.

Carnegie, M. E., & Osborne, E. M. (1962). Integration in professional nursing. *Crisis, 9,* 47–50.

Chambers, L. A. (1957). *America's tenth man.* New York: Twayne Pub.

Cofer, A. B. (1974). Autobiography of a black nurse. *American Journal of Nursing, 74,* 1836–1838.

Coles, A. B. (1969). The Howard University School of Nursing in historical perspective. *Journal of the National Medical Association, 61,* 105–118.

Coles, A. B. (1972). The status of black nurse power. *Urban Health, 1,* 32–33. passim.

Cornely, P. B. (1934). A study of negro nursing. *Public Health Nurse, 34,* 449–451.

Creelman, L. (1958). Nursing in the African region. *International Nursing Review, 5,* 19–20.

Cunningham, M. E. (1994). Afrocentrism and self-concept. *Journal of National Black Nurses Association, 7*(1), 15–24.

Dannett, S. (1966). *Profiles of negro womanhood* (Vol. 1). 1619–1900. Philadelphia: Goodway.

Dannett, S. (1966). *Profiles of negro womanhood, twentieth century,* (Vol. II). Philadelphia: Goodway.

Davis A. (1987). *Architects for integration and equality: Early black American leaders in Nursing.* New York: Teachers College, Columbia University, Unpublished doctoral dissertation.

Davis, L. (1974). The minority practitioner in nursing. *Current Issues in Nursing Education,* New York: National League for Nursing.

Davis, M. (1982). *Contributions of black women to America.* Columbia, SC: Kenday Press.

Dell, M. A., & Halpin, G. (1984, April). Predictors of success in nursing school and on State Board Examinations in a predominately black baccalaureate nursing program. *Journal of Nursing Education, 23,* 147–150.

De Vooght, J. & Walker, K. (1989). Community mental health care in Grenada. *International Nursing Review, 36,* 22–24.

DeYoung, L. (1976). *The foundations of nursing.* St. Louis: C. V. Mosby.

Diploma schools. (1973). For Negro schools, nearly a century. *RN, 36,* 67–68.

Dodson, D. W. (1953). No place for race prejudice. *American Journal of Nursing, 53,* 164–166.

Doona, M. E. (1986). Glimpses of Mary Eliza Mahoney. *Journal of Nursing History, 1,* 20–34.

Doswell, W. M. (1989, January). Nursing research needs of black Americans: 1989 and beyond. *Journal of National Black Nurses Association, 3,* 45–53.

Elmore, J. A. (1976). Black nurses: Their service and their struggle. *American Journal of Nursing, 76,* 435–437.

Fauset, A. H. (1938). *Sojourner Truth: God's faithful pilgrim.* Chapel Hill, NC: University of North Carolina Press.

Feldbaum, E. A. (1980). *The nursing profession and black nurses.* College Park, MD, University of Maryland.

Fernandez-Santiago, M. (1994). Cultural diversity in an undergraduate nursing curriculum: An overview. *Journal of Cultural Diversity, 1,* 13–15.

Freedman's school administered by U.S. Public Health Service. (1941). *American Journal of Nursing, 41,* 102.

Gaskin, F. C. (1986, January). Detection of cyanosis in the person with dark skin. *Journal of National Black Nurses Association, 1,* 52–60.

Gunter, L. M. (1961). The effects of segregation on nursing students. *Nursing Outlook, 9,* 74–76.

Hagans, I. R. (1986, July). The black nurse as advocate. *California Nurse, 84,* 3.

Harris, L. (1986, February). Has affirmative action in nursing been successful in North Carolina? *Journal of National black Nurses Association, 1,* 71–78.

Harris, L. O. (1972). Where is the Black nurse? *American Journal of Nursing, 72,* 282–284.

Harvey, L. H. (1970). Educational problems in minority group nurses. *Nursing Outlook, 18,* 48–55.

Haupt, A. C. (1935). A pioneer in negro nursing. *American Journal of Nursing, 35,* 857–859.

Heisler, A., & Marr, G. (1954). Intergroup relations. *American Journal of Nursing, 72,* 1341–1343.

Heisler, A. (1956). Promoting the intergroup relations program. *American Journal of Nursing, 56,* 588–589.

Herrmann, E. K. (1985). *Origins of tomorrow: A history of Belizean nursing education.* Belize, Central America: Ministry of Health.

Heymann, M. (1993). Early postnatal assessment of the newborn in the developing country: Malawi. *Association of Black Nursing Faculty Journal, 4,* 90–94.

Hine, D. C. (1982). The Ethel Johns Report: Black women in the nursing profession, 1925. *Journal of Negro Education, 67,* 212–228.

Hine, D. C. (1982). From hospital to college: Black nurse leaders and the rise of collegiate nursing schools. *Journal of Negro Education, 51,* 222–237.

Hine, D. C. (Ed.). (1985). *Black women in the nursing profession, a documentary history.* New York: Garland.

Hine, D. C. (1988). They shall mount up with wings as eagles: Historical images of black nurses, 1890–1950 In *Images of Nurses: Perspectives from History, Art, and Literature,* Anne Hudson Jones (Ed.). Philadelphia, University of Pennsylvania Press. 177–196.

Hine, D. C. (1989). *Black women in white: Racial conflict and cooperation in the nursing profession, 1890–1950.* Bloomington & Indianapolis, Indiana University Press.

Hine, D. C. (1989). Black women in the nursing profession, A documentary history. In Reverby, S. (Ed.) *The history of American nursing.* New York: Garland Publishing.

Holleran, C. A. (1993). The many labors of the International Council of Nurses. *Nursing and Health Care, 14,* 206–207.

Holt, R. (1944). The negro nurse: A study in professional relations. *RN, 7,* 39–40, 72–80.

Iveson, J. (1984). A pin to see a peep show . . . Mary Seacole. *Nursing Mirror, 158,* 13, 36.

Jegede, S. A. (1975). Cultural approach to nursing in Africa. *Nigerian Nurse, 7,* 6–8.

Jones, S. H. (1992). Improving retention and graduation rates for Black students in nursing education: A developmental model. *Nursing Outlook, 40,* 78–85.

Kalisch, B. J., Kalisch, P. A., & Clinton, J. (1981). Minority nurses in the news. *Nursing Outlook, 29,* 49–54.

Kandandara, J. (1993). Quality through management. *International Nursing Review, 40,* 140–143.

Kangori, S. W. (1972). University education for nurses at the University of Nairobi. *Kenya Nursing Journal, 1,* 42–43; 52.

Kiereini, E. M. (1983). Evolution of health care in developing countries: The challenges for the nurse. *Kenya Nursing Journal, 11,* 15–21.

Kiereini, E. M. (1988). WHO's role in the development of nursing in the African region. *International Nursing Review, 35,* 65–66.

Kiereini, E. M. (1990). AIDS impact on women and children in Africa. *International Nursing Review, 37,* 373–376.

Kisseih, D. A. (1968). Development of nursing in Ghana. *International Journal of Nursing Studies,* (Volume B), 207.

Kisseih, D. A. (1969). Responsibilities of the nurse in developing countries. *Ghanaian Nurse, 5,* 22–28.

Kupperschmidt, B. (1988, May). Culturally sensitive nursing care for black clients. *Oklahoma Nurse, 33,* 9, 18.

Landauer, S. (1970). Recent nursing developments in the English-speaking Caribbean. *International Nursing Review, 17,* 172–183.

Lerner, G. (Ed.). (1973). *Black women in white America: A documented history.* New York: Vintage Books.

Lewis, M. C. (1981). A Black perspective: Afro-American men in nursing. *Nursing Leadership, 4,* 31–33.

Long, O., & Bolton, L. B. (1986, February). The National Black Nurses' Association's response to the Secretary's Task Force Report. *Journal of National Black Nurses Association, 1,* 24–26.

Luckraft, D. (Ed.). (1976). *Black Americans: Implications for black patient care.* New York: American Journal of Nursing Co.

Macqueen, E. M. (1974). Public health nursing in Kenya. *Kenya Nursing Journal, 3,* 21–22.

March, G. (1957). Ten green years, nursing organization in Jamaica—1946–1956. *International Nursing Review, 4,* 27–32.

Marshall-Burnett, S. (1981). A brief reflection on the life of Mary Seacole 1805–1881. *Jamaica Nurse, 21,* 14–15.

Matula, H. (1987). Mary Elizabeth Carnegie's research on black history and black nurses. *Society of Nursing History Gazette, 7*(2), 1–2.

McPherson, J. M. (1975). *The Abolitionist Legacy: From Reconstruction to the NAACP.* Princeton, NJ, Princeton University Press.

Memorial for first black nurse unveiled. (1973). *Missouri Nurse, 42,* 4.

Miller, H. S. (1968). *The history of Chi Eta Phi Sorority, Inc.* Washington, DC: The Association for the Study of Negro Life and History.

Miller, H. S. (1986). *America's first black professional nurse: A historical perspective.* Atlanta: Wright Publishing Co.

Miller, H. S. (1988). *Mary Mahoney,* Chi Eta Phi Sorority. Washington, D.C.

Miller, H. S., & Mason, E. D. (Eds.). (1983). *Contemporary minority leaders in nursing: Afro-American, Hispanic, Native American Perspectives.* Kansas City: American Nurses' Association.

Miller, M. H. (1972). On blacks entering nursing. *Nurses Forum. 11,* 248–263.

Mosley, M. O. (1992). *The development of Black community health nursing in the northeastern United States, 1906–1934: Contributions of Elizabeth Tyler and Edith Carter.* Unpublished doctoral dissertation. Teachers College, Columbia University, New York.

Negro nurses in Liberia commended. (1946). *American Journal of Nursing, 46,* 799.

Newell, H. (1951). *The history of the National Nursing Council.* New York: The Council.

Ngcongco, V. N., & Stark, R. D. (1990). Family nurse practitioners in Botswana: Challenges and implications. *International Nursing Review, 37,* 239–243.

Nichols, L. (1954). *Breakthrough on the color front.* New York: Random House.

Nkongho, N. (1994). Family theraphy and the Iglo family system. *Journal of Cultural Diversity, 1,* 4–7.

Nondo, C. S. (1991). Support workers in Zimbabwe. *International Nursing Review, 38,* 177–188.

Northrup, H. R. (1950). The ANA and the negro nurse. *American Journal of Nursing, 50,* 207–208.

Olade, R. A. (1990). A survey of nursing research in Nigeria. *International Nursing Review, 37,* 299–302.

Onyejiaku, E. E., et al. (1990). Evaluation of a primary health care project in Nigeria. *International Nursing Review, 37,* 265–270.

Osborne, E. M. (1949). Status and contribution of the negro nurse. *Journal of Negro Education, 18,* 364–369.

Osei-Boateng, M. (1992). Nursing in Africa today. *International Nursing Review, 39,* 175–180.

Piero, P. (1974). Black-white crises. *American Journal of Nursing, 74,* 280–281.

Pratt, W. (1970). The challenge of nursing in developing countries. *International Nursing Review, 17,* 158–169.

Prestwidge, K. J. (1989). *Bibliography of African-Americans, Native Americans, Hispanics in engineering, science and the health professions.* Flushing, NY: Huespin Publication.

Prestwidge, K. J. (1990). *Women in science, engineering, and the health professions: A bibliography.* Flushing, NY: Huespin Publication.

Rann, E. L. (1916). The Good Samaritan Hospital of Charlotte, North Carolina. *Journal of the National Medical Association, 56,* 223–225.

Reid, U. V. (1990). An economic model for nurse manpower planning in the Caribbean—Part I: The issues. *International Nursing Review, 37,* 335–339.

Reid, U. V. (1990). An economic model for nurse manpower planning in the Caribbean—Part II: Strategies. *International Nursing Review, 37,* 377–379.

Reid, U. (1993). Human resources in nursing: Determining requirements and skills. *International Nursing Review, 40,* 119–123.

Report, Official Newsletter, New York State Nurses Association. (1993, January/February). Estelle Massey Riddle blazed the trail for Black nurses. *24,* 1, 6.

Rice, F. (1994). Folk medicine: Observations and examples. *Journal of Cultural Diversity, 1,* 26–27.

Riddle, E. (1934). What price quotas. *Public Health Nursing, 36,* 389–393.

Robinson, A. D. (1994). Attitudes toward nursing home residents among order of three cultural groups. *Journal of Cultural Diversity, 1,* 16–18.

Robinson, A. M. (1972). Black nurses tell you: Why so few blacks in nursing. *RN, 35,* 33–34 passim.

Rosenkretter, M. M., Reynolds, B. J., Cummings, H., & Zakutney, M. A. (1993). The Barbados project: An experience in collaboration and neutrality. *Nursing and Health Care, 14,* 528–532.

Ruffin, J. E. (1974). Issues for the black nurse today: Competence and commitment. *Current Issues in Nursing Education.* New York: National League for Nursing.

Rutledge, A. L., & Gass, G. Z. (1967). *Nineteen negro men: Personality and manpower retraining.* San Francisco: Jossey-Bass.

Sage. (1985). Photographic essay. *A scholarly journal on black women, 2*(2), 4–9.

Sajiwandani, J. (1985). The direction of nursing in Zambia: Where are we heading? *Zambia Nurse, 13,* 12–16.

Sands, R. F. (1988). Enhancing cultural sensitivity in clinical practice. *Journal of the National Black Nurses' Association, 2,* 54–63.

Schorr, T. M., & Zimmerman, A. (Eds.). (1988). *Making choices, taking chances: Nurse leaders tell their stories.* St. Louis: C. V. Mosby.

Scott, E. J. (1919). *The American Negro in the World War.* Washington, DC: The Author.

Seacole, M. (1857). *Wonderful adventures of Mrs. Seacole in many lands.* WJS (Ed.). London: James Blackwood.

Seivwright, M. J. (1981). The Florence Nightingale of Jamaica. *Jamaican Nurse, 21,* 16–17.

Shapiro, C. (1948). The negro nurse in the U.S. *RN, 12,* 32–35.

Sloan, P. E. (1978). *A history of the establishment and early development of selected nurse training schools for Afro-Americans, 1886–1906.* Unpublished doctoral dissertation, Columbia University Teachers College, New York.

Sloan, P. E. (1985). Early black nursing schools and responses of black nurses to their educational programs. *Western Journal of Black Studies, 9,* 158–172.

Smith, G. R. (1979). *Liberation through a professional association: A case study of the national black nurses' association.* Unpublished doctoral dissertation, University Graduate School—Midwest, University for the Experimenting Colleges and University, Cincinnati, OH.

Smith, J. C. (1992). *Notable black American women.* Detroit: Gale Research, Inc.

Staupers, M. K. (1970). The black nurse and nursing goals. *Journal of the National Medical Association, 62,* 304–305.

Tate, B. L., & Carnegie, M. E. (1965). Negro admissions, enrollments, and graduations-1963. *Nursing Outlook, 13,* 61–63.

The ANA and YOU. (1941). New York: American Nurses' Association.

The Negro public health nurse. *Public Health Nurse, 34,* 452–454.

Tomes, E., & Nicholson, A. D. (1979). *Black nursing pioneers, leaders, organizers (1770–1980).* Washington, DC: The Association for the Study of Afro-American Life and History.

Tomes, E. K., & Shaw-Nickerson, E. (1986). Predecessors of modern black nurses: An honored role. *Journal of the National Black Nurses' Association, 1,* 72–78.

Tucker-Allen, S. (1994). Cultural diversity and nursing education: An organizational approach. *Journal of Cultural Diversity, 1,* 21–25.

Upvall, M. J. (1992). Nursing perceptions of collaboration with indigenous healers in Swaziland. *International Journal of Nursing Studies, 29,* 27–36.

Vaughan-Richards, G. A. (1968). A review of nursing education in Nigeria. *Nigerian Nurse, 1,* 25–27.

Vernon, C. (1969). The Florence Nightingale of Jamaica; the story of Mary Seacole. *Jamaica Nurse, 9,* 19, 22.

Ward-Murray, E. M. (1990). *The development of nursing education: Barbados.* Unpublished doctoral dissertation, Teachers College, Columbia University, New York.

Watson, C. (1984). Hidden from history: Mary Seacole, the black nurse famous in her day for her work in the Crimea. *Nursing Times, 80,* 16–17.

Williams, B. S. (1976). Historical review of ethnic nurse associations. In Branch, M. F., & Paxton, P. P. (Eds.). *Providing Safe Nursing Care for Ethnic People of Color.* New York: Appleton-Century-Crofts.

Williams, B. S. (1986). Guest editorial: The challenge to black nurses. *Journal of National Black Nurses Association, 1*(2), 11–15.

Wilson, E. H. (1943). *Hope and dignity.* Philadelphia: Temple University Press.

Winder, A. E. (1971). Why young black women don't enter nursing. *Nursing Forum, 10,* 56–63.

Yamba, R. (1990). Primary health care in relation to nursing education in Zambia. *Zambia Nurse, 15,* 3–7.

Yearwood, A. C. (1983). *The effective and ineffective behaviors of black and white nurse leaders: An executive development program.* Unpublished doctoral dissertation, Teachers College, Columbia University.

Yergan, L. (1956). Mission in Liberia. *Nursing Outlook, 4,* 564–566.

Zrnizrm, E. B. (1985). Nursing in the Zambia flying doctor services. *Zambia Nurse, 13,* 11–12.

Appendix A

Black Deans and Directors of Baccalaureate and Higher Degree Programs in Nursing, December 31, 1994

Alabama

Dr. Margie N. Johnson, Tuskegee University, Tuskegee
Dr. Roberta O. Watts, Jacksonville State University, Jacksonville
Dr. Sheila P. Parham-Davis, Oakwood College, Huntsville

Arkansas

Corliss Dickerson (Interim), University of Arkansas at Pine Bluff

Delaware

Dr. Mary P. Watkins, Delaware State College, Dover

District of Columbia

Dr. Dorothy Powell, Howard University, Washington
Dr. Elizabeth Clanton, University of the District of Columbia, Washington

Florida

Dr. Bobbie Jean Primus-Cotton, Bethune-Cookman College, Daytona Beach
Dr. Margaret W. Lewis, Florida A&M University, Tallahassee
Mrs. Laurel Boyd, University of West Florida, Pensacola

Georgia

Dr. Lucille B. Wilson, Albany State College, Albany
Dr. Marlene Mitchell-Tibbs, Columbus College, Columbus

Illinois

Dr. Lucille Davis, Chicago State University, Chicago
Dr. Francesca A. Armmer, Bradley University, Peoria
Dr. Annie Lawrence, Governors State University, University Park

Iowa

Dr. Geraldene Felton, University of Iowa, Iowa City

Kentucky

Dr. Cora Newell-Withrow, Berea College, Berea

Louisiana

Dr. Enrica Singleton, Dillard University, New Orleans
Dr. Janet Rami, Southern University-Baton Rouge, Baton Rouge

Maryland

Dr. Doris Starks, Coppin State College, Baltimore
Dr. Eleanor Walker, Bowie State University, Bowie

Massachusetts

Dr. Brenda S. Cherry, University of Massachusetts, Boston

Michigan

Dr. Regina Williams, Eastern Michigan University, Ypsilanti
Dr. Bernardine Lacey, Western Michigan University, Kalamazoo

Mississippi

Dr. Frances Henderson, Alcorn State University, Natchez

Missouri

Mrs. Juanita Roth, Southwest Missouri State University, Springfield

New Jersey

Dr. Dolores Brown-Hall, Thomas Edison State College, Trenton

New York

Dr. Pearl Skeete Bailey, York College, Jamaica
Dr. Bertie M. Gilmore, Medgar Evers College, Brooklyn

North Carolina

Dr. W. Kaye McDonald, North Carolina Central University, Durham
Dr. Beverly Malone, North Carolina A&T State University, Greensboro
Dr. Ernestine Small, Winston-Salem State University, Winston-Salem
Dr. Virginia Adams, University of North Carolina at Wilmington
Dr. C. DaCosta Hunte, Fayetteville State University, Fayetteville

Oklahoma

Dr. Carolyn Kornegay, Langston University, Langston

Pennsylvania

Dr. Cynthia F. Capers, LaSalle University, Philadelphia

South Carolina

Dr. Debra L. Austin, South Carolina State College, Orangeburg

Tennessee

Dr. Virginia W. Adams (Interim), East Tennessee State University, Johnson City

Texas

Dr. Dollie Brathwaite, Prairie View A&M University, Houston

Virginia

Dr. Bertha Davis, Hampton University, Hampton

Appendix B

Charter Members National Association of Colored Graduate Nurses[*]

Mrs. Dara Yarborough Allen	Georgia
Mrs. Sadie Poole Bomar	New York
Mrs. Rosa Williams–Brown	Florida
Edith Carter	New York
Mrs. Eva Davis Felton	District of Columbia
Martha Franklin	Connecticut
Mary I. Grant	New York
Clara M. Harris	New York
Mrs. Pattie Reeves Holmes	Georgia
Mrs. Margaret A. Johnson	Florida
Mrs. Nancy Lois Kemp	Pennsylvania
Mrs. Minnie B. Kelly Lee	Virginia
Mrs. Mary Clark Lemus	Virginia
Annie L. Marin	New York
Mrs. Jane Hammond Nelson	New York
Mrs. Frances Robinson Quinn	Virginia
Charlotte A. Rhone	North Carolina
Mrs. Eleanor Christie Selah	Pennsylvania
Mrs. Theodore B. Strickland	New Jersey
Viola Symons	Ohio
Mrs. Adah B. Thoms	New York
Mrs. Mary Tucker	Pennsylvania
Mrs. Viola Ford Turner	South Carolina
Mrs. Louise Walters	New York
Mrs. Octavia Walters	New York
Mrs. Effie Brooks Watkins	New York

---

[*]Source: Staupers, M. K. (1961) *No Time for Prejudice*. New York: Macmillan.

Appendix C

Mary Mahoney Award Recipients, 1936–1994

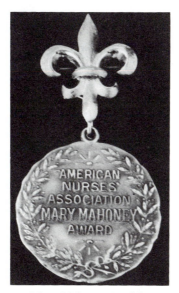

Mary Mahoney Medal.

1936	Adah B. Thoms	1942	Ruth Logan Roberts
1937	Nancy Louis Kemp	1943	Ludie A. Andrews
1938	Carrie E. Bullock	1944	Mable C. Northcross
1939	Petra A. Pinn	1945	Susan E. Freeman
1940	Lula G. Warlick	1946	Estelle Massey Riddle Osborne
1941	Ellen Woods Carter	1947	Mabel Keaton Staupers

1949	Mary E. Merritt	1972	Mary Mills
1951	Eliza F. Pillars	1974	Fostine G. Riddick Roach
1952	Marguerette Creth Jackson	1976	Carolyn McCraw Carter
1954	May Maloney (White)	1978	Mary S. Harper
1956	Mildred Ann Vogel (White)	1980	Mary Elizabeth Carnegie
1958	Fay O. Wilson	1982	Lillian Holland Harvey
1960	Marie Mink	1984	Verdelle Bellamy
1962	Mildred Adams (White)	1986	Elnora Daniel
1964	M. Elizabeth Pickens (White)	1986	Mary Malone (White)
1964	Alice M. Sundberg (White)	1988	Hattie Bessent
1966	Katharine Ellen Faville (White)	1990	Ethelrine Shaw-Nickerson
1968	Helen S. Miller	1992	Bertha Gipp (Native American)
1970	Vernice D. Ferguson	1994	Dorothy Ramsey

Appendix D

Charter Members, Chi Eta Phi Sorority[*]

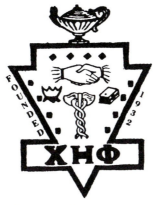

Chi Eta Phi logo.

Aliene C. Ewell
Clara Beverly
Gladys Catching
Bessie Cephas
Henrietta S. Chisolm
Susan Freeman

Ruth Garrett
Olivia Howard
Mildred Lucas
Lillian Mosely
Clara Royster
Katherine Turner

---

[*]Source: *Directory, Chi Eta Phi Sorority.* Washington, D.C., The Sorority, 1983.

Appendix E

Honorary Members, Chi Eta Phi Sorority

Ella W. Allison
Nancy Lois Ruth Anderson
Ludie Andrews
Hattie Bessent
Hazle W. Blakeney
Amanda C. Blount
Linda Burnes Bolton
Rose Lee Brady*
Delores F. Brisbon
Edith P. Brocker
Hazel W. Johnson Brown
Olivette Kalfa Caulker
Mary Elizabeth Carnegie
Lillian Carter (White)*
Anna B. Coles
Alida C. Dailey*
Elnora Daniel
Blythe Davis*
Anne Davis Drice
Rhetaugh G. Dumas
Vernice Ferguson
Sylvia Flack
Lula P. Foster*

Florence Gipe (White)*
Ann Papino Glenn*
Hazel A. Goff (White)*
Camille Masco Goldsmith
Charles E. Hargett
Mary S. Harper
Ruth W. Harper (White)
Paula C. Hollinger
Theoria Houston*
Virginia Hunter
Jennie Jergenson
Alma Vessells John*
Alleah B. King*
Bernardine Lacey
Lena Lavette
Artherene Sermons Lee
Katherine Lepper*
Mary Eliza Mahoney*
Beverly Malone
Grace Sata Matsunaga (White)
Charlotte K. May
Mary Mills
Barbara Nichols

*Deceased.

Estelle Massey Osborne*
Bettye Phillips
Edith V. Plump
Betty Phillips
Isabelle Ryer*
Marion B. Seymour*
Daisy Schley*
Gloria R. Smith
Myrtis Snowden
Reva Speaks*
Mabel K. Staupers*

Ivy K. Tinkler
Sharon McBride Valente
Thelma Vines
Lula Warlick*
Lois M. Walters
Bessie Whitman*
Betty Smith Williams
Marian Willingham*
Margaret A. Wilson
Catherine Worthy*

---

*Deceased.

Appendix F

Charter Members, National Black Nurses' Association*

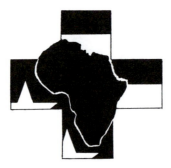

NBNA logo.

Betty Jo Davison	Winifred Riddle
Mary Harper	Gloria Rookard
Florrie Jefferson	Janice Ruffin
Phyllis Jenkins	Lauranne Sams
Mattie Kelly	Ethelrine Shaw-Nickerson
Geneva Norman	Betty Williams

*Source: Smith G.R. (1979). *Liberation Through a Professional Association: A Case Study of the National Black Nurses Association.* Unpublished doctoral dissertation, 1979.

300

Appendix G

Founding Members, Association of Black Nursing Faculty in Higher Education

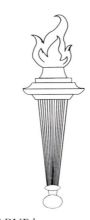

ABNF logo.

Sonia Baker
Doris E. Bell
Lucille Davis
Bevelyn Edmonds
Barbara Haynes
Linda B. Hureston
Katie McKnight
Georgia B. Padonu

Meryl Price
Sandra Sayles-Cross
Iris Shannon
Eva D. Smith
Ruby Steele
Sallie Tucker-Allen, Founder
Sandra Millon Underwood

Appendix H

Black Fellows Inducted in the American Academy of Nursing

AAN logo.

1973   Dr. Rhetaugh Dumas
(Charter Fellow)
Dr. Geraldene Felton
(Charter Fellow)

1974   Dr. Juanita Fleming
Dr. Myrtis Snowden

1975   Dr. Lucille Davis
Vernice Ferguson

1976   Dr. Mary Elizabeth Carnegie
Dr. Virginia Ford

1977   Fostine Riddick Roach
Dr. Iris Shannon
Dr. Gloria Smith

1978   Dr. Mary Harper

Dr. Barbara McArthur
Estelle Massey Osborne
(Honorary Fellow)*
Dr. Oliver Osborne
Dr. Ora Strickland

1979   Dr. Elnora Daniel
Dr. Faye Gary
Dr. Laurie Gunter

1980   Dr. Betty Smith Williams

1981   Dr. Irene D. Lewis
Dr. Barbara Logan
Dr. Ethelrine Shaw–
Nickerson
Dr. Patricia Sloan

*Deceased

Note: Because AAN records do not indicate race, Fellows presented here are those identified as black by the author, who apologizes for any omissions.

1982	Dr. Beverly Bonaparte
	Dr. Marie Bourgeois
	(Honorary Fellow)
1984	Dr. Carolyn McCraw
	Carter
	Dr. Hazel Johnson-Brown
1986	Barbara Nichols
1987	Dr. May Louise Wykle
1988	Dr. Beverly Malone
1990	Clara L. Adams-Ender
	Dr. M. Linda Burnes-Bolton
	Dr. Juanita Hunter
	Dr. Bernardine Lacey
	Dr. Cora Newell-Withrow
	Dr. Jeanette O'Neal Poindexter
	Dr. Dorothy Ramsey
1991	Dr. Frieda Butler
	Dr. Bertha Davis
	C. Alicia Georges
	Dr. Virginia Hunter
	Dr. Dorothy Powell
	Dr. Lovetta Smith
	Dr. Sallie Tucker-Allen

	Dr. E. Juanita Lee
1992	Dr. Cynthia Barnes-Boyd
	Dr. Willa Doswell
	Dr. Martha Jean Foxall
	Dr. Fannie Gaston-Johannson
	Dr. Loretta Sweet Jemmott
	Dr. Eva D. Smith
	Dr. Rosalyn Jones Watts
1993	Verdelle Bellamy
	Dr. Barbara Holder
	Dr. Ruth Johnson
	Jean Marshall
	Dr. Cornelia Porter
	Dr. Hilda Richards
	Dr. Beverly Claire Harris Robinson
	Dr. Bess Stewart
1994	Daisy Alford
	Dr. Janice Brewington
	Dr. Mamie Montague
	Dr. Willar White-Parson
	Dr. Joyce Gizer
	Beverly Jones
	Dr. Charlie Jones-Dickson

---

*Deceased

Chronology

1854–1856 — Mary Seacole, a black woman, nursed in the Crimean War with Florence Nightingale

1861–1865 — Black women nursed in the Civil War—Sojourner Truth, Harriet Tubman, Susie Taylor, to name a few

1865 — Freedmen's Bureau established by Congress, March 3

1879 — Mary Mahoney, America's first black trained nurse, graduated from New England Hospital for Women & Children, Boston, MA.

1883 — Sojourner Truth, abolitionist and Civil War nurse died, September 26, Battle Creek, Michigan

1886 — Spelman Seminary (renamed Spelman College), Atlanta, Georgia, started first nursing program for blacks. Led to a diploma

1893 — Nursing program (diploma) established at Howard University, Washington, D.C.

1896 — American Nurses' Association (ANA) founded; membership derived from alumnae associations, hence blacks eligible then

— Supreme Court Decision, Plessy v. Ferguson, established the "separate but equal" doctrine

1898 — Namahyoke Curtis, a black untrained nurse, assigned by War Department as a contract nurse in Spanish-American War

— Anita Newcomb McGee, M.D., organized army nursing service

1900 — Jessie Sleet Scales, first black public health nurse

1901 — Army Nurse Corps established under Army Reorganization Act, with a nurse in charge

1903   —Nurse Practice Acts secured by state nurses' associations: New York, New Jersey, North Carolina, and Virginia

1906   —Elizabeth Tyler Barringer, first black public health nurse on staff of the Henry Street Visiting Nurse Service, founded in New York by Lillian Wald

1908   —National Association of Colored Graduate Nurses founded by Martha Franklin

        —Navy Nurse Corps authorized by Navy Appropriations Act of 1908

1909   —First convention of National Association of Colored Graduate Nurses (NACGN) held in Boston

        —Lillian Wald was among the 40 persons who signed the call to conference, which led to the establishment of the National Association for the Advancement of Colored People (NAACP), February 12

        —Ludie Andrews, at her own expense, sued the Georgia State Board of Nurse Examiners to secure black nurses the right to take state board examination and become licensed; succeeded in 1920

1912   —At the invitation of Lavinia Dock, NACGN sent a representative to International Congress of Nurses (ICN) in Cologne, Germany. Mrs. Rosa Williams Brown; Adah B. Thoms, and Ada Senhouse represented Lincoln School for Nurses

1913   —Harriet Tubman, Civil War nurse, died in Auburn, New York, March 10

1914   —Booker T. Washington, founder of Tuskegee Institute, initiated National Negro Health week to inspire public and private agencies to join forces to improve the health of Negro people. Black nurses in all areas of work and education participated in projects to call attention to the many health needs of black people

1916   —Membership in ANA derived from state nurses' associations; the southern states and the District of Columbia barred black nurses, hence barred them from ANA

1918   —Eighteen black nurses admitted to the Army Nurse Corps after armistice of World War I, and assigned to Camp Sheridan, Ohio, and Camp Grant, Illinois

— Frances Reed Elliott Davis, first black nurse accepted in the American Red Cross Nursing Service; her pin read "1-A," with the letter "A" designating "Negro"

— NACGN organized a nursing registry to place black nurses for private duty, staff nursing, and as directors of nursing

1920 — NACGN incorporated in State of New York

1921 — Nursing Service, Veterans Bureau established

1923 — Newly constructed Veterans Hospital at Tuskegee, Alabama, dedicated. Until 1941, this was the only VA facility where black nurses were assigned

1926 — Mary Mahoney, America's first black trained nurse, died, January 4; buried in Everett, Massachusetts

— Annual observation of Negro History week (now black history month) initiated by Carter G. Woodson to raise consciousness of African-Americans re their worth and draw attention of others to what they had contributed to American culture

1928 — NACGN began publishing *National News Bulletin* as its official organ

1929 — Adah B. Thoms published *Pathfinders,* the first historical account of black nurses

1931 — Estelle Massey Osborne, first black nurse in USA to earn a master's degree—Teachers College, Columbia University, New York

1932 — Chi Eta Phi Sorority, Inc., a national sorority, composed of black registered nurses, organized in Washington, D.C., by Aliene Carrington Ewell, October 16

1934 — First regional conference by NACGN convened at Lincoln School for Nurses, New York

— Headquarters for NACGN established at 50 West 50th Street, New York City, in the same building with the three major national organizations—American Nurses Association (ANA), National League of Nursing Education (NLNE), and National Organization for Public Health Nursing (NOPHN)

1935 — NACGN organized the National Citizens Committee for Nursing Education and Service

1936 — St. Philip Hospital School of Nursing, a segregated unit of the Medical College of Virginia at Richmond, inaugurated a new course in public health nursing for Negro graduate nurses—one year in length leading to a certificate

1939   —Biracial National Advisory Council of NACGN established. Ruth Logan Roberts, first chairperson

1940   —NACGN invited by the three major nursing organizations to become a member of the Nursing Council on National Defense which, in 1942, became the National Nursing Council for War Service

1941   —U.S. Army established a quota of 56 black nurses for admission to the Army Nurse Corps, January

—Florida State Nurses Association voted to delete the word "white" from its constitution

—National Association of Colored Graduate Nurses began campaigning in March for the removal of the quota of 56 that had been established for black nurses in the Army. By the end of World War II, 512 black nurses had been commissioned in the army, and three units had served overseas

—First black nurse to enter the military service during World War II—Lt. Della Raney Jackson, April. She was promoted in 1942 to chief nurse and then major, Army Nurse Corps

—Midwifery School for Negro nurses inaugurated at Tuskegee Institute, Alabama

1943   —Estelle Massey Riddle Osborne appointed consultant, National Nursing Council for War Service

—Adah B. Thoms died at Lincoln Hospital in New York, February 21

—The Honorable Frances Payne Bolton, Congresswoman from Ohio, introduced in Congress a new amendment to the Nurse Training Bill that barred racial bias, June. With this new amendment a legal fact, 3,000 black students were enrolled in the U.S. Cadet Nurse Corps; black specialists were appointed to USPHS, Children's Bureau of the Department of Labor, and the Federal Security Agency as consultants, advisors, and staff members

—Susan E. Freeman, chief nurse of first black overseas unit, Liberia

1944   —A telegram from Truman Gibson of the War Department in July read: "Negro nurses will be accepted without regard to any quota. They will be used both in this country and abroad should they apply for commissions in the regular manner"

1945 — U.S. Navy dropped the color bar against black nurses, January 25

— Frances F. Gaines, President of NACGN, appointed to the Postwar Planning Committee of the American Nurses' Association—first black nurse to serve on an ANA committee

— NACGN invited by Joint Board of Directors of ANA, NLNE, and NOPHN in February to join these organizations in a proposed study of the structure of the national nursing organizations

— First black nurse commissioned in the U.S. Navy as ensign, Phyllis Daley, March

1946 — Mabel K. Staupers elected to Board of Directors of the National Nursing Council, March 1

— ANA House of Delegates in convention adopted unanimous resolution for the elimination of discrimination against racial groups

— Alma Vessells John appointed Executive Secretary, NACGN June 27, succeeding Mabel K. Staupers, who resigned after 12 years of service

— President Truman created the landmark Committee on Civil Rights, December 5

1947 — Alma Vessells John appointed to the National Commission on Children and Youth, Children's Bureau, Department of Labor, February

— Grace Higgs, President of the Florida Association of Colored Graduate Nurses named to the Board of Florida State Nurses Association as a courtesy member without voice or vote, February

1948 — Ensign Edith DeVoe, one of four black nurses commissioned in the U.S. Navy during World War II, sworn into the regular navy (Nurse Corps), January 6

— First Lt. Nancy C. Leftenant, first black to become a member of the Regular Army Nurse Corps, March. She had joined the Reserve Corps, February, 1945

— Estelle M. Osborne, first black to be elected to the Board of Directors, ANA. Nominated by the Oregon delegation, she received the second highest number of votes cast; served a four-year term

— House of Delegates at ANA convention voted individual membership to all black nurses excluded from any state association with the proviso that when a state admitted black members, they would give up individual membership

— Georgia Brown McKenzie appointed auxiliary instructor, VA hospital, Castle Point, New York. First black nurse promoted beyond staff level at any integrated VA facility

— President Truman issued two executive orders mandating an end to racial discrimination in federal employment and equal treatment in the armed services, July 26

1949 — Estelle M. Osborne represented ANA as delegate to the International Congress of Nurses, Stockholm, Sweden, June

— NACGN members in convention in Louisville, Kentucky, August, voted to dissolve the organization—ANA-NACGN Liaison Committee suggested functions and responsibilities be absorbed by ANA

— Mary Elizabeth Carnegie, first black nurse elected to the Board of Directors of a state nurses association. The state was Florida, and she received the highest number of votes of any candidate for that office. Reelected in 1950 for a three-year term

1950 — ANA House of Delegates adopted an intergroup relations program to work for full integration of nurses of all racial groups in all aspects of nursing

— Esther McCready instituted legal proceedings to gain admission to the University of Maryland School of Nursing

— First issue of the annual *Glowing Lamp,* official organ of Chi Eta Phi

1951 — Estelle M. Osborne, first black, elected to the Board of Directors of the American Journal of Nursing Company (AJN Co.). At that time she was on the faculty of New York University

— National Association of Colored Graduate Nurses dissolved, January

— Mabel Staupers received the National Association for the Advancement of Colored People's Spingarn Medal for "spearheading the successful movement to integrate Negro nurses into American nursing life as equals." The medal was given at the 42nd convention of the NAACP in Atlanta, Georgia. Staupers was the fourth woman to receive it. The other three were: Mary Talbert, Mary McLeod Bethune, and Marian Anderson

1952 — ANA assumed from NACGN the presentation of the Mary Mahoney Award. That year, it went to Marguerette Creth Jackson

— First black nurse elected to Board of National League for Nursing (NLN). Willie Mae Johnson Jones, Montclair, New Jersey Public Health Nursing Service

— Governor Pyle of Arizona appointed Muriel Cheesman Island to the State Board of Nurse Examiners, first for a black in any state

1953 — Rita E. Miller Dargan, first black nurse to serve on the Basic Board of Review of the NLN Accrediting Service

— NLN Board voted unanimously to reaffirm its position that all activities of NLN including visual aids and radio spot announcements shall include all groups regardless of race, color, religion, and sex

— Mary Elizabeth Carnegie, first black nurse appointed to editorial staff of the *American Journal of Nursing*, July 23

1954 — Estelle M. Osborne appointed Assistant Director for General Administration of the NLN, February 1. She retired in 1966 as associate general director

— Supreme Court decision, *Brown v. Board of Education* (Topeka, Kansas), asserted that "separate educational facilities were inherently unequal," thus nullifying the Plessy v. Ferguson separate but equal decision, May 17

1955 — Norfolk Division, Virginia State College, only black school to participate in experimental study to establish associate degree programs. Hazle Blakeney, director of Norfolk Program

— Elizabeth Lipford Kent, first black nurse to earn a Ph.D.

1956 — Larcie Levi Davis from New York was the first black nurse to receive a NLN Fellowship Award for doctoral study. The fellowships, administered by NLN until 1963, were made available through a grant from the Commonwealth Foundation

— Mary Elizabeth Carnegie joined the editorial staff of *Nursing Outlook* as associate editor, September, after having served three years with the *American Journal of Nursing* as assistant editor

— Estelle M. Osborne, assistant director for General Administration of the NLN, was one of 150 delegates to the fourth annual conference of the National Women's Advisory Committee of the Federal Civil Defense Administration, October

1961 — Mabel K. Stauper's book, *No Time for Prejudice,* published— history of NACGN

1962 — Lillian Harvey began a two-year term on the 12-member Expert Advisory Committee for the Professional Traineeship Program of the USPHS

1964 — Margaret E. Bailey, first black nurse to be promoted to lieutenant colonel, U.S. Army, July 15

— Medical Committee for Human Rights, which included nurses, sent a team to Mississippi to provide medical assistance to civil rights workers, July

— On July 2, President of United States, Lyndon B. Johnson, signed the Civil Rights Act of 1964. Title VI prohibits discrimination in federally supported programs and institutions. Black nurses and students benefited

— President Lyndon B. Johnson signed into law, September 1, the Nurse Training Act of 1964, thereby making it possible for many black nurses to get federal funding for their education

1966 — First grants awarded by the Sealantic Fund to selected nursing programs to reach out for Negro and other disadvantaged youth to prepare them for entering and completing baccalaureate programs in nursing

1967 — Warren Hatcher, first black man nurse to earn a Ph.D. A graduate of Mills School for Men at Bellevue Hospital in New York, his doctorate from New York University was in public administration

—Lawrence Washington, the first man (who happened to be black) to receive a regular army commission in the Army Nurse Corps. This was the result of PL 89-609 passed September 30, 1966, by the 89th Congress, which authorized commissions in the Regular Army for men nurses

1968 —Chi Eta Phi Sorority, Inc., organized and chartered a chapter in Monrovia, Liberia, West Africa. Twenty-one neophytes were pledged under Supreme Basileus Leota Brown

—Helen Miller wrote and published *History of Chi Eta Phi*

1970 —Mary Harper and Lauranne Sams on ANA Commission on Nursing Research

1971 —National Student Nurses' Association received its first contract of $100,000 from the Division of Nursing, then Department of Health, Education, and Welfare, to employ a program director and staff for its Breakthrough to Nursing Project for the recruitment of minority students and men to schools of nursing, June

1972 —Ethelrine Shaw-Nickerson elected third vice-president of ANA. ANA developed a strong affirmative action program with Shaw-Nickerson as chairman of the Task Force. She also served as first chairperson of the Commission (now Cabinet) on Human Rights—1976–1980

—Juanita Fleming elected to Executive Committee, ANA Council of Nurse Researchers

—National Black Nurses' Association incorporated

—Colonel Hazel W. Johnson-Brown received the Anita Newcomb McGee Award, given by the Daughters of the American Revolution (DAR) to the nurse chosen by the Surgeon General as the U.S. Army Nurse of the Year

1973 —American Nurses' Foundation published the *International Directory of Nurses With Doctoral Degrees,* January. Forty-six blacks identified

—Of the 36 charter fellows named by the ANA Board of Directors to the American Academy of Nursing (ANA), January 31, two were black— Rhetaugh Dumas and Geraldene Felton

—Mabel K. Staupers received the NLN Linda Richards Award at Convention, Minneapolis

—Chi Eta Phi, in cooperation with ANA, restored the gravesite of Mary Mahoney, first black graduate nurse

—Mary Elizabeth Carnegie appointed editor, *Nursing Research,* September 4

1974 —ANA received a grant in July from the National Institute of Mental Health to initiate a fellowship program to help minorities earn Ph.Ds. Dr. Ruth Gordon was first project director

1975 —Eleanor Acham Lynch appointed director, Department of Test Construction, NLN, January

—Lillian G. Stokes received the NLN Lucile Petry Leone Award for excellence in teaching. She had achieved recognition by her peers at Indiana University School of Nursing as an innovator of teaching techniques. She was the first Black to earn this award

—First Distinguished Ludie Andrews Award presented by the National Grady Nurses Conclave held in New York, August 11, to Theresa Dixon of Detroit. The award, presented by Mabel K. Staupers, was initiated by Pecola Rodriquez

1976 —Cleophus Doster from California elected President of the National Student Nurses' Association. First black and man

—Clara L. Adams-Ender, first woman in the U.S. Army to be granted the Master of Military Art and Science degree, June 10.

—Evelyn K. Tomes received one of six grants from the American Nurses' Foundation to collect information on black nurses. Her research project was "Black Nurses—An Investigation of Their Contributions to Health Services and Health Education"

—Three black nurses inducted into ANA Hall of Fame: Mary Mahoney, Martha Franklin, and Adah B. Thoms

1977 —Dedication of the M. Elizabeth Carnegie Nursing Archives at Hampton University, Hampton, Virginia, October 7. Patricia Sloan, historiographer, is director of the Archives

—American Nurses' Association received a grant from the National Institute of Mental Health, July 1, to help minority nurses pursue doctoral study in the area of psychiatric/mental health nursing

1978   —Charles Hargett, first man nurse to receive the Mabel K. Staupers Award; presented by Omicron Chapter, Chi Eta Phi Sorority, New York

—Original art work of the U.S. commemorative postage stamp honoring Harriet Tubman, Civil War nurse and freedom fighter, presented to Hampton University, April 15, for placement in the M. Elizabeth Carnegie Archives

—Barbara Nichols, first black nurse to be elected president of the ANA and re-elected in 1980

—Estelle Osborne first black nurse to be inducted as honorary fellow in the American Academy of Nursing (ANA)

—Master's program in nursing at Hampton University accredited by the NLN. This was the first master's program at a historically black institution

—Mary Elizabeth Carnegie first black elected President, AAN

1979   —Brigadier General Hazel Johnson-Brown became first black chief of the Army Nurse Corps

—Barbara Sabol appointed by Governor John Carlin of Kansas as secretary, Department on Aging—a cabinet-level post

1980   —Vernice Ferguson appointed Deputy Assistant Chief Medical Director for Nursing Programs of the Veterans Administration. Her immediate position before was Chief, Clinical Center, Nursing Department, National Institutes of Health

—Nita Barrow knighted Dame of St. Andrew by order of Her Majesty, Queen Elizabeth II

—Patricia Sloan appointed Ombudsman and consultant to Executive Director, ANA

1981   —Estelle Massey Osborne died, December 12, in California

1982   —Cleophus Doster, past president, National Student Nurses' Association, elected to honorary membership

—Irmatrude Grant, first black nurse to receive the Ann Magnussen Award for Volunteer Service to the Red Cross, May 26

—Fostine Riddick, first black nurse to be appointed to the Board of Trustees of a major academic institution— Tuskegee University, Alabama

—Freddie Johnson, first graduate of the ANA Registered Nurse Fellowship Program, died, November 3. Dr. Johnson was an associate professor and assistant director of research at the University of Nebraska College of Nursing in Omaha

1983 — Barbara Nichols appointed secretary of Wisconsin's Department of Regulation and Licensing, a cabinet-level post

— Barbara Sabol appointed secretary, Department of Health and Environment of Kansas—a cabinet-level post

— Gloria Smith appointed Director of the Michigan Department of Public Health, March 1, by Governor Jim Blanchard—the first for a nurse. For 10 years, Dr. Smith had been dean of the College of Nursing, University of Oklahoma, Oklahoma City

— Three black nurses honored by the University of Pennsylvania School of Nursing May 7 for national contributions to the profession—Mabel K. Staupers, Mary Harper, and Mary Elizabeth Carnegie

— Colonel Clara Adams-Ender, U.S. Army Nurse Corps, received the Roy Wilkins Meritorious Award for her service in seeking and achieving new milestones as a professional and a role model, July 14. Award presented at the annual convention of NAACP in New Orleans

— Lieutenant Colonel Joyce Johnson-Bowles received the Anita Newcomb McGee Award

1984 — Estelle M. Osborne inducted into ANA Hall of Fame

— Vernice Ferguson elected honorary fellow, Royal College of Nursing of the United Kingdom, September 12

— Ora Strickland, first black chairperson of the Board of Directors of the American Journal of Nursing Company, the leading publisher of nursing periodicals and multimedia educational programs

— Lillian Epps Johnson, civilian nurse at Langley Air Force Base Regional Hospital, Virginia, received the Congressional Award for Exemplary Service to the Public

1985 — M. Elizabeth Carnegie honored by Nurses House with the first Emily Howland Bourne Award for her achievements as a leader, educator, consultant, editor, and author

— Vernice Ferguson elected President, Sigma Theta Tau International, Honor Society of Nursing

1986 — Ethelrine Shaw-Nickerson elected President, American Nurses' Foundation

—Dame Nita Barrow, Permanent Mission of Barbados to the United Nations

1987 —Honorary Doctor of Laws bestowed upon M. Elizabeth Carnegie by Hunter College, City University of New York

—Recognition Award to M. Elizabeth Carnegie from Mugar Library Associates, Boston University, Boston, Massachusetts

—Barbara Sabol appointed New York State's Executive Deputy Commissioner of Social Services

1988 —Juanita Hunter recipient of ANA Honorary Human Rights Award

1989 —National Black Nurses Association initiated annual celebration of black Nurses Day, February 1

—Mabel K. Staupers died, September 30 at age 99

—Gloria Smith appointed by Secretary Louis Sullivan of Health and Human Services as chairperson, National Commission on the Nursing shortage

—Nancy Leftenant Colon (retired Air Force nurse) elected National President, Tuskegee Airmen, Inc. August, at 18th annual convention, Washington, D.C.

1990 —Congress proclaimed March 10 as Harriet Tubman Day in the USA, honoring her as the brave, black woman freedom fighter

—Dame Nita Barrow, public health nurse educator and stateswoman, appointed Governor General of Barbados, West Indies

—Geraldene Felton named to four-year term as commissioner-at-large by the Commission on Institutes of Higher Education, North Central Association of Colleges and Schools

—Geraldene Felton appointed to the Special Medical Advisory group of the Veterans Administration—the only nurse on the 22-member panel

—Barbara Sabol named by Mayor David Dinkins to head New York City's Human Resources Administration—the first nurse to run the giant agency

—Dr. Juanita Fleming and Dr. Linda Burnes-Bolton named to the 17-member National Advisory Council for Health Care Policy, Research and Evaluation. The council advises

Secretary of the U.S. Department of HHS and Administrator of the Agency for Health Care Policy and Research

—Dame Nita Barrow received the R. Louis McManus Award for Distinguished Service to Nursing by the Department of Nursing Education Alumni, Teachers College, Columbia University, New York, June

—Ellie Mack elected to Board of Directors, American Cancer Society

1991 —Brigadier General Clara Adams-Ender, retired Chief of the Army Nurse Corps, appointed Commanding General, Fort Belvoir, Virginia (first woman to command an Army Post) and Deputy Commanding General, District of Columbia Military District

—Dr. Gloria Smith appointed Coordinator of Health Programs and Program Director, W. K. Kellogg Foundation, Battle Creek, Michigan

—Mary Elizabeth Carnegie awarded honorary Doctor of Public Service, Marian College, Indianapolis, Indiana

—Dr. Betty Smith Williams received the NAACP Legal Defense and Education Fund Black Women of Achievement Award

—Dr. Gloria Essoka, Associate Professor, Hunter-Bellevue School of Nursing, New York, appointed visiting professor, Kamuzu College of Nursing of Malawi, Africa

1992 —Dr. Grace Carolyn Brown appointed President, Roxbury Community College, Boston, Massachusetts

—Dr. Hilda Richards appointed Chancellor, Indiana University Northwest, Gary

—Eddie Bernice Johnson (D–Texas) elected to House of Representatives, first nurse ever elected to U.S. Congress. She had been a State Senator

—Dr. Mary Elizabeth Carnegie received the American Academy of Nursing Media Award for portraying a positive image of nurses in her book, *The Path We Tread*

—Dr. Mary Elizabeth Carnegie received *American Journal of Nursing* Book of Year Award for *The Path We Tread*

—Lois Jean Moore appointed President and Chief Executive Officer of the Harris County Hospital District, the largest district in Texas

—Barbara Sabol, Administrator and Commissioner, New York Human Resources Administration, elected Fellow of the National Academy of Public Administration

1993 — Gwendolyn Braxton, Assistant Academic Vice-President, Delaware State University, Dover, among 12 nurses appointed to review President Clinton's National Health Care Reform Proposal

—Dr. Loretta Sweet Jemmott appointed to Advisory Committee, National Institute of Nursing Research

—Deloris Williams, Springfield, Massachusetts, Public Health Commissioner, elected to four-year term as Trustee, National Conference of Local Health Officers

—New York Governor Mario M. Cuomo proclaimed 1993 as Black History Year in the state

—Vernice D. Ferguson received the President's Medal from The Catholic University of America, Washington, D.C.

1994 —Dr. Mary Elizabeth Carnegie received Honorary Doctor of Science, Indiana University Southeast, New Albany

—Dr. Mary Elizabeth Carnegie received Honorary Doctor of Humane Letters from Thomas Jefferson University, Philadelphia, Pennsylvania

—Dr. Mary Elizabeth Carnegie received Lillian D. Wald Spirit of Nursing Award from Visiting Nurse Service of New York

—Barbara J. Sabol became President of the University Research Corporation and Center for Human Service, Bethesda, MD

Index

Other Books of Interest from NLN Press

Book Title	Pub. No.	Price	NLN Member Price
□ **In Women's Experience** *Edited by Patricia Munhall*	14-2612	$37.95	$34.35
□ **African American Voices** *Edited by Ruth Johnson*	14-2631	32.95	29.95
□ **Peace and Power: A Handbook of Feminist Process, 3rd Edition** *Edited by Charlene Wheeler &* *Peggy Chinn*	15-2404	16.95	14.95
□ **Annual Review of Women's Health, Volume II** *Edited by Beverly McElmurry &* *Randy Spreen Parker*	19-2669	37.95	34.35
□ **First Words: Selected Addresses from the National League for Nursing 1894-1933** *Edited by Nettie Birnbach &* *Sandra Lewenson*	14-2410	38.95	34.95
□ **Legacy of Leadership** *Edited by Nettie Birnbach &* *Sandra Lewenson*	14-2514	39.95	35.95